Energy Medicine

This book is dedicated to Nora

And to fond memories of Candace

For Elsevier

Content Strategist: Shelly Stringer
Content Development Specialist: Carole McMurray
Project Manager: Julie Taylor
Designer: Christian Bilbow
Illustration Manager: Ceil Nuyianes

SECOND EDITION

Energy Medicine

The Scientific Basis

JAMES L. OSCHMAN, PhD
Nature's Own Research Association
Dover
New Hampshire
USA

ELSEVIER

Edinburgh London New York Oxford Philadelphia St Louis Sydney Toronto

ELSEVIER

First edition 2000
Second edition 2016

ISBN 978-0-443-06729-7

Notices

ELSEVIER your source for books,
journals and multimedia
in the health sciences

www.elsevierhealth.com

  Working together
to grow libraries in
developing countries

The
Publisher's
policy is to use
paper manufactured
from sustainable forests

www.elsevier.com • www.bookaid.org

Printed in Great Britain
Last digit is the print number: 12

CONTENTS

There is no harm in doubt and skepticism, for is thru these that new discoveries are made.
RICHARD FEYNMAN (LETTER TO ARMANDO GARCIA J, DECEMBER 11, 1985)

Those who have taken upon them to lay down the law of nature as a thing already searched out and understood, whether they have spoken in simple assurance or professional affectation, have therein done philosophy and the sciences great injury. For as they have been successful in inducing belief, so they have been effective in quenching and stopping inquiry; and have done more harm by spoiling and putting an end to other men's efforts than good by their own.
FRANCIS BACON (NOVUM ORGANUM, 1620)

It is necessary to think in a new way about science.

*Once the hope of mankind, modern science has now become the object of such mistrust and disappointment that it will probably never again speak with its old authority. The crisis of ecology, the threat of atomic war, and the disruption of the patterns of human life by advanced technology have all eroded what was once a general trust in the **goodness** of science ... Even among scientists themselves there are signs of a metaphysical rebellion. Modern man is searching for a new worldview ... For several centuries Western civilization has operated under the assumption that man can understand the universe without understanding himself.*
JACOB NEEDLEMAN (A SENSE OF THE COSMOS, 2003)

Look at the step-by-step process by which we come to understand the world around and within us. Energy is a huge part of this. Our personal ability to understand and manipulate the energies of nature gives us direct experience of the most vital aspects of life. However, because of historical confusions and vested interests our culture and our education have obscured the nature of energy and thereby denied us the opportunity to explore what is arguably the most important part of our nature and of our health. The resulting confusion has spilled over into our healthcare system, which is in a crisis that threatens our prosperity and national security. To ignore energy is to deny the application to our health and welfare of one of the greatest areas of human inquiry – physics. This book has the goal of bringing the physical and biomedical sciences into cooperation as we look to the future of our healthcare system.
JAMES L. OSCHMAN (2014)

For a number of years before I actually had the profound pleasure of meeting Dr Oschman, I kept hearing about him from energy therapists of many types. Here was a real scientist, a cellular biologist and physiologist with impeccable credentials, who dared to associate with Rolfers, acupuncturists and other bodyworkers in a bold search to establish the nature of the real science underlying energy medicine. Dr Oschman's quest was to explain and document what he had learned with clarity and scholarship in such a convincing way that old paradigm naysayers would be forced to listen and join the dialog. Now he has succeeded by providing us with a breakthrough text which maps out an elegant theory of the human body and how it is impacted upon by energy medicine. This is a theory fully compatible with classical physiological and electromagnetic principles, as well as electronics and modern physics, a theory which doesn't need to invoke 'subtle energies' or other mysterious forces which currently lack a scientific rationale.

For years I had lectured and written on the power of healing techniques considered at best unorthodox and at worst quackish, which I had experienced in my own body as powerful and having merit despite the strong resistance and irrational dismissal by most of conventional medicine and my own inability to explain them in the conventional biological paradigm. Feeling 'energy moving' is a common denominator in many of these techniques and I constantly experienced this from my first encounter with acupuncture over twenty-five years ago to my recent interaction with Dr Oschman at the AMTA (American Massage Therapy Association) meeting to design scientific experiments to demonstrate the efficacy and mechanism of action of massage therapy. There in South Carolina, when Dr Oschman proceeded to 'pull' some energy away from my 'stagnant' liver, I felt the appropriate movement before he had even described it. Thus in scientific parlance I was blind to the anticipated outcome, as when years earlier my young son, unaware of the reflexology chart, had accurately reeled off six or seven places in his body to where he had felt 'something move' from the six or seven points of his feet I had manipulated in accordance with that chart. These types of mini-experiment on myself and family over the years had convinced me that there is something so compelling that energy medicine should be taken seriously and studied, not squelched and ignored simply because the reigning paradigm – until now – had no theories to explain it.

How exciting then that Dr Oschman's research has provided a brilliant, concise simple explanation for the sense shared in many diverse energy therapies that claim that energy must move in the body. Today most bodyworkers and body psychotherapists take as a fact the twin neo-Freudian and neo-Reichian concepts that trauma is absorbed and stored in the body and can be unblocked by some corrective energy flow. I have understood for some time that therapeutic massage can be so much more than increasing the blood circulation in sore muscles; our concept of the psychosomatic network (Pert 1999) envisions memories stored in the body (the subconscious mind) in the form of alterations at receptor molecules which transduce chemical changes into ionic fluxes and thus the propagation of electromagnetic waves throughout the network which joins the nervous system, immune cells, gut, glands, skin, etc.

Dr Oschman carefully traces the history of ideas from several fields which support his vision of the body as a liquid crystal under tension capable of vibrating at a number of frequencies, some in the range of visible light. Based upon these revolutionary, but well-supported ideas, I am most excited about the new possibilities of bringing about a rigorous understanding of the nature of emotions on an energetic level. In emphasizing emotions as the mind–body bridge, I have been struck by the ability to span the physical realm of internal communication via ligands and receptors and the spiritual realm of external communication among people, animals and the rest of nature.

It will be most interesting to begin to gain more experimental proof of the external energetic patterns emitted from the hands of healers, the approach Dr Oschman was recommending in South Carolina. We can then start to attempt to measure and understand the energetic forces that act together on seemingly separate creatures which in reality must be continually subjected to unifying emotional(?) forces which drive them to interact more like molecules in solution.

It is not difficult now to imagine different emotional states, each with a predominant peptide ligand-induced 'tone' as an energetic pattern which propagates throughout the bodymind, a 'vibratory flow' which can restore communication among 'blocked', diseased or unintegrated body parts. I too have moved beyond the 'lock and key' model of receptor/ligand binding to the notion of vibrating receptors and ligands which attract at a distance as they resonate at the same frequency. Dr Oschman's new paradigm vision of the human body allows me at last to be able to begin to understand how different emotional states, by triggering the release of various peptide ligands, trigger sudden, even quantum, shifts in consciousness accompanied by concomitant shifts in behavior, memory and body posture. Perhaps we can now begin to imagine how physical 'adjustments' of spinal joints that house peptidergic nerve bundles, therapies that emphasize emotional expression and feeling within the body, and hands on healings where practitioners claim to be able to feel energetic differences and emit appropriate corrective energies share common energetic mechanisms.

The publication of *Energy Medicine – The Scientific Basis* by Jim Oschman is a milestone in the history of medicine which will open hearts and minds to new hypotheses and experimental approaches toward understanding important modes of healing previously thought to be too mysterious to be approached scientifically. Also, we may begin to have a new paradigm vision of the human body as a dynamic shape-shifting bundle of multiple personalities, not merely layered, but capable of sudden and dramatic transformations able to be stabilized in new healing states of mind and body. Bravo!

Candace B. Pert

Reference

Pert, C., 1999. Molecules of Emotion: The Science Behind Mind–Body Medicine. Simon & Schuster, New York.

This book is about a subject that scientists have always found extremely controversial and confusing. For centuries, concepts of 'life force' and 'healing energy' have been virtually off-limits for consideration by serious and respectable scientists. Therapeutic approaches employing healing energy have been regarded with a great deal of skepticism. The legacy of this history is that there are many who will not even open a book such as this.

Why, then, would a serious and thoughtful scientist dare to take on this subject? Those willing to read on will find that there are extraordinarily good reasons. Stated simply, times have changed dramatically. Both scientists and energy therapists around the world have made discoveries that have forever altered our picture of human energetics. Individually, most of these discoveries have not been perceived as major breakthroughs or milestones. But it now appears that the seemingly disparate experimental results and experiences and concepts are converging. A promising new branch of academic inquiry and clinical research is opening up. Approaches that have appeared in competition or conflict are actually supporting each other.

The book is the outcome of an invitation by Dr. Leon Chaitow and his editorial team at the *Journal of Bodywork and Movement Therapies*, published by Churchill Livingstone, an imprint of Harcourt Publishers. I was asked to clarify and come to terms with the word *energy* as it is utilized both in science, in the various branches of bodywork and movement therapies, and in healthcare generally (Magnetic Resonance Imaging scans for example). Was 'energy' a concept that could be explained in terms acceptable to a scientific and intellectually critical mind?

I had already researched this topic for about 15 years: The invitation from Dr. Chaitow gave me an opportunity to gather together many more pieces of a fascinating puzzle.

In the process of writing the journal articles, I noticed similarities between the discoveries of modern medical researchers and the daily observations of 'hands-on' energy therapists. In essence, these traditionally very different approaches to the body are beginning to validate one another.

To be specific, and to anticipate Chapters 6 and 15, oscillating magnetic fields are being researched at various medical centres for the treatment of bone, nerve, skin, capillary, and ligament damage. Virtually identical energy fields can also be detected around the hands of suitably trained therapists. There is an inescapable conclusion.

Medical research is demonstrating that devices producing pulsing magnetic fields of particular frequencies can stimulate the healing of a variety of tissues. Therapists from various schools of energy medicine can project from their hands fields with similar frequencies and intensities. Research documenting that these different approaches are efficacious is mutually validating. Medical research and hands-on therapies are confirming each other. The common denominator is the pulsating magnetic field, which is called a biomagnetic field when it emanates from the hands of a therapist.

In addition, Dr. Chaitow asked me to describe how the evolving concepts might impact specific clinical practices. The inclusion of clinical aspects added a valuable focus to the articles. An appreciation of current energy medicine research enables students and practitioners of all therapeutic disciplines to find a common ground for discussion. Complementary therapies complement each other. Phenomena that previously seemed disconnected could supplement one another, leading to a better understanding of the living body than would be achieved by any single approach. I thank Dr. Chaitow for having the foresight to set this rewarding process in motion.

This book gives me the opportunity to include details that could not be fitted into the journal articles because of space constraints. It also enables me to bring the story up to date with discoveries that have been made since the articles were written. In this book, I have expanded on important topics that were only mentioned in the journal articles, such as emerging information on the physics underlying energy and the roles of energy in consciousness. Finally, it is possible to include a wealth of technical information and quotations that was not appropriate for the journal. This material will be of particular interest to the professional scientist wishing to critique the ideas presented here. Some of this information is technical, and non-technical readers can skip it if they wish.

Only passing reference is made to the ways that various energy techniques are practiced and to the extensive and growing research that supports their claims of clinical efficacy. The reader interested in these topics can consult the appropriate schools that teach clinical techniques and the relevant clinical literature. My inquiry is an attempt to use the latest scientific research to answer the question 'If it works, then how does it work?' An understanding of mechanisms is crucial, because successful clinical trials have much more impact if there is a logical explanation of how a method works. Moreover, therapists benefit enormously from knowledge of mechanisms, because it helps them explain and even enhance their work.

I have received treatments from practitioners of many of the techniques described, and I am convinced that these experiences have helped me become more aware of myself and of my personal energy system. However, I am not an advocate of any one method over another. I have lectured at various schools of bodywork and movement therapy around the world but am not on the faculty of any of them. The aim here is not to promote any particular method but to help understand the mechanisms involved and connect the phenomena with medical science. We have much to learn from each other if we can learn to use a common language.

I thank all of the clinicians who have challenged me to explain their insights and observations. Peter Melchior started me on this journey, by telling me details of important scientific research – such as that of Dr. Harold Saxton Burr – that I had never encountered during my academic education. Dr. Chaitow and the staff of Churchill Livingstone did an excellent job of producing the series for the *Journal of Bodywork and Movement Therapies*, and Graeme Chambers efficiently and professionally rendered the artwork. I particularly thank the production editors, Lynn Percy and Ewan Halley, and the copyeditor, Sally Livitt, for their careful work in preparing the manuscripts for publication in the journal, and Stephanie Pickering for her thorough editing of the book manuscript. I am indebted to the many scientists and therapists who have alerted me to important discoveries so that I can include them in this book. And I am especially appreciative of the role of my dear wife, Nora, who knows more about energy than I ever will. She discussed every aspect of this work with me and gave me the freedom and encouragement to wander deeply into the minutest nooks and crannies of living structure and energy.

James L. Oschman
Dover, New Hampshire, 2000

In science, the acceptance of new ideas follows a predictable, four-stage sequence. In Stage 1, skeptics confidently proclaim that the idea is impossible because it violates the Laws of Science. This stage can last for years or for centuries, depending on how much the idea challenges conventional wisdom. In Stage 2, skeptics reluctantly concede that the idea is possible but that it is not very interesting and the claimed effects are extremely weak. Stage 3 begins when the mainstream realizes not only that the idea is important but that its effects are much stronger and more pervasive than previously imagined. Stage 4 is achieved when the same critics who previously disavowed any interest in the idea begin to proclaim that they thought of it first. Eventually, no one remembers that the idea was once considered a dangerous heresy.

RADIN (1997)

Our medicine is always a work in progress. There are many unanswered questions. This book is written from a firm belief that the study of energetics is our best hope for solving the mysteries of life and healing. Looking at medicine through the lens of energetics is like opening the front door in springtime and allowing the fresh air and the scent of spring flowers to come in. For energy medicine has gone through a cold winter of confusion and misunderstanding, and that season is now behind us.

The study of energy medicine will give you a clearer picture of the world around and within you. Some of the science presented here may seem a bit daunting, but there is no reason for anyone to shy away from it. The information can make a huge difference for your personal health and happiness and your comprehension of nature and healthcare should you need it. The author should be able to explain the subject with clarity so that anyone can understand it and with accuracy that most scientists will verify. I say 'most scientists' because there is no subject that all scientists agree upon. In some cases these disagreements are extremely interesting, and I will strive to present both sides of critical or controversial issues. In some places you will find new insights that have arisen during the process of preparation of the book and working through the evidence. You will also discover that energy is a multi-disciplinary subject that touches upon every aspect of what it is to be alive and on every aspect of health and medicine. Prepare yourself for an interesting and enjoyable journey!

One of the most exciting recent discoveries is the mechanism by which living systems are so incredibly sensitive to energy fields in their environment. These energy fields can be produced by therapeutic medical devices, the hands of therapists, or by technologies such as radio, TV, radar, cell phones, Wi-Fi, and countless other technologies. There is no longer a question about whether the wireless devices we have incorporated in our lives can affect our health. We now have reached the stage where we know why these technologies create problems for many people and how to deal with the issue (see Chapters 3, 16 and 17).

Research and clinical experiences from around the world have enabled energy medicine to take its place among the dominant academic disciplines, on a par with physics, philosophy, astronomy, pharmacology, orthopedics, and so on. As an academic discipline, energy medicine is a mature and multi-disciplinary endeavour and is firmly supported by, and supports, the other well-established disciplines.

We now know that many of the most common health disorders and diseases are partly or entirely energetic in nature and are therefore difficult to prevent or treat when energy is left out of the equations of life and healing. This fact is documented by one of the most significant advances

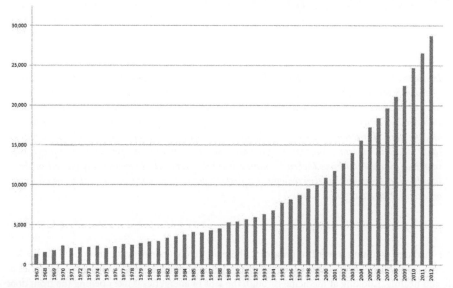

Figure P-1   Peer-reviewed studies of inflammation, 1967–2014, data from the National Library of Medicine database, Pub Med (as of December 25, 2014).

in biomedicine that took place during the years since the publication of the first edition of this book. Specifically, the study of inflammation has become one of the most active areas of biomedical research, with nearly 450,000 peer-reviewed studies completed during the period 1967–2014 (see Figure P-1). Each of these studies represents an enormous investment in time and money and expertise to achieve acceptance in a peer-reviewed journal. This growing body of research can be summarized with the statement that many and perhaps all of the chronic diseases and disorders that plague modern society, and that are the most costly in terms of money and human suffering, have a common cause, and that cause is best described in terms of energetics. While there are literally hundreds of thousands of well-controlled studies correlating virtually every chronic disease with inflammation, much less is known about the reasons for these correlations. The author has been personally involved in research that is revealing the reasons for these correlations and the roles of energy medicine in preventing and treating inflammatory conditions. This will be described in chapter 17, which details what we have learned about the energetic aspects of inflammation and how many of the hands-on, energetic, and movement therapies are able to produce dramatic effects with gentle, natural and completely non-invasive approaches. One of these approaches is extremely simple and can be done by anyone. This is connecting the body with the earth.

During the same period that research on inflammation took off, beginning in 1967, there has been an increase in the frequency of use of the term 'energy medicine' in books published in the English language (Figure P-2). Skepticism or not, energy medicine is here to stay and is a key part of the medicine of the future. The learning curve is steep because of important and fascinating new knowledge being gained by the combination of basic science and hands-on therapies. Yes, the author believes that the insights of therapists who touch patients every day represent important *data* about how the human body functions in health and disease.

Experience has shown that a logical explanation helps patients understand, accept, and take advantage of treatments that have previously seemed mysterious. Some patients simply cannot respond to a treatment that is beyond their conceptual framework. This is a fascinating energetic phenomenon in itself that has implications for our growing interest in the effects of concepts and consciousness and intention on the healing response.

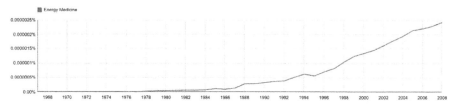

Figure P-2 Increasing use of the term "energy medicine" in books published in the English Language between 1967 and 2012.

Being conversant in the language of science helps alternative practitioners, medical doctors, and patients communicate with each other. Physicians are increasingly being asked by patients for an educated opinion about various CAM therapies. The science of energetics provides a common language with the potential to demystify and unite virtually all of the diverse branches of medicine.

Articulating this common language is my passion, and my goal is to present the technical information as clearly as possible without losing scientific accuracy. It can be challenging for readers who lack a science background to wend their way through the concepts described here. In spite of this, many physicians and other health care workers have shown me tattered copies of the first edition, with lots of highlighting, underlining, notes sticking out, worn out covers. Many have told me, 'I struggled with unfamiliar concepts, but it was worth it, for I really needed this information and now I use it every day'. And, 'I had to read it three times, but it is sinking in, and it is really important to me'. I truly admire these individuals for recognizing the value of ideas that are at first unfamiliar, but whose mastery is crucial to the evolution of their life and profession. And I, too, often have to read scientific articles several times before they make sense.

Readers will notice that I have kept equations to a minimum. There are parts of science that are regarded as explainable only through careful study of the mathematics. On the other hand, one of my mentors, the great Danish physiologist, Hans Ussing (1911–2000), himself a master of the application of mathematics to physiology, told me that anyone who develops an equation to explain his or her results should also be able to explain his or her discoveries in plain language. I have therefore sought out such explanations to make things easier for all of us.

There is nothing more satisfying for an author or a teacher than watching the significance of a new idea or a clearer picture of human structure and function being grasped by either a novice or a skilled practitioner. Often these concepts enable people to push beyond what they have thought is possible and to demonstrate their discoveries to their colleagues. Often insights about human energy systems enable them to find ways of doing the work they have learned and practiced with more effectiveness and less effort. In the last decade many advances have taken place as a result of practitioners' growing appreciation of the science of energy.

Several key points summarize the scientific advances that have taken place since the first edition of this book. First, no new science challenges the main conclusions reached in the first edition. In fact, new discoveries are showing that living systems are even more sensitive to the energies in their environment than we had previously suspected. This is important because serious health conditions can be produced by minute fields in the environment – fields that are so tiny that it is a real stretch for many to believe that they are possible. Second, the study of the relationships between living systems and both the Earth's surface and sunlight have led to new appreciations of the profound health significance of those energetic relationships. Finally, study of the effects of energetic contact with the surface of the Earth has added a new dimension to our understanding of how the immune system functions in health and disease.

Readers will undoubtedly notice and wonder about the repeated references and quotations from Albert Szent-Györgyi. I make no apology for this. Albert Szent-Györgyi has been acknowledged by many as one of the most brilliant scientists of the twentieth century. Moreover, he was passionate about the importance of energy in relationship to health and disease. And he was continually baffled that nobody understood the important direction he was trying to point out. He could see clearly that our myopia about energy was a major contributor to our myopia about cancer and other major chronic diseases. Curing cancer was his foremost passion because he had lost two beloved members of his family to the disease. He was bewildered that he was repeatedly denied funding for his cancer research. I had the extreme good fortune to know this remarkable man, to work in the laboratory across the hall from his Institute of Muscle Research at the Marine Biological Laboratory in Woods Hole, Massachusetts. Szent-Györgyi's institute eventually became the centre of a worldwide network of scientists under the auspices of the National Foundation for Cancer Research. Consequently, I met and became friends with many distinguished scientists from around the world who came to visit Szent-Györgyi and work in his laboratory. For the study of energy medicine, the writings of Albert Szent-Györgyi and his colleagues are among the clearest and most important available. Other scientists who have contributed at his level can be counted on the fingers on one hand, and their work will also be presented here. Some of their names: Harold Saxton Burr, Robert O. Becker, W. Ross Adey, Fritz Albert Popp, Marco Bischoff, Emilio Del Giudice, Cyril Smith, and Mae-Wan Ho. While a journalist and not a scientist, Lynne McTaggart has made an enormous contribution by describing key advances in energetics in ways that anyone can understand. Her two books, *The Field* (2008) and *The Bond* (2011) document some of the remarkable new discoveries that are being applied to modern medicine.

After many years of study of the writings of Albert Szent-Györgyi and his colleagues, it is now clear to me that they were engaged in the search for a fundamental system that is of vital importance for health and healing. Lack of recognition of the importance of this pioneering work, and consequent lack of funding for research, prevented the completion of these efforts. It is exciting to report that modern discoveries in the fields of cell biology and biophysics enable us to understand where these investigations were headed.

During the writing of the first edition, a number of therapists published fascinating descriptions of the ways their work was being incorporated into hospitals and clinics. Among these are the fascinating books of Julie Motz (1998) and her physician colleague, Mehmet Oz (1998). Others have written compelling books about their personal experiences with energy healing (e.g. Brennan, 1987; Collinge, 1998; Egidio, 1997). More recently, a number of books have documented how energy medicine is entering mainstream medicine both through departments of physical therapy (Charman, 2000) and rehabilitation medicine (Davis, 2009). Donna Eden and her colleague David Feinstein have made practical applications of energy medicine widely available through their lectures and workshops around the country and around the world. Their trainings are enabling many to have rewarding careers in energy medicine. They have now published a series of books, beginning with Eden and Feinstein (1999). A growing number of books have energy medicine in their titles, attesting to the increasing significance of energetics for a wide variety of clinicians. Energy medicine techniques have been catalogued in an *Encyclopedia of Energy Medicine* (Thomas, 2010). I mention these sources because I believe the experiences they describe, extraordinary as they may sometimes seem, lay a strong foundation for the medicine of the future.

One of the most exciting areas of energy medicine is the field known as energy psychology. Those who suffer from emotional trauma and abuse can be just as debilitated as those who have a chronic disease or physical injury. Indeed, it now appears that many if not most chronic illness can be traced to a traumatic or emotional event in a patient's life. To free a person from the consequences of long-standing emotional pain and agony can be immensely rewarding for all concerned. Energy psychology has become one of the fastest growing and most exciting branches of complementary medicine Chapter 12 discusses energetic aspects of the subconscious mind and intuition.

In conclusion, there was a time when many were reluctant to use the terms *Energy Medicine* and *Energy Psychology*, and their skepticism was justified because of the lack of appreciation of the roles of energetics in regulating vital physiological processes, including healing. Another issue was the widespread misuse of scientific language when talking about energetics. Growing familiarity with the language and concepts of energy medicine as well as of modern physics has forever changed this perspective and has taken the theory and practice of biomedicine to a new level.

James L. Oschman
Dover, New Hampshire, 2014

References

Brennan, B.A., 1987. Hands of Light. A Guide to Healing Through the Human Energy Field. Bantam Books, Toronto.

Charman, R.A. (Ed.), 2000. Complementary Therapies for Physical Therapists. Butterworth-Heinemann, Oxford.

Collinge, W., 1998. Subtle Energy. Where Ancient Wisdom and Modern Science Meet. Warner Books, New York.

Davis, C.M., 2009. Complementary Therapies in Rehabilitation. Evidence for Efficacy in Therapy, Prevention, and Wellness. 3rd Edition. Slack Incorporated, Thorofare, NJ.

Eden, D., Feinstein, D., 1999. Energy Medicine. Tarcher, New York, NY.

Egidio, G., 1997. Whose Hands Are These? A Gifted Healer's Miraculous True Story. Warner Books, New York.

McTaggart, L., 2008. The Field: The Quest for the Secret Force of the Universe. Harper Perennial, New York.

McTaggart, L., 2011. The Bond: How to Fix Your Falling-Down World. Atria, New York.

Motz, J., 1998. Hands of Life: From the Operating Room to Your Home, an Energy Healer Reveals the Secrets of Using Your Body's Own Energy Medicine for Healing, Recovery, and Transformation. Bantam Books, New York.

Oz, M., 1998. Healing from the Heart: a Leading Heart Surgeon Explores the Power of Complementary Medicine. Dutton, New York.

Radin, D.I., 1997. The Conscious Universe. Harper Edge, San Francisco.

Thomas, L., 2010. The Enclycopedia of Energy Medicine. Fairview Press, Minneapolis, MN.

ACKNOWLEDGEMENTS

My involvement in energy medicine began when Rolfer Peter Melchior described the work of Harold Saxton Burr from Yale University School of Medicine, who had spent decades researching the energy fields of living things. Burr's discoveries were fascinating, but I was left with two burning questions: why did I never learn about this remarkable work during my lengthy academic education? And what do modern medical researchers think of his excellent work, published in some 93 articles between 1932 and 1956? Eventually it became clear that the energy therapies had been left behind during the period of explosive growth in pharmaceutical medicine and the race to find 'a pill for every disease'. And the answer to the second question is that medical researchers simply do not think about energy. One reason: medical education gives little attention to physics and biophysics, subjects that are at the foundation of energy medicine and that are beginning to contribute to mainstream medicine.

Thus began my detailed investigation of biological energy from every possible perspective. As described in the Preface to the First Edition, Leon Chaitow and his editorial team at the *Journal of Bodywork and Movement Therapies* accelerated the process by commissioning a series of articles aimed at clarifying the term 'energy' as it is used both in science and in the various branches of medicine. Eventually Churchill Livingstone published the first edition of this book, leading to invitations to present to students at many schools of complementary and alternative and integrative medicine. Meeting the teachers and innovators in therapies from A to Z (Acupuncture to Zero Balancing) enabled me to connect my academic background in physics, biophysics and biology with remarkable discoveries that were being made every day by therapists devoted to healing with diverse forms of energy. To acknowledge each of these individuals would fill many more pages. I shall simply give a big 'thank you' to all who have given me an incredibly enriching education about aspects of medicine that cannot be found in any medical texts.

The journey was nourished and sustained by my close colleague, Nora Oschman, who discussed every idea from her perspective as a naturalist – a sensitive observer of living nature. You will find her insights 'between the lines' of every page of this book and in our many other articles on new ways of looking at energy and consciousness.

The chapter on Acupuncture contains some previously unpublished work of Joie Pierce Jones (1941–2013), who was professor of radiological sciences at the University of California at Irvine. I will always be grateful to Joie for fascinating conversations – his work was simply extraordinary. He pioneered a variety of new and innovative developments in ultrasonic imaging, tissue characterization, acoustical microscopy and non-contact ultrasonic imaging, and applied them to the study of Acupuncture and Pranic Healing. I am also thankful that Joie's wife, Becky Jones, encouraged the publication of his remarkable gifts to the Acupuncture profession, documented in Chapter 14.

Atty. Judy Kosovich, from Washington DC was inspired to write valuable appendices on the legal and ethical aspects of energy medicine. The result is a unique access to resources needed by those who develop therapeutic devices based on energy. Midge Murphy, JD, Ph.D. also prepared a valuable resource entitled *Legal Issues in the Practice of Energy Therapies: Empower Your Practice & Reduce Your Potential Liability with Essential Risk Management Strategies*. We did not have space to re-publish her important material here, but it is available on her web site: http://www.midgemurphy.com/. Every practitioner needs to know how to construct their practice in a way that minimizes the risks inherent in offering innovative energy-oriented methods to the public. While energy medicine and energy psychology are gaining recognition and visibility, they are still perceived as being 'suspect', 'unproven', and 'on the fringe' by legal authorities, including licensing boards, regulatory agencies, and the Federal Trade Commission. Because of our current legal and regulatory system, both licensed and non-licensed practitioners using energy techniques and organizations offering training in these methods face significant challenges, and need the vital information that Dr. Murphy has compiled for them.

Finally, the editorial staff at Elsevier has made a remarkable contribution to the field of energy medicine through their careful editing and illustrating of this book. While much of this went on 'behind the scenes', I worked most closely with Julie Taylor, who called attention to a million or so glitches in the manuscript and managed the entire project, and with Rajkumar Raj who dealt with the challenging task of obtaining permissions for the illustrations. Carole McMurray and Shelly Stringer provided crucial guidance and extra encouragement when it was needed.

Look at the step-by-step process by which we come to understand the world around and within us. Energy is a huge part of this. Our personal ability to understand and manipulate the energies of nature gives us direct experience of the most vital aspects of life. However, because of historical confusions and vested interests our culture and our education have obscured the nature of energy and thereby denied us the opportunity to explore what is arguably the most important part of our nature and of our health. The resulting confusion has spilled over into our healthcare system, which is in a crisis that threatens our prosperity and national security. To ignore energy is to deny the application to our health and welfare of one of the greatest areas of human inquiry – physics. This book has the goal of bringing the physical and biomedical sciences into cooperation as we look to the future of our healthcare system.

JAMES L. OSCHMAN (2014)

Scientific medicine is unfinished – it is in a continuing state of evolution. This book celebrates one of many turning points in that evolutionary process as it summarizes a fresh perspective from which every aspect of medicine can be reviewed and richly renewed. In essence, a major gap in biology is being filled. The new discoveries are not being developed within any particular discipline or by a particular method. Instead, fundamental observations are being made in a wide variety of areas using a vast array of techniques. After all, like it or not, any approach to the body utilizes energy in one form or another, and energy has many dimensions. An open-minded consideration of energetics has the potential to improve the treatment of serious disorders and diseases and injuries that do not respond to clinical methods based on concepts that leave energy out of the picture.

The author has been immersed in this subject long enough, and has talked to enough experts in the field, to have a clear picture of the basic principles. The concepts presented here will equip the reader to evaluate and appreciate the current breakthroughs as well as lay a substantial foundation for discoveries that will undoubtedly take place well into the future. Researching this subject has led to several concepts that are significant for all branches of medicine, surgery, and healthcare in general. These developments are important for government and hospital administrators, physicians, nurses, complementary and alternative therapists, and for every patient. The book contains a wealth of detail about concepts that may seem new and unfamiliar to some readers. Before diving in, it is important to have the big picture of the major conclusions and their significance. This background material is presented at the beginning to inspire the reader to work through unfamiliar technical details so the exciting developments can be understood. The author is committed to making the science as understandable yet scientifically accurate as possible.

Energy medicine has two main branches, which, in turn, have two secondary branches. None of these perspectives is independent of the other – each informs the others. One branch is represented by the world of devices and technologies utilizing various forms of energy (light, sound, magnetism, electricity, electromagnetism, heat, vibration, and so on). Equally important is the second branch, the manual therapies, employing many of the same forms of energy, but from natural sources, such as the human hand and natural radiations or from substances found in nature. Both of these branches of energy medicine are further divided into two categories. These can be termed local and distant healing. The latter is the most controversial branch of energy medicine, because there are many who are certain that prayer and distant healing cannot be effective because they have no scientific basis. This is not accurate, for there are logical theories to explain distant healing. Some therapists practice these methods daily and report continuous success. Quantum physics is mentioned in several places (e.g. Chapter 2) as it can help readers understand that some of the most important discoveries in the history of science are beginning to provide entirely plausible and rational concepts that can explain such phenomena, although these concepts, too, are controversial.

...our present thinking about quantum mechanics is infested with the deepest misconceptions.
                                                              GULL, LASENBY AND DORAN (1993)

The fact that a concept is controversial should never be taken as a reason to dismiss it out of hand. The history of science has repeatedly shown, for example, that agreement of experts, even unanimous agreement, is not a reason to accept or reject a scientific idea. The disagreements, in fact, are some of the most fascinating topics for study.

One observation about the seemingly very different energetic approaches is that they can inform each other in important ways. The most significant of these is that any discovery about the energetics of living systems, whether made by the use of a sophisticated scientific or medical instrument or through sensitive touch and careful direct observation of patients, informs all who are seeking a better understanding of how living systems really function. As concrete examples of this, there are several individuals whose practice of hands-on energy therapies of various kinds has led to the development of valuable diagnostic and/or treatment technologies. These are the individuals who can see or palpate the benefits of introducing particular forms of energy in particular ways, a skill that enables them to refine their devices. And there are those whose process is the reverse – seeing and understanding how a particular medical device works provides them with a clearer picture of what they can accomplish with their hands. These are some of the most fascinating and clinically significant stories of discovery that can be told.

Now we turn to the fundamentals of energy medicine. Several examples of important phenomena will be presented. Taken together, these insights reveal more rapid and subtle communications and energy flows than those described in conventional physiology and biochemistry texts.

The first concerns the various kinds of biofields, which have been subject of much skepticism. These are the energies that move about rapidly within and around any organism. After a long period when science regarded such energy fields as fiction or illusion, modern scientific investigations conducted at respected research facilities has shown that energy fields are both real and profoundly important. These discoveries are summarized in Chapter 8.

The most well-documented energy fields are the bioelectrical flows produced during the functioning of organs such as the heart, brain, and muscles. They are known in clinical medicine by the technologies that measure them – the electrocardiogram, electroencephalogram, and electromyogram. Less well known are the fields produced by the retina, nerves, lungs, ovaries, and other organs and glands. In general, these electrical fields arise as consequences of the movements of electrical charges associated with virtually all physiological or regulatory processes taking place in the body. Indeed, there is evidence that every event within the organism is associated with measurable electrical activity. In many cases, this activity occurs before, during, and after a particular function is carried out. Post-process electrical activity is part of the feedback system by which the body recognizes that the function has taken place.

It is not always appreciated that the well-established laws of physics require that the flow of charges produced by any process within the body must produce magnetic fields in the surrounding space. Hence the electrical activity of the heart, the largest electrical field generator in the human body, must produce a biomagnetic field that extends into the space around the body. The detection and measurement of this biomagnetic field stands as one of the major advances in the science related to complementary and alternative medicine and helps the skeptical physician and researcher understand the basis for many of these popular therapies. While much more research is needed on this fascinating topic, when energy therapists talk about healing through field interactions, they are talking about real, measurable and well-documented phenomena.

Over the last few decades, scientists have developed more than adequate measurable and logical connections between biological energy fields and generally accepted scientific knowledge. Methods have been developed to measure subtle but important energy fields within and around the human body. A few decades ago these fields were considered nonexistent by academic medicine. Not only are we documenting the presence of such fields, but researchers are understanding how fields are generated and how they are altered by disease and disorder. We shall see that measurements of the biofields around the human body are now being used in Western medical diagnosis to make treatment decisions. We are also beginning to understand the biophysical mechanisms that enable both complementary therapists and conventional physicians to detect and manipulate energy fields for the benefit of the patient.

Below the level of measurable energetic interactions lies an area known as subtle energies. These are energies that we know must be present because of observable clinical effects, even though no energy can be measured with conventional instruments. Quantum physics is helping us understand the nature of the physical forces that underlie electricity, magnetism, and electromagnetism. This is actually what quantum physics is all about. We now know, for example, that what we refer to as matter is a phenomenon that arises from subtle quantum processes. Stephen Hawking (2011) has edited a compendium of the key papers on this subject with the title, *The Dreams That Stuff Is Made of: The Most Astounding Papers on Quantum Physics and How They Shook the Scientific World*. Papers in Hawking's book are authored by the luminaries in the field: Max Planck, Albert Einstein, Ernest Rutherford, Niels Bohr, Werner Heisenberg, Erwin Schrödinger, Paul A. M. Dirac, Wolfgang Pauli, Max Born, Boris Podolsky, Nathan Rosen, David Bohm, John Bell, Leopold Infeld, Robert Oppenheimer, Hans Bethe, Richard Feynman, Freeman Dyson, George Gamow, and others. Milo Wolff (2008) and others have written convincingly about a wave theory of matter.

Entanglement is the concept that all objects in the universe interact with each other via a substructure of space itself, the quantum vacuum. Nobel Laureate Erwin Schrödinger coined the term entanglement, and he was convinced that this was *the* characteristic of quantum systems that shows how completely different they are from classical Newtonian systems. The story of entanglement is the story of quantum physics itself. And quantum physics is regarded as the most successful theory in the history of science.

Applying quantum physics to energy medicine is somewhat hazardous because the field has many conflicting interpretations. This means that any interpretation that is used to develop a logical argument will have its supporters and its opponents. This does not mean we should not go out on a limb and look at these fascinating ideas. All ideas and interpretations in any field are tentative.

Biological coherence is an important quantum phenomenon that is helping us understand many processes that would be otherwise mysterious. These profound interactions are described in Chapters 11 and 16.

The models we use to visualize microscopic structures are extremely useful, because they provide the basis for our conceptions of processes that are essentially invisible. Two important examples are our pictures of the structure of atoms, and of cells. Figure 1 shows the classical structure of the atom as it is often depicted in texts (left) and a more contemporary model that is rarely referred to in the more recent literature (right).

A second source of confusion concerns the structure of the cell (Figure 2). The conventional model of the cell shown at the left has the various organelles more or less floating about in a liquid cellular 'soup'. The cell is also apparently floating in the connective tissue or extracellular matrix. The more contemporary model shown on the right includes the cytoskeleton and nuclear matrix and shows the integrins that connect the cytoskeleton with the extracellular matrix or connective tissue. Further details can be found in Chapter 10. Various versions of the atom and cell models

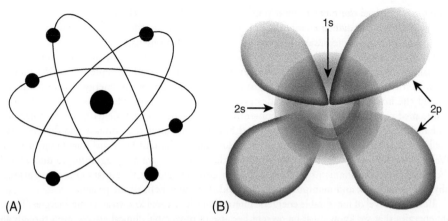

Figure 1 Images of one of the most important and fundamental units found in nature: the atom. The atom visualized here is carbon, with 6 electrons orbiting around a central nucleus (A). This kind of image derives from two articles published by the Danish physicist, Niels Bohr (1913a,b). This image has come to symbolize the 'atomic age'. (B) A more contemporary model of carbon has the 6 electrons in 'orbitals', which are volumes in space that the electrons tend to occupy. The 1s and 2s orbitals can contain 2 electrons; there are three 2p orbitals that can contain up to two electrons each, but only two are shown here because an individual carbon atom has only one electron in each of two 2p orbitals, bringing the total to six electrons. It is the presence of "unfilled orbitals" that enables carbon to form electron-sharing bonds with other carbon atoms or with many other kinds of atoms to create the world of organic chemistry. This quantum character of carbon has enabled this atom to be the fundamental building block of living matter.

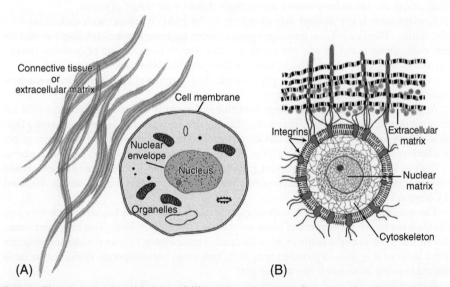

Figure 2 The conventional model of the cell (A) has the various organelles more or less floating about in a liquid cellular 'soup'. The cell is has no connections to the connective tissue or extracellular matrix. The more contemporary model (B) includes the cytoskeleton and nuclear matrix and also shows the integrins that connect the cytoskeleton with the extracellular matrix, connective tissue and fascia. Further details can be found in Chapter 10 Various versions of the model shown to the left appear repeatedly in textbooks. The model is hopelessly out of date and gives a completely inaccurate picture of the fundamental building block of living matter. The drawing to the right shows a more modern and holistic picture of the cell as will be discussed in more detail in Chapters 9 and 10.

shown to the left in these two illustrations appear repeatedly in textbooks. Both of these models are hopelessly out of date and give the beginning student a completely inaccurate picture of two of the most important and fundamental units found in nature. Progress in medicine requires reference to the more accurate and up-to-date images of both the atom and the cell shown on the right in Figures 1 and 2. Moreover, these updated images are vital to our understanding of energetics.

In the absence of an accurate picture of atoms and cells, the beginning student and the experienced researcher alike are simply unable to comprehend the speed and subtleties of energy and information transfer that are vital to living processes.

For a long time, the body has been regarded as a bag of electrolytes in which molecules carrying energy and information move from place to place by random diffusion. Similarly, cellular biochemistry has been based on the idea that molecules diffuse randomly from place to place, eventually encountering enzymes that modify them in specific ways, after which the enzymatic products diffuse away, eventually encountering the next enzyme in the reaction sequence (Figure 10.5). Control of physiological processes and biochemical reactions is similarly envisioned in terms of dissolved agents such as hormones or drugs or reactants that diffuse from place to place and that can interact at different stages of the regulatory/biochemical sequences (Figures 3.11 and 16.6). Several scientists have pointed out that such schemes are far too slow to account for the speed and subtlety of actual living processes. From the perspective of energy medicine, the regulatory and biochemical processes described in most texts are artefacts of the way tissues are studied. Most of biochemistry, for example, is based on fragments of cells and pieces of organelles that have been isolated and purified and suspended in solvents in a test tube (Figure 10.4). Another approach is to extract, dehydrate, and purify molecules and then crystallize them. The study of such preparations has led to important new knowledge, but the techniques used to prepare them alter them from their natural states. This means that one must always be cautious when extrapolating information from study of these materials to the intact cell or intact animal. Isolated and purified materials may be easier to study than intact living tissues, but the processing always leads to preparations that have little or no relationship to the way they are in the intact organism.

Another problem has been the way biochemists have regarded water. For a long time it has been thought that water acts as an inert solvent, a medium in which important molecules are dissolved and wander about. We now know that the relationship of water with living molecules is intimate and profoundly important (Figures 3.14 and 14.5). No biochemical or physiological processes can occur without water.

A third important area concerns resonance, a physical phenomenon whose therapeutic significance should not be underestimated. Resonance explains why molecules do not have to touch to interact (Figures 3.11 and 16.6).

The first edition of the book has had an appeal to those who are seeking the ideas and information that will lead to improved patient care, and to thoughtful patients who seek to increase their understandings of how their bodies function in health and disease. As these words are being written, the number of therapeutic options for patients is increasing rapidly, and determining which modality will work for them can be a confusing and daunting process. Education in this direction is important because it is increasingly obvious that a clear picture of what is happening inside one's own body can be profoundly important in the healing process and/or in simply getting the most out of life. In other words, an understanding of energetics can help anyone at any stage of one's life.

This book tells two stories. One is the story of the emergence of a new and tremendously exciting branch of academic medicine. Behind this emerging science is the equally fascinating tale of why the whole subject has been so confusing and controversial in the past. This second narrative accounts for the paradox of the enduring and widespread academic skepticism and myopia about therapeutic approaches that are based on concepts of energy, at the same time that these methods appear to be benefiting many people. The medicine of the future will recognize and incorporate these methods as a significant advance over present procedures that emphasize reducing symptoms rather than treating causes.

Many therapists who work daily and successfully with human energy systems have felt alien-ated from the sciences that provide the logical and rational foundation for conventional medicine. Some of their most remarkable and important experiences, and those of their clients, seem to defy analysis from current scientific perspectives. A close look at energy medicine resolves this unnecessary confusion and controversy.

Energetics is a rich multi-disciplinary topic. Following the flows of energy through the body is a lesson in every domain of science, ranging from cosmological and geophysical to inter-organism interactions (the ecological level) to physiology, biochemistry, molecular biology, pathology, and behaviour, as well as organs, tissues, cells, molecules, atoms, subatomic particles, and the space between all of the parts. Energetics provides a rich and fascinating and exciting perspective for exploration. Not only does energy teach us about the minutest parts of the living body, but energetic interactions also account for the important properties that arise from the relations be-tween the parts and the environment. One of these properties we call wholeness, the integration that enables the parts to work together successfully. While there has been tension between holistic and reductionist philosophies, energy medicine joins these two perspectives into a seamless whole.

Energetic medicine is pointing in an obvious direction. Most of us prefer a personal philoso-phy and a medicine that enables us to get over our physical or emotional sicknesses or injuries or psychological confusions immediately, if not sooner. The phenomenon of spontaneous healing or remission is a dramatic indication of our innate potential to recover from the most devastat-ing conditions. Clinical experience has shown that rapid and spontaneous remissions can and do happen, even for the most advanced cancers or for the most catastrophic of injuries (see *The Spontaneous Remission Project*, Hirschberg and O'Regan, 1993). This fact shows that, under the appropriate conditions, disease fighting and repair processes in the body can be very powerful. Energy medicine is helping us understand how this is possible.

Spontaneous healing is rare and unpredictable, but there are enough well-documented examples of individuals quickly and permanently recovering from 'terminal' and 'incurable' conditions to stimulate research into how this can happen. Some medical researchers are attempting to induce spontaneous remissions 'on demand' by triggering the body's own defences against cancer and other diseases. While there are few answers, it does appear that 'all the circuitry and machinery is there; the problem is simply to discover how to turn on the right switches to activate the process' (Weil, 1995). When we discuss circuits and switches, we are talking about energy flows. I have personally seen enough instances of both conventional and complementary practitioners 'turning the right switches' or 'jump-starting the healing process' to know that an understanding of 'spontaneous' healing may not be as far away as we might think. Modern research, complemented by the observations of energy therapists, is teaching us about where to look for the 'circuits' and the 'switches'.

The confusion and hostility surrounding energy therapies has contributed significantly to our current medical crisis and the disruptive division between so-called conventional and comple-mentary therapies. In the past, the most remarkable success stories of complementary therapists (as well as healings in the religious context) were often dismissed because there was no logical explanation. The practitioners themselves usually could add little in the way of clarification. By bringing recent science into the picture, we are finding the missing links in our images of the human body in health and disease.

References

Bohr, N., 1913a. On the Constitution of Atoms and Molecules, Part I. Philosophical Magazine 26 (151): 1–24.

Bohr, N., 1913b. On the Constitution of Atoms and Molecules, Part II. Systems Containing Only a Single Nucleus. Philosophical Magazine 26 (153): 476–502.

Gull, S., Lasenby, A., Doran, C., 1993. Imaginary Numbers are not Real – the Geometric Algebra of Spacetime. Cited by Close RA http://www.verumversa.com/ClassicalWaveTheoryOfMatter.pdf, accessed 1-20-13.

Hawking, S., 2011. The Dreams that Stuff is Made of: The Most Astounding Papers on Quantum Physics and How They Shook the Scientific World. Running Press, Philadelphia, PA.

Hirschberg, C., O'Regan, B., 1993. Spontaneous Remission: An Annotated Bibliography. Institute of Noetic Sciences, Petaluma, CA.

Weil, A., 1995. Spontaneous Healing: How to Discover and Enhance Your Body's Natural Ability to Maintain and Heal Itself. Alfred A Knopf, New York.

Wolff, M., 2008. Schroedinger's Universe and the Origin of the Natural Laws.

CHAPTER 1

Introducing and Defining Energy and Energy Medicine

Preconceived notions are the locks on the doors to wisdom.
Merry Browne

It is never too late to give up our prejudices.
Henry David Thoreau

… help me not to despise or oppose what I do not understand.
William Penn

Prejudice is the child of ignorance.
William Hazlitt

Chapter Summary

The purpose of this chapter is to remind readers of how much they already know about energy from their daily experiences of the energetic world within and around them. All of our sensory systems are energy sensors. Before reading further, you might take a few minutes to tune into your own sensory systems, one at a time, to remind yourself of what we usually take for granted – our ability to create a three-dimensional awareness of the world around us using a variety of senses. For example, if you close your eyes and listen, you will find yourself at the centre of a world of sounds. Because of our binaural sound detecting system, we often know the direction from which each sound is coming and can perhaps estimate our distance from its source. Also, listen carefully for a very high-pitched sound that seems to be inside your head. A search of the web shows that many people hear this. Some feel that is tinnitus or some hearing problem. However, it is often a normal part of the operation of the brain, a phenomenon referred to by Stone (1986) as the 'ultrasonic core'. In *Human Tuning*, Beaulieu (2010) describes how day-to-day stresses can change the sound in the head and how the normal condition can be restored with tuning forks. It is not generally known that the ears produce sounds as part of the hearing mechanism. These are called otoacoustic emissions, and they are generated from within the inner ear. They were first demonstrated by Kemp (1978).

Again, with your eyes closed, tune into your thermal body – your awareness of the temperature of the different parts of your skin surface – and your touch body – your awareness of the various pressures on different surfaces of your skin. This can include the places where you experience the weight of your body in contact with surfaces – your gravity body.

To derive full benefit from the contents of this book, set aside previous notions about the subjects of energy and energy medicine and the ways nature works. Simply look at the information with an open mind and with 'new eyes'. The following quotations may encourage this process. Some of the emerging concepts in energy medicine may surprise the educated person because they are different from what they learned in school. When possible, conventional academic texts and journals are cited here. However, some of the most vital and important aspects of the subject will not be found in any medical texts or peer-reviewed scientific journals and therefore cannot be verified from conventional sources. Other information comes from recent research and little-known but very reliable sources and simply has not yet been incorporated into mainstream academic inquiry. Still other sources are ancient healing practices that have not been explored by modern medicine for one reason or another, in spite of the wisdom they have to contribute. Please take a step back from what you have learned about biology and medicine. About half of what we have been taught about nature is wrong or out of date, and the other half is half-wrong. The half-wrong concepts are the most deceptive because they create an illusion that we understand something or have a complete picture when we really do not. Every simple or partial answer can conceal a set of important, unanswered, and, often, unasked questions. In this way, potentially productive lines of inquiry can be closed down, as Francis Bacon stated in 1620 (see the frontispiece of this book).

Forms of Energy in Nature and Their Sensation

We begin with a discussion of the forms of energy found in our environment that we sense with our so-called 'five senses'. Sensation is not, as we shall see, what we usually think it is. Humans actually have far more than five senses. One scholar (Murchie, 1978) recognized 48 senses and trimmed his list to 32:

- Sight, including polarized light and seeing without physical eyes, such as the heliotropism or sun sense of plants.
- The sense of one's visibility or invisibility, related to the ability to either advertise or camouflage one's presence through control of pigmentation, luminescence, transparency, screening, and other means.
- Sensitivity to nonvisible radiations, such as radio waves, X-rays, and gamma rays.
- Temperature sense, related to the ability to insulate, hibernate, or estivate. In the human, this sense has separate receptors and nerves. Animals estivate to escape elements of their environment, such as living in hot, desert climates where water is scarce; behaviour is oriented around staying as cool as possible during the day and collecting moisture at the rare times it is available.
- Electromagnetic sense, including awareness of magnetic polarity, such as organisms that migrate along the magnetic field of the earth.
- Hearing, including sonar and the detection of infra- and ultrasonic frequencies beyond human awareness.
- Pressure awareness, including underground and underwater, as in the lateral line organ of fish and the Earth tremor sense of burrowers, as well as a barometric sense.
- Touch, including on the surface of the skin and the awareness of muscular motion, tickling, vibration as found in spiders; awareness of heartbeat, blood circulation, breathing, and other bodily functions.
- The sense of weight and balance.
- The sense of space or proximity.
- Coriolis sense, or the awareness of the Earth's rotation.
- Smell.
- Taste.
- Appetite, hunger, and the urge to obtain food.
- Humidity sense, including thirst, evaporation control, and the ability to find water or evade a flood.
- Pain, including external, internal, mental or spiritual distress, or a combination of these, and the impulse to weep.
- Fear, including the dread of injury or death, or attack or suffocation, falling, bleeding, disease, and other dangers.
- The procreative urge, including sex awareness, courting, mating, nesting, brooding, parturition, maternity, paternity, and raising the young.

Many, if not all, of the sensory systems are vibration detectors. Vibration, in turn, is one of the most important characteristics of the energies within and around us. In other words, virtually all energies are rhythmic – they are rarely constant, but vary from time to time, often coming in pulses or oscillations. Even heat, which is usually a scalar quantity (having magnitude but not direction), resolves into the rate of vibration of atoms or molecules. We are burned when we come in contact with a hot object because the atoms in the object are vibrating rapidly and transfer their violent momentum to our tissues, damaging them. Finally, we will see how the simple definitions of energy used in physics can help us understand the nature of both energy and energy medicine.

The 'Five Senses'

Energy comes in different forms, and we are familiar with many of them because we sense energies all the time to interpret what is going on within and around us and to track our interactions with the world around us. We are taught that there are five senses: sight, hearing, taste, touch, and smell (Figure 1.1). Each of these senses involves organs with specialized cells that have receptors for specific kinds of energy. These cells transduce or convert the vibrations into a local 'generator' or 'receptor' potential, which is then converted into trains of action potentials that are conducted through nerves to the brain, which integrates and interprets the incoming information to create our ever-changing picture of the energy world around us and of our place and movements within that world.

Sight is the most sophisticated sense in humans. In terms of our evolutionary history, smell is probably the oldest of the senses – the simplest and most ancient bacteria and protozoa have chemical senses that enable them to move toward nourishment and away from toxic environments. Given the length of time olfaction has been exposed to the evolutionary process, it may be a far more sophisticated sense than we usually realize. In terms of neuroscience, the sense of smell is a 'first responder' because of the short pathways between the olfactory bulb in the nose and the limbic system and hippocampus. Animals can usually react to and interpret an odour before they can see its source. The reason for this is that it takes from one-quarter to one-half second for the

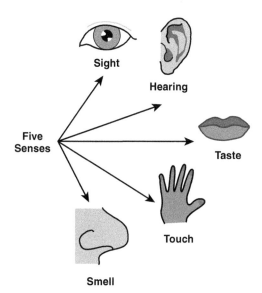

Figure 1.1   The traditional 'five senses' enable us to detect the energies present in our environment.

brain to form a visual image in the visual cortex and even longer for the brain to interpret the image. Our sense of smell is virtually instantaneous.

At a fundamental level, many of our senses detect different forms of vibration. Light and sound are obviously vibrational or frequency phenomena, although they travel through different media. Light moves through so-called empty space (later we will see that space has a structure, see Figure 13.11), whereas sound requires a medium such as air or water. The mechanisms involved in taste and smell are not as well understood. While there is debate on the topic, it seems likely to this author that taste and smell are also vibratory senses, although this is not the conventional view (see Burr, 2004 for a perspective on the arguments about the nature of olfaction). Touch involves four kinds of sensations that can be identified: cold, heat, contact, and pain. Heat and cold are obviously vibrational senses; contact and pain are more challenging to explain. For complementary and alternative therapies, the study of the physiology and energetics of touch are of profound importance.

Touch has a vibrational aspect. One of the ways we can determine what we are touching is by moving our fingers over it. Most objects can be identified by their texture. Different textures, in turn, set up qualitatively different vibrations in touch receptors gliding over a surface. These vibrations are encoded into neural impulses that are conveyed to the brain where they are interpreted. Our fingertips have remarkable capabilities for the detection of minute differences in surface textures and contours.

Beyond the Five Senses

In 1907, Charles Scott Sherrington introduced the terms *proprioception, interoception,* and *exteroception.* The *exteroceptors* are the organs responsible for detecting information from outside the body – the traditional five senses. The *interoceptors* give information about the internal organs. *Proprioception* is awareness of movement derived from muscular, tendon, and articular (joint) tensions and pressures. Joint receptors are located in the capsules of joints. Stretching the capsule deforms the endings, leading to a receptor potential, and the extent of the depolarization determines the frequency of the action potentials that are generated. It is now recognized that joint angle is sensed from composite signals from joint receptors, muscle length receptors, and skin receptors. Much of the research on this topic has focused on the finger and hand sensors, which are of particular interest to hands-on therapists who rely on their hands and fingers for sensation and dexterous movements (Johnson, 2004). *Kinesthesia* is often used interchangeably with *proprioception,* although kinesthesia places greater emphasis on motion. The kinesthetic sense enables us to touch the tip of our nose with our eyes closed or to reach to and scratch a part of our body that is itchy.

The proprioceptive sense also includes information from sensory neurons located in the inner ear (motion and orientation) and in the stretch receptors located in the muscles and joint-supporting tendons and ligaments (stance). Humans therefore have awareness of balance and motion that can involve the coordinated use of a number of sensory organs. Our sense of balance results from the complex interaction of visual inputs, the proprioceptive sensors (those that are affected by gravity and the stretch sensors found in muscles, skin, and joints), the inner ear vestibular system, pressure sensors on the soles of the feet, and the central nervous system.

Synesthesia

Some people experience a fascinating phenomenon called synesthesia, or 'mixing of the senses', in which one type of sensory stimulation evokes the sensation of another. For example, hearing a sound may produce a sensation of a color, or a shape may be sensed as a smell or taste. Synesthesia is hereditary, occurring in about 1 out of 1000 individuals. The most common forms of synesthesia link numbers or letters with colors. Examples of synesthesia have been documented in many interesting books and articles, such as *The Man Who Tasted Shapes* (Cytowic and Cole, 2003) or *The Man Who Mistook His Wife for a Hat* (Sacks, 1998).

There are other forms of energy that are less visible or palpable, but we know them to be part of our world: electricity, magnetism, chemical energy, and electromagnetism.

A Magnetic Sense?

Many therapists who work with the human energy system report a sort of magnetic sense when they bring their hands close to the surface of another person's body. The sensation is comparable to the experience of holding a magnet in each hand and bringing the magnetic poles toward each other. With practice, many therapists are able to use this phenomenon to locate areas in the patient's body that are chronically disturbed or painful. Likewise, magnetic therapy involves projecting magnetic fields from the therapist's hands to encourage energy flow and healing in a part of a patient's body.

Until recently, there was little science to support the concept of a magnetic sense. However, a recent report describes a plausible mechanism for sensing and projecting biomagnetic fields with the human hand (Irmak, 2010). The proposed mechanism involves Merkel cells found in the skin. These cells (Figure 1.2) contain pigment granules composed of neuromelanin, which is an iron-containing magnetic material. In the presence of a magnetic field the melanin-containing granules, which are called melanosomes, will tilt. According to the Irmak hypothesis, cytoskeletal filaments can couple this movement to mechanically gated ion channels in the Merkel cell surface (Figure 1.3A). According to Irmak, this system can also work in reverse, i.e., the Merkel cells can also produce a biomagnetic field, as shown in Figure 1.3B.

The Merkel cell hypothesis can be placed in the context of another fascinating but little-known concept of the role of melanin as a system-wide organizing molecule (Barr et al., 1983). On the basis of an extensive review of the biology of neuromelanin, these authors proposed that there are two whole-body 'melanocentric systems' that play key roles in development, tissue repair, and a variety of other regulations. This investigation synthesized a vast amount of research on melanin to provide a basis for a system that can explain many of the phenomena taking place in energy medicine and a wide range of complementary and alternative therapies.

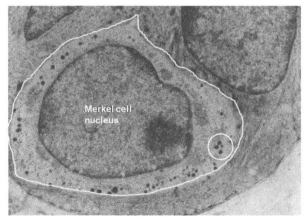

Figure 1.2 A Merkel cell in the epidermis. The cell (outlined in white) is a magnetic receptor because of the melanin granules (indicated by the small oval) that contain melanin, a magnetic material. *(From Bloom and Fawcett, A Textbook of Histology, 12th edition, Chapman & Hall, New York, with permission.)*

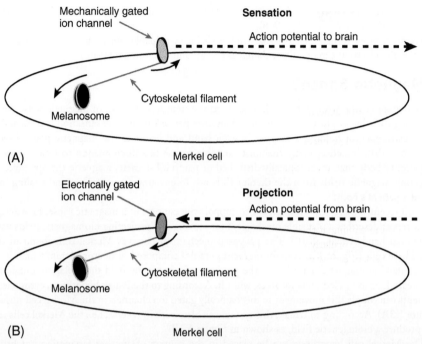

Figure 1.3   Possible basis for an ability to sense and project magnetic fields, based on Irmak (2010). The melanosome contains a magnetic material called neuromelanin and acts like a tiny magnet. (A) Magnetic sense: A biomagnetic field causes the melanosome to rotate, and a cytoskeletal filament tugs on a mechanically sensitive ion channel in the cell membrane. When the channel opens, it creates a receptor potential that is transmitted via sensory neurons to the brain. (B) Magnetic projection: An action potential from the brain causes an electrically gated ion channel in the membrane to rotate. The movement is conveyed to the melanosomes via a cytoskeletal filament such as a microtubule or micofilament, causing the melanosome to rotate and produce a magnetic field.

Individual melanin molecules are not magnetic, but many such molecules can accumulate to form granules that bind iron or other metals. This occurs in Merkel cells in the skin and in pigmented neurons in the region of the brain known as the substantia nigra. The binding of neuromelanin to iron is of interest due to its role in brain aging and Parkinson's disease.

Double et al. (2003) and Kincade (2006)

Melanin is also a semiconductor. The significance of this will be discussed in more detail in Chapters 10-12, 15, and 17.

A 'Sixth Sense'

One can also find references to a 'sixth sense', which refers to any supposed sense or means of perception, such as intuition, remote sensing, telepathy, clairvoyance, and so on, other than the conventional five senses mentioned above. Such phenomena have been discussed in scholarly texts such as Radin (1997), and many people view them as both real and important. As with other controversial topics such as prayer and distant healing, these phenomena can be discussed in terms of energetics, especially in terms of quantum physics. A basis for subtle and often unconscious sensory phenomena arises from consideration of quantum coherence, which will be discussed in Chapters 13 and 16.

Defining Energy and Energy Medicine

An excellent definition of energy comes from physics: *Energy is the ability to do work*. Everyone knows what it feels like to not have any energy and therefore not feel like doing anything. When one or another of our living energy systems is not operating optimally, we simply do not feel energetic; we do not feel right. From the perspectives emerging from energy medicine, such conditions can be described in terms of energetic circuits within the body. When these circuits are compromised or imbalanced, we are unable to utilize our personal energy normally. A variety of names have been given to such conditions when they become chronic, including 'chronic fatigue syndrome' and 'myalgic encephalomyelitis'. Fatigue (also referred to as exhaustion, lethargy, languidness, languor, lassitude, and listlessness) describes a range of common conditions, usually associated with physical and/or mental weakness, varying from a general state of lethargy to specific work-induced burning sensations in one's muscles. Bodywork and movement therapists regularly observe that some patients have visible structural imbalances that can be corrected by various approaches and that the result is a great increase in personal energy. Physical fatigue is the inability to continue functioning at the level of one's normal abilities. It is widespread in everyday life, but usually becomes particularly noticeable during heavy exercise. Mental fatigue is another common experience. Lack of energy can arise because of dehydration, malnutrition, exhaustion, depression, and other causes. Recent work on grounding or earthing has added another dimension to our understanding of human energetic systems – electron deficiency (see Chapter 17 for more details). This book will provide readers with a better understanding of their personal energy systems that will often enable them to escape or avoid such conditions.

In physics and other sciences, the term, "energy" (from the Greek ενεργός energos, "active, working") is a physical quantity that represents a measurable property of objects and systems. The English scientist, Thomas Young (1773–1829), was the first to use the term "energy" in 1807. The concept had emerged out of the earlier idea of vis viva *(from the Latin for* living force*) which the German Gottfried Wilhelm Leibniz (1646–1716) introduced as the essential property that is conserved during natural processes (see Smith, 2006).*

Energy is always conserved, that is energy can be converted from one form to another in a natural process, but the total amount of energy always remains the same. In other words, energy can never be created nor destroyed. This is a law of physics known as the law of conservation of energy. It is an exact law and no exceptions have been found. An early general statement of the law is in Mohr (1837): "Besides the 54 known chemical elements there is in the physical world one agent only, and this is called Kraft *[energy or work]. It may appear, according to circumstances, as motion, chemical affinity, cohesion, electricity, light and magnetism; and from any one of these forms it can be transformed into any of the others."*

In the International System of Units (SI), work is measured in joules (symbol: J). It is a measure of heat, electricity and mechanical work. The rate at which work is performed is power. The SI unit of power is the watt (W), which is equal to one joule per second. Other, non-SI units of power include ergs per second (erg/s), horsepower (hp), and foot-pounds per minute. One unit of horsepower is equivalent to 33,000 foot-pounds per minute, or the power required to lift 550 pounds one foot in one second, and is equivalent to about 746 watts. Other units include those used to measure the energy in food, calories or kilocalories; heat or Btu per hour (Btu/h); and tons of refrigeration (12,000 Btu/h).

A scientific definition of energy medicine:

Energy medicine is defined as the diagnostic and therapeutic use of energy, whether detected by or produced by a medical device or by the human body.

Energy medicine recognizes that the human body utilizes various forms of energy for the internal communications that maintain and organize vital living systems and for powering processes such sensation, digestion, circulation and movement. Energy medicine involves the use energies of particular intensities and frequencies and other characteristics that stimulate the repair of one or more tissues, or that enable built-in healing mechanisms to operate more effectively. Such energies can come from the environment, from another human being or from a medical device.

The term *life force* has been controversial for more than a century. Some scholars have regarded the discussion in the first edition of this book to have brought that controversy to an end.

We now know that the living organism is designed to both adapt to and utilize many different kinds of forces and that healing processes involve the operation of many kinds of communications. There is no single 'life force' or 'healing energy'. Instead, there are many systems in the body that take in, store, release, conduct, and utilize various kinds of energy and information. Different energetic therapies focus on different aspects of this multiplicity, and each of these therapies presents a valuable set of clues and testable hypotheses about how human energy systems work.

Modern biomedicine focuses almost exclusively on chemical energy. Biochemists have a detailed model of how the food we eat is used to manufacture molecules that can store, transport, and release chemical energy at places where energy is required, such as in nerves, muscles, glands, and organs. The adenosine triphosphate (ATP) molecule produced by mitochondria is envisioned as a primary intermediate in energy metabolism. The discovery of ATP and its interactions has been one of the great accomplishments of modern biochemistry and molecular biology. An equally detailed picture has emerged of molecular signals that regulate many physiological processes. For example, a host of molecules known as cytokines regulate the immune system as it carries out the diverse protective and defensive processes that are essential to life (Figure 1.4). Neuropeptides and neurohormones connect nerve cells with the tissues they influence and play huge roles in modulating emotions. These molecules are ancient in terms of evolution and are actually produced by virtually every cell in the body (Pert, 1999).

The physiological, biochemical, anatomical, and energetic systems in the body interdigitate – indeed, they are embedded within each other. Effective therapeutic work on one system inevitably affects the composite. Stated differently, organization and functional integration are contagious – when one physiological system begins to function optimally, neighbouring systems improve as well. This is the reason we have such a diversity of alternative therapies: Each approach may focus on a different energy system but can have a multitude of beneficial effects. For example, body-workers and movement therapists may focus on the structural and kinetic systems in the body, and the benefits of their work will spill over into the neural, immune, and emotional realms. Energy psychologists are often able to resolve old traumatic experiences, which frequently leads to spontaneous healing of serious diseases. Subtle aromas, homeopathic remedies, or gentle touch often shifts the entire organism to a new level of functioning.

Energy medicine is a rich and fascinating multidisciplinary topic with a broad scientific and practical agenda. Following the flows of energy through the body is a lesson in every domain of biology, ranging from cells and their molecular and atomic components to tissues, organs, organ systems, and the environment at all levels of scale. Not only does energy medicine teach us about the minutest parts of the living body, but energetic interactions also account for the important properties that arise from the relations between the parts. One of these properties we call *wholeness*, the integration that enables the parts to work together, whether it is to heal a scratch or a broken bone, recover from cancer, or set an Olympic record.

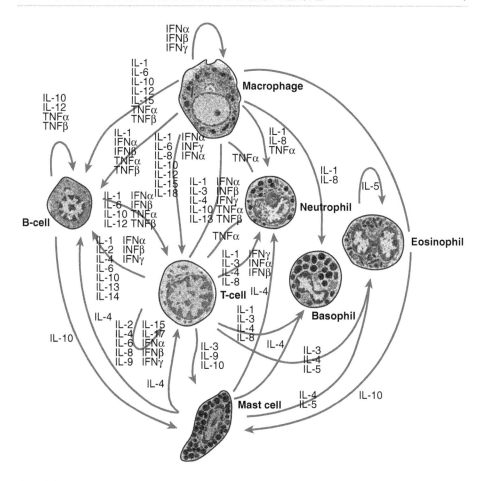

Figure 1.4 The cytokine network and other regulatory systems are usually described in terms of molecular signals that can diffuse from place to place and that can thereby regulate systemic processes such as the immune response. Energy medicine recognizes the vital roles of such molecular signalling and adds another dimension: resonant electromagnetic or photonic signalling between the signalling molecules and receptors on cell surfaces. Molecular resonance will be discussed in more detail in Chapters 3 and 9.

Research in a variety of fields has demonstrated that living cells and tissues are designed to both adapt to and utilize many different kinds of forces. We have also learned that that healing processes involve the operation of many kinds of communications. There is no single 'life force' or 'healing energy'. Instead, science recognizes many systems in the body that take in, store, release, conduct, and utilize various kinds of energy and information. Different energetic therapies focus on different aspects of this multiplicity, and each of these therapies presents a valuable set of clues and testable hypotheses about how human energy systems work.

References

Bacon, F., 1620. Novum Organum. In: Thomas Fowler, (Ed.), Book II of Instauratio magna. McMillan and Co., Clarendon Press, Oxford, 1878, The New Organon.

Barr, F.E., Saloma, J.S., Buchele, M.J., 1983. Melanin: the organizing molecule. Medical Hypotheses 11, 1–40.

Beaulieu, J., 2010. Human Tuning: Sound Healing with Tuning Forks. BioSonic Enterprises Ltd, Stone Ridge, NY.

Burr, C., 2004. The Emperor of Scent: A True Story of Perfume and Obsession. Random House, New York, NY.

Cytowic, R.E., Cole, J., 2003. The Man Who Tasted Shapes. Bradford Books, MIT Press, Cambridge, MA.

Double, K.L., Gerlach, M., Schünemann, V., Trautwein, A.X., Zecca, L., Gallorini, M., Youdim, M.B., Riederer, P., Ben-Shachar, D., 2003. Iron-binding characteristics of neuromelanin of the human substantia nigra. Biochem. Pharmacol. 66 (3), 489–494.

Irmak, M.K., 2010. Multifunctional Merkel cells: their roles in electromagnetic reception, finger-pring formation, Reiki, epigenetic inheritance and hair form. Medical Hypotheses 75, 162–168.

Johnson, K., 2004. Closing in on the neural mechanisms of finger joint angle sense. Focus on quantitative analysis of dynamic strain sensitivity in human skin mechanoreceptors. J. Neurophysiol. 92, 3167–3168.

Kemp, D.T., 1978. Stimulated acoustic emissions from within the human auditory system. J. Acoust. Soc. Am. 64, 1386–1391.

Kincade, K., 2006. FEL reveals links between melanin structure and Parkinson's. Laser Focus World 42 (12), 33.

Mohr, K.F., 1837. Ansichten über die Natur der Wärme. Ann. der Pharm. 24, 141–147.

Murchie, G., 1978. The Seven Mysteries of Life. An Exploration in Science and Philosophy. Houghton Mifflin Company, Boston, MA, pp. 178–180.

Pert, C.B., 1999. Molecules of Emotion: The Science Behind Mind-Body Medicine. Simon & Schuster, New York, NY.

Radin, D.I., 1997. The Conscious Universe. The Scientific Truth of Psychic Phenomena. HarperCollins, New York, NY.

Sacks, O., 1998. The Man Who Mistook His Wife for a Hat: and Other Clinical Tales. Touchstone, Clearwater, FL.

Sherrington, C.S., 1907. On the proprioceptive system, especially in its reflex aspect. Brain 29, 467–485.

Smith, G.E., 2006. The *Vis Viva* dispute: a controversy at the dawn of dynamics. Phys. Today 59 (10), 31–36.

Stone, R., 1986. Polarity Therapy. The Complete Collected Works. vol. 1. CRCS Publications, Sebastopol, CA, Page 10.

Young, T., 1807. Lectures on natural philosophy. London. Lecture VIII, p. 78. See Fechner, G.T. (1878). Ueber den Ausgangswerth der kleinsten Absweichungssumme. Hirzel, S., p. 650; also see Kelland, P., 1845. A course of lectures on natural philosophy and the mechanical arts, a new edition with references and notes, in two volumes, by Young, T., Talyor and Walton, London.

CHAPTER 2

Basic Physics and Biophysics, Part I: Electricity and Magnetism

If you wish to understand the universe, think of energy, frequency, and vibration.

Nikola Tesla

Chapter Summary

Every morning millions of people around the world awake to a tone or to music coming from an alarm clock or clock radio. In rural areas, the wake-up call may be the sound of a rooster or birds singing. Often the day begins with flipping a light switch, pressing a button on a coffee maker, turning on the stove to make breakfast, and starting the car. For some of us, starting the car takes place after we have unlocked the car door, either by turning the car key in the lock, or by pressing a button that unlocks the door with a radio signal. Each of these everyday events involves various forms of energy, conversions of energy from one type to another, the movement of energy from one place to another, and an incredible phenomenon called resonance. *Resonance* is the remarkable phenomenon that enables us to hear the rooster and see the light from a star – light that may have begun its journey to Earth long before we were born. Each of these events can teach us a piece of the story of energy medicine because the human body depends on electricity and resonant interactions, and all of these phenomena have profound medical implications.

This chapter explores the basic physics that enables us to turn on a light and the biophysics that enables us to see that light. In discussing these events we will have to take a close look at such things as electrons, electric currents, and radio waves. If you are confused about these subjects, there is no reason for concern – some of the greatest minds in history have puzzled over what an electron really is, what magnetism is, how currents actually flow through wires, or how sound, light, and radio signals travel through space. This chapter will present some of the tentative and often-debated conclusions those great minds have reached about the nature of these everyday phenomena. The important point is that the story of energy medicine and how our bodies sense and use energy can best be understood and communicated with the basic information and vocabulary from the disciplines of physics and biophysics. This is the scientific background and language needed to comprehend energy medicine and to learn more about how our bodies work. Some parts of the story are a bit technical, and they have been separated into boxes so it is easy for the reader to skip them.

An Academic Discipline

This book, and especially this chapter, point towards a new academic discipline called *energy medicine*. This new discipline is as scientifically and philosophically sound and detailed as any other academic discipline and is having a profound impact on medicine. The reason for this is that energetics provides the intellectual glue, the fabric that can connect all of the other disciplines together into a coherent biomedicine.

This is not a chapter on physics, nor is it a chapter on biology. It is about the interface between these two disciplines. The whole book and all the exciting vistas of energy medicine described here hinge on the information in this chapter. Basic physics principles will be presented followed by a brief introduction to their therapeutic implications with references to the chapters where these implications will be explored in more detail. The simple vocabulary that follows constitutes a precise language that can be used to create a wide-ranging conversation about energy medicine.

We will discuss some of the basic laws of physics and how they apply to living things. Some of these laws of physics are extremely reliable – they have always worked since they were described well over a century ago. We experience them every day when we start our car or take an elevator. Electric generators and motors work because of two laws of physics described in this chapter. If the car does not start or the elevator does not go up or down, it is not because there is an error in the laws of physics – it is because of some gap in the circuitry. Energy medicine discusses the circuitry within our bodies – the realm of biophysics – how problems in the circuitry can give rise to disease and disorder and how the circuits can be repaired.

Some Vocabulary

Our exploration of the basics tells us that the clock radio that wakes us in the morning brings the sound of music to us from a distant source via electromagnetic signals. Our radio transduces or converts these electromagnetic signals into sound waves that travel through the air to our ears. Our ears transduce these sounds into electrical events within our nervous system. A description of these processes introduces the basic energy vocabulary that will be used throughout this book. You can refer back to these definitions and the other topics in this chapter as needed during your exploration of energy medicine.

- *Transduction* is a process or mechanism that converts signals from one form to another or converts one type of energy to another. An electronic device or a biological process that does this is called a *transducer*. Our eyes transduce patterns of light into chemical messages in retinal cells that are transduced into nerve impulses. Our ears transduce sound waves into nerve impulses. Touch receptors in our skin transduce the touch from another person into nerve impulses, and so on.

- *Resonance* refers to the tendency of any object to oscillate or vibrate at maximum amplitude at certain frequencies, known as the system's *resonant* or *natural frequency*. A bell, a violin string, a vocal cord, or an eardrum will have a certain resonant frequency depending on its physical characteristics (e.g., elasticity) and its geometry. Resonance also refers to the coupling that can take place between two systems with similar resonant frequencies. When one system vibrates, the other one vibrates at the same frequency, even though they are separated by some distance. Hence the resonance between the vibrations of a speaker's vocal cords and the hair cells in a listener's cochlea enables us to hear.

- Objects with similar form will tend to resonate. One name for this is the *tuning fork effect*. Consider a tuning fork tuned to A, 440 cycles per second (Hz), the international 'concert pitch' used to tune orchestras. A sharp blow to the tuning fork will cause all other nearby objects with the same resonant frequency to vibrate. This includes other tuning forks tuned to A, as well as the violin's second string and the first string of the viola. This example of resonance involves sound waves moving through the air.

- Radio transmitters set up electrical oscillations of particular frequencies in an electrical conductor referred to as a *transmitting antenna*. These electrical oscillations create electromagnetic fields that travel through space and set up corresponding oscillations in another electrical conductor called a *receiving antenna*. The transmitting and receiving antennas are similar in geometry, enabling them to resonate. The receiving antenna is connected to an electronic circuit that converts (transduces) the electromagnetic oscillations into sound waves that travel through the air to our ears. We need to know about electromagnetic

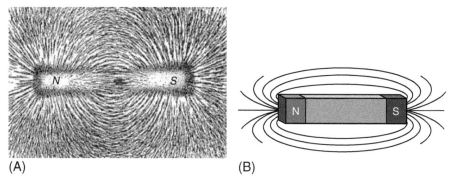

(A)   (B)

Figure 2.1 The English physicist Michael Faraday referred to the patterns traced out in metal filings near a magnet (A) as magnetic curves. Later he called them lines of force. (B) Imaginary lines in space that show the nature of the field. The notation has been widely used to describe magnetic interactions (right) and other energetic relationships between objects.

resonance because it also takes place between molecules in the body to produce important regulatory effects.

- The speaker in the radio or the vocal cords in the rooster vibrate, and both of these phenomena create sound waves that travel through the air and eventually cause our eardrum to vibrate. These mechanical vibrations or oscillations of our eardrum are conducted through the structures within our ears and eventually cause tiny hairs within our cochlea to vibrate. Our ears transduce the sound waves into electrical signals that are conducted to our brains via nerves. At the end of this process is the *auditory cortex*, which enables us to hear the sound.

- Energetic interactions between objects are often visualized by means of 'lines of force'. Several examples of this notion will appear in this and subsequent chapters. The concept of lines of force is thought to have begun with the early research of the English chemist and physicist Michael Faraday (1852), who described the curved patterns traced out in metal filings near a magnet (Figure 2.1A). Initially, he referred to these as magnetic curves and later called them magnetic lines of force (Figure 2.1B) or simply lines of force (Fisher, 2004). These geometric shapes provide a convenient way of visualizing energy linkages between objects, including electrical, magnetic, gravitational, and electromagnetic interactions. Lines of force have made possible sophisticated mathematical and experimental concepts and theories that will be discussed in this chapter.

Electric, Magnetic, and Electromagnetic Fields

Electric charge is a fundamental property of some subatomic particles such as electrons and protons. A stationary electric charge is surrounded by a spherical electric field (Figure 2.2). This electric field influences other electrically charged objects. There are two ways of describing the influences of fields and the ways they interact with each other. One perspective is that objects have properties that modify the space around them such that another object entering that space will have a force exerted upon it. A second perspective does not require the concept of force: Objects have properties that modify the space around them such that another object entering that space will experience a change in its motion. In the case of the electron, shown in Figure 2.2, the lines of force reveal the direction of motion a positive test charge would experience when brought into the space around the electron. Specifically, since opposite charges attract, the positive test charge will be drawn towards the center of charge of the electron.

With regard to the image of the electron shown in Figure 2.2, recognize that the view of the electron as a point in space is but one of several models of the electron and other charged particles.

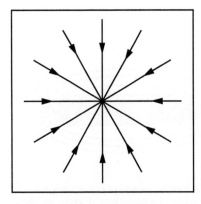

Figure 2.2   The electric field of a stationary electric charge. Note that the charge is imaged as a point in space. This is a simplification that has made it easier to calculate charge interactions. However, there are other valuable perspectives on the nature of the electric charge that will be discussed in this chapter.

WHAT IS AN ELECTRON?

Much of the discussion that follows will concern the behaviour of electrons and other charged particles. We shall see that when a charge moves, magnetic fields are produced. And we will also see that the opposite is true: Magnetic fields alter the motions of nearby charges. These principles are profoundly important for energy medicine. Many of the techniques used in energy medicine look like New-Age hocus-pocus until they are viewed through the discerning eyes of the physicist and biophysicist. Hence this chapter is an introduction to the worldview from these perspectives.

It is necessary to look at the nature of these particles in some detail because many of the seemingly remarkable phenomena in energy medicine will remain inexplicable without reference to the behaviour of these fundamental particles. What is being presented in this section goes deep – to the fundamental properties of all matter in the universe. Readers may wish to postpone reading this section until their curiosity has built up from the concepts presented in later sections of the book, and they feel motivated to dig deeper.

Understanding the basic physics and quantum aspects of charged particles is a continuing challenge for scientists from every field of inquiry. Many of the fundamental questions have not been answered completely. Other questions have several answers, with great minds disagreeing about which is correct. This must not stop us from looking at the pieces of the puzzle we understand or think we understand. As we look at these concepts, we must keep in mind that all of the information is subject to change as more discoveries are made. Some of the more extraordinary conclusions that have been reached are not agreed upon by all physicists. For example, there is abundant evidence for non-locality, i.e., at a fundamental level, all of the particles in the universe are dependent on and continuously interacting with all of the other particles in the universe. All parts are continuously in relationship and communication. Some physicists and quantum physicists regard this concept as preposterous; others observe phenomena every day in their laboratories that can only be explained in this way.

> *At root what is, is no longer THINGS but what happens BETWEEN things, these are the terms of the reality contemporary to us – and the terms of what we are.*
>
> OLSON (1983)

Hence there is disagreement about what an electron actually is. This is not surprising, since electrons are far too small to be seen with any microscope. We do have sophisticated tools that allow us to infer what an electron may be like, and the nature of these tools tells us much about the nature of physical reality – but not everything.

The issue takes us to our fundamental conceptualization of the structure of the material world. Indeed, a number of distinguished scientists have concluded that there is no matter as such. They suggest that what we refer to as matter is actually a local condensation of energy.

In Quantum Field Theory (QFT), "... there are no particles; there are only fields and field quanta ... everything is fields; ... reality consists only of fields and interactions between fields."

BROOKS (2010)

and

Matter, which is you and me and all three-dimensional things, are regions where the field is extremely intense. We are beings of energy.

WALKER (2002)

Some people are uncomfortable with these ideas:

To some, the real disappearance of matter seems as disturbing as the loss of life and ruin of the city, for associated with the word 'matter' in most people's minds is the word 'reality.'

CONANT (1981)

Many texts refer to electrons as particles that can be mathematically treated as though they are points in space. Treating an electron as a point in space greatly simplifies the mathematical treatments of charge and field effects. However, while simplifications can be very useful, it must always be remembered that the analytical process began with a simplification that may be an approximation of reality and not reality itself. Therefore, some of the subsequent conclusions may be distorted accordingly. Philosophers of science have developed a useful perspective on this phenomenon and refer to *meaning invariance*. It is a problem that occurs again and again in science. It is always essential to examine tentative assumptions about nature that were temporarily useful but that have gradually come to be taken as facts. Philosopher of science Paul Feyerabend (1981) wrote that situations arise when a solution to a problem will be considered acceptable only if it does not disturb the meanings of certain key terms and assumptions and all of the work that has been done that is based on those assumptions. Meaning invariance can make problems insoluble. In other words, we are discouraged from discussing a wave model of the electron because doing so might require revision of countless calculations and conclusions based on the point or particle assumptions, conclusions that have been applied throughout the field of physics. On the same subject, Northrop (1959) comments: 'One of the basic problems in the unification of scientific knowledge is clarifying the relation between the concepts used in the early stages of development of the field and those which come later. In the context of the structure of matter, and a wide range of other scientific issues, meaning invariance poses deep problems'.

An alternative model of the structure of the electron emerges from an energy-wave model. Such a model has its roots in statements from the most important physicists. For example,

Physical objects are not in space, but...objects are spatially extended. In this way the concept 'empty space' loses its meaning... The particle can only appear as a limited region in space in which the field strength or the energy density is particularly high...

EINSTEIN (1954)

Milo Wolff (2009) has written eloquently about a wave model. His model resolves many of the confusions and paradoxes of the particulate model. The basic conclusion is that every electron

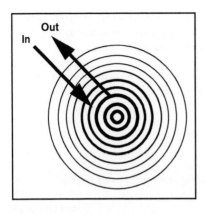

Figure 2.3   Wave model of the electron based on the work of Milo Wolff. The electron exists because of the interactions of 'in-waves' coming from all other electrons and 'out-waves' that extend to all other electrons in the universe. *(From Wolff, M., 1993. Fundamental laws, microphysics, and cosmology. Physics Essays 6(2):181–203.)*

exists because of its interactions with all other electrons in the universe. The electron exists because of the interactions of 'in-waves' coming from all other electrons and 'out-waves' that extend to all of the other electrons (Figure 2.3). Wolff and his colleagues have prepared dramatic animations showing the in- and out-waves and their interactions that produce standing waves. This concept, including the nature of these in- and out-waves, can provide tentative explanations for some of the otherwise mysterious phenomena taking place in energy medicine. For example, the effects of prayer and distant healing, considered by many to be scientifically unsupportable, are a logical consequence of the wave model of matter proposed by Wolff.

WHAT IS CHARGE?

We would like to know the source of the electron's electric charge because it is fundamental to electricity, magnetism, and electromagnetism; is part of many physical laws; and is fundamental to countless biological processes. Indeed, it is the attraction of the opposite charges of the electron and proton that holds the universe together. Charge is so fundamental that one would think it would be well understood. Unfortunately, we do not really know how charge arises. We do know that the proton gets its charge from the charged particles (quarks) it is made of. Of course, then the question becomes: Why are quarks charged? And are there also quarks in electrons? Apparently not. So far, electrons have resisted all attempts to find any hint of internal structure. We also know that the proton is 1836 times more massive than the electron. How can these two particles, the electron and the proton, with such a huge difference in mass, have identical charges? Again, we simply do not know what charge is, so we cannot answer this basic question. It is an important question because the charges of electrons and protons in an atom exactly cancel each other so that atoms can be electrically balanced or neutral.

MAGNETISM FROM ELECTRICITY: AMPÈRE'S LAW

If you are frustrated by the lack of precision of our knowledge at the basic level of electrons and protons, it will be comforting to know that the behaviour of these objects at larger scales is very reliable and predictable. They are so predictable that their behaviour is described by very well established physical laws. Laws are defined as scientific generalizations that are observations based on the behaviour of natural processes that are repeated again and again for many years. By definition, physical laws are statements about phenomena that are consistent: There have never been repeatable contradicting observations to refute them. Hence laws are solid enough that they are accepted universally within the scientific community.

There are two physical laws that are of immense importance to energy medicine. The first is Ampère's law, developed in 1826 by André-Marie Ampère (1775–1836). As a physical law, it is very reliable – no exceptions have been found in well over 150 years of physics research.

Ampère's law was devised to quantify an accidental discovery made in 1820 by Hans Christian Ørsted (1777–1851). While giving a physics demonstration at the University of Copenhagen, Ørsted noticed that electric currents flowing from a battery and through a wire caused nearby compass needles to wiggle when the battery was switched on and off (Figure 2.4). The momentous conclusion was that electric currents can create magnetic fields in the surrounding space. The phenomenon was so reliable that Ørsted became convinced that magnetic fields radiate from all around a wire carrying an electric current. In other words, electricity gives rise to magnetism. The unit of magnetic induction, the oersted, has been named in honour of Ørsted's fundamental contribution to the field of electromagnetism.

Ørsted's findings influenced the French physicist André-Marie Ampère (Figure 2.5) to devise a single mathematical formula to represent the magnetic forces between current-carrying conductors. One reason Ampère's law is so important for energy medicine is that it explains the origin of the biomagnetic field surrounding the human body. As will be described in Chapter 5. See Figure 5.17, the various organs in the body generate electrical currents that flow through the tissues and therefore generate magnetic fields both within and around the body.

The strongest electrical field is produced by the heart and generates a current that flows through the circulatory system, which is a good conductor. In accord with Ampère's law, this current produces the strongest biomagnetic field of the body (Figure 2.6). This point is important because of the skepticism about energy fields around the body that are described and used by

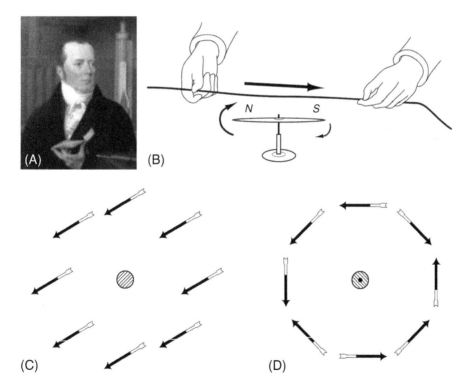

Figure 2.4 In 1820, Hans Christian Ørsted (A) accidentally discovered that passing a current through a wire would cause nearby compass needles to rotate (B). Electricity can give rise to magnetism! This has become a basic law of physics called *Ampère's law*. In the absence of an electric field, all of the compass needles point towards the north pole (C). When a current passes through a wire (D), the compass needles orient themselves in a circle around the wire. In this illustration the wire is represented as the dot in the center of the compass needles, and the current is flowing towards the viewer.

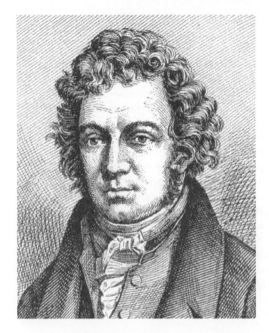

Figure 2.5 André-Marie Ampère (1775–1836).

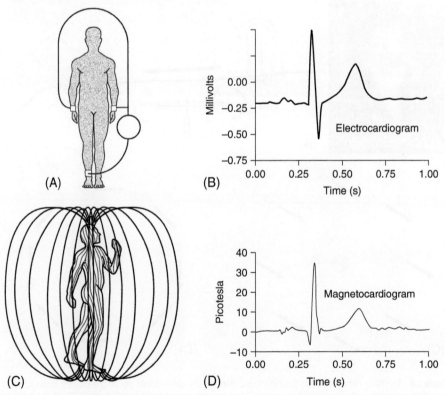

Figure 2.6 The strongest electrical field is produced by the heart and generates an electrical field that is conducted throughout the body via the circulatory system (A), which is a good conductor. The electrical field of the heart is recorded in the electrocardiogram (B). In accord with Ampère's law, this current produces the strongest biomagnetic field of any organ, and the field is radiated into the space surrounding the body (C). Modern devices can record the biomagnetic field of the heart, which is called a magnetocardiogram (D). Biomagnetic fields are discussed in detail in Chapter 8.

various complementary and alternative medicine (CAM) practitioners. The laws of physics require the production of a biomagnetic field around the body as a result of the electrical activity of the heart and other organs. In Chapter 8 we will see the methods that have been used to measure these biomagnetic fields.

ELECTRICITY FROM MAGNETISM: FARADAY'S LAW OF INDUCTION

About 11 years after Ørsted's important discovery in Denmark, another important finding took place simultaneously in England and America. Electromagnetic induction is the reverse of Ampère's law, i.e., magnetic fields can cause currents to flow through conductors. Electromagnetic induction was discovered by the English chemist and physicist, Michael Faraday in 1831, and, independently and at the same time, by an American scientist, Joseph Henry (Figure 2.7). The resulting law of physics is known as Faraday's law of induction because Faraday published his results before Henry. Note from Figure 2.7C the inductive effect with a single loop of wire. Coils with larger numbers of turns increase the inductive effect. This is mentioned because many of the tissues in the human body have a helical aspect to them, and therefore have the possibility of utilizing the phenomenon discovered by Faraday and Henry. The unit of capacitance, the farad, is named after Michael Faraday. Capacitance will become significant and will be defined when the oscillator is described.

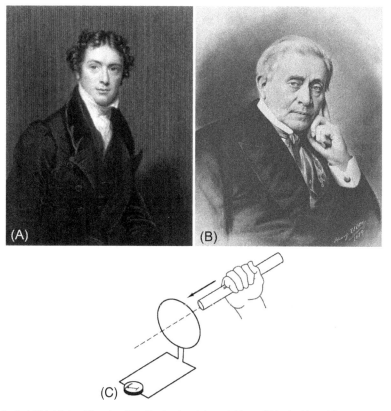

Figure 2.7 In 1831, Michael Faraday (A) in England and Joseph Henry (B) in the United States independently discovered that a moving magnetic field will induce a current flow through a wire without touching it (C). Magnetism can be converted into electricity.

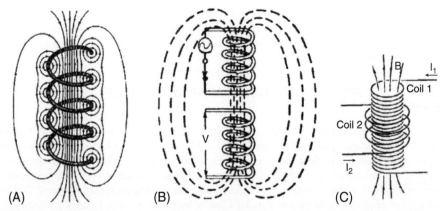

Figure 2.8 Coils are used to create to intensify magnetic fields. (A) Simple coil known as a solenoid. (B) Transformer made with two coils in series. A voltage across the lower coil induces a current flow in the upper coil. (C) Transformer with one coil wound around another. Transformers can be used to couple one electrical field to another (B) or to change one voltage to another (C). If coil 1 in (C) is the primary coil, the voltage in the secondary coil, coil 2, will be lower. This is called a step-down transformer. If coil 2 is used as the primary coil, the voltage in the secondary coil, coil 1, will be higher.

The unit of inductance, the henry, is named after Joseph Henry. Again, inductance will be defined in connection with the oscillator. Henry's work on the electromagnetic relay was the basis of the electrical telegraph, invented independently by Samuel Morse and Charles Wheatstone. Induction and coils provide the basis for important devices such as solenoids, which produce much stronger magnetic effects than a straight wire, and transformers composed of two coils, a primary and a secondary, which can step voltages up or down (Figure 2.8). We shall see that induction also explains how the electrical fields from the hands of a therapist, which are caused in part by the electric field of the heart flowing through the circulatory system, can induce the flows of microcurrents in the tissues of a patient and how certain energy medicine devices can likewise induce currents in tissues. These phenomena will be discussed in more detail in Chapter 15.

Ampère's Law and Faraday's Law of Induction in Action: Energy Medicine Devices and Energy Therapies

Explaining these two laws of physics lays a foundation for understanding a variety of energy therapies performed either with medical devices or with the human hand. These approaches will be discussed in detail in Chapter 15 For this chapter it is sufficient to point out that extensive research has shown that pulsing magnetic fields will induce current flows in the tissues of a patient and that these current flows can be therapeutic. A classic and thoroughly researched example is provided by the use of pulsed magnetic fields to stimulate the healing process in two serious, debilitating, and expensive medical conditions known as delayed union of fracture (improper healing within 6 months) or fracture nonunion (failure of union after 6 months). In the early 1980s, Brighton Friedenberg & Black (1979), Bassett (1982) and others demonstrated that fracture nonunions could be stimulated to heal using tiny electric and magnetic fields. In his last scientific paper, orthopedic surgeon and medical researcher C.A.L. Bassett explained:

> *Jump starting a car with a dead battery creates an operational machine; exposure of a nonunion to PEMFs can convert a stalled healing process to active repair, even in patients unhealed for as long as 40 years!*
>
> BASSETT (1995)

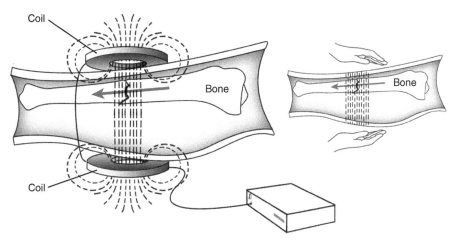

Figure 2.9 Pulsing magnetic fields generated by coils can 'jump start' the healing process in two medical conditions, delayed union of fracture (improper healing within 6 months) or fracture nonunion (failure of union after 6 months). Inset shows comparable situation produced by fields induced from the hands of a therapist.

Figure 2.9 shows the system developed by Bassett and colleagues using coils placed near a bone fracture to induce current flows through a fracture site. Research has shown that the induced field must be small or it will not work (Rubin et al., 1989). The strength of the field employed in medical devices is comparable to that produced from the hands of therapists. The evidence for this profound statement will be presented in Chapter 15.

References

Bassett, C.A.L., 1995. Bioelectromagnetics in the service of medicine. In: Blank, M. (Ed.), Electromagnetic Fields: Biological interactions and Mechanisms. Advances in chemistry Series, vol. 250. American chemical Society, Washington, DC, pp. 261–275 (chapter 14).

Brighton, C.T., Friedenberg, Z.B., Black, J., 1979. Evaluation of the use of constant direct current in the treatment of non-union. In: Brighton, C.T. (Ed.), Electrical properties of bone and cartilage. New York: Plenum Press:519–545.

Brooks, R.A., 2010. Fields of Color: The theory that escaped Einstein. Published by Rodney A. Brooks, Boston, MA, Chapter 7.

Conant, J.B., 1981. Quoted from Readings from Nadeau, R.L., Readings from the New Book on Nature: Physics and Metaphysics in the Modern Novel, page 48.

Einstein, A., 1954. Relativity. The special and general theory. In: Appendix 05 in the Fifteenth enlarged edition. Routledge, New York, NY.

Feyerabend, P., 1981. Realism, Rationalism and Scientific Method: Philosophical Papers, vol. 1. Cambridge University Press, Cambridge, UK, p. 185.

Fisher, H.J., 2004. Faraday's Experimental Researches in Electricity: The First Series. Green Lion Press, p. 22.

McFall, P., 2006. Brainy young James wasn't so daft after all. The Sunday Post, 23 April.

Northrop, 1959.

Olson, C., 1983. The Maximus Poems. Butterick, G.F. (Ed.). University of California Press, Berkeley.

Rubin, C.T., McLeod, K.J., Lanyon, L.E., 1989. Prevention of osteoporosis by pulsed electromagnetic fields. J Bone Joint Surg Am. 71 (3), 411–417.

Walker, M.J., 2002. Healing Massage: A Simple Approach. Delmar Cengage Learning.

Wolff, M., 2009. Schrödinger's Universe. Einstein, Waves & the Origin of the Natural Laws. Outskirts Press, Parker Co.

Figure 2.9 ...

References

...

CHAPTER 3

Basic Physics and Biophysics: Electromagnetism and Resonance

All objects in the universe, from the very smallest to the very largest, are continuously vibrating. Since matter is composed of charged particles such as electrons and protons, all vibrating matter is emitting electromagnetic fields. To be more specific, a stationary charge is surrounded by an electric field and a moving charge produces magnetic fields (Ampère's circuit law, Chapter 2).

Vibrating matter resembles a pendulum or a child on a swing – its position goes from stationary to rapid motion and back to stationary again. Its field goes from purely electric to purely magnetic and back again, in repeating cycles. James Clerk Maxwell (Maxwell, 1865) synthesized Ampère's circuit law and Faraday's law of induction (see Chapter 2) to create a classical electromagnetic theory. Electromagnetic waves move through space at the speed of light, with the electric fields perpendicular to the magnetic fields. The wavelength is the distance between peaks of the field.

Electromagnetic fields play a huge role in our daily lives, because they are involved in technologies such as cellular phones, electronic car keys, garage door openers, radio, television, police and military communications, radar, and so on. The key to the operation of all of these technologies, and to the use of energy fields in clinical medicine, is resonance – the phenomenon that enables electromagnetic fields produced in one place to affect things at a distance.

The Power of Resonance

The astonishing effectiveness of resonance can be appreciated from the long distance communications involved in the U.S. space program. Launched in 1972, Pioneer 10 explored the asteroid belt, Jupiter, and the outer planets in our solar system and then continued its journey beyond Pluto and Neptune. In 1973, Pioneer 10 became the first manmade object to leave the solar system, where it began to collect information on the interstellar wind and cosmic rays coming from deep space. On the thirtieth anniversary of its launch, NASA sent a message to the spacecraft, which was then 7.4 billion miles away from Earth. The message was sent from a radio telescope in the desert east of Los Angeles, and a radio telescope in Spain received a response 22 h and 6 min later. Pioneer 10 used two radio transmitters, coupled to two amplifiers producing 8 W of power, comparable to a very small light bulb. Pioneer's last, very weak signal was received on 23 January 2003. Its radioisotope power source finally decayed, and it no longer had enough power to send additional transmissions to Earth. The last transmission took place when Pioneer 10 was 7.6 billion miles away (NASA, 2009).

This is the extraordinary power of resonance. In this chapter we begin to explore the nature of radio and other resonant electromagnetic communications and their implications for living systems and energy medicine.

Importance of Frequency

Very weak energy fields at the appropriate frequencies can be profoundly therapeutic. Other frequencies can produce pathophysiological responses. While it may go against intuition, it appears that, within limits, it is not the strength of the signal that determines whether it will be beneficial or harmful, but instead it is the frequency. Resonance is the reason for this frequency specificity. Biological effects, like molecular resonances, are very frequency specific. This is vital for a wide range of energy therapies using frequencies applied to the human body, whether these signals come from medical devices, the human voice, or the human hand, herbs or aromas, music, or other modalities.

For a long time scientists were very suspicious about the idea that very tiny energy fields could have any biological effects. Recent research has resolved this issue by identifying the likely mechanisms involved. This information will be detailed in Chapter 16, where we explore health effects of the electromagnetic environment.

The biophysical question is how very tiny electromagnetic fields can have such profound effects. A recent study (Pall, 2013) points out that the answer to this question has been hiding in plain sight in the scientific literature for a long time. Modern science is so highly focused and specialized that few have taken the time to read and evaluate the relevant literature. Martin Pall has done this for us.

An example of a therapeutic effect was discussed in the last chapter in relation to bone repair facilitated by exposure to tiny pulsing fields. The fact of this therapeutic success in increasing osteoblast differentiation and maturation is difficult to challenge, because it has been the subject of so many studies. Pall lists these studies, and they are reproduced here in the box because the critical or skeptical reader will want to look at these articles.

Studies Demonstrating the Effectiveness of Low Level Pulsing Electromagnetic Fields in Stimulating Bone Repair (From Pall, 2013)

Ryabi JT 1998 Clinical effects of electromagnetic fields on fracture healing. Clin Orthop Relat Res. 355(Suppl. l):S205–15.

Oishi M Onesti ST 2000 Electrical bone graft stimulation for spinal fusion: a review. Neurosurgery. 47:1041–55.

Aaron RK Ciombor DM Simon BJ 2004 Treatment of nonunions with electric and electromagnetic fields. Clin Orthop Relat Res. 10:579–93.

Goldstein C Sprague S Petrisor BA 2010 Electrical stimulation for fracture healing: current evidence. J Orthop Trauma. 24(Suppl. 1):S62–5.

Demitriou R Babis GC 2007 Biomaterial osseointegration enhancement with biophysical stimulation. J Musculoskelet Neuronal Interact. 7:253–65.

Griffin XL Warner F Costa M 2008 The role of electromagnetic stimulation in the management of established non-union of long bone fractures: what is the evidence? Injury. 39:419–29.

Huang LQ He HC He CQ et al. 2008 Clinical update of pulsed electromagnetic fields on osteroporosis. Chin Med J. 121:2095–9.

Groah SL Lichy AM Libin AV et al. 2010 Intensive electrical stimulation attenuates femoral bone loss in acute spinal cord injury. PM R. 2:1080–7.

Schidt-Rohlfing B Silny J Gavenis K et al. 2011 Electromagnetic fields, electric current and bone healing – what is the evidence? Z Orthop Unfall. 149:265–70.

Griffin XL Costa ML Parsons N et al. 2011 Electromagnetic field stimulation for treating delayed union or non-union of long bone fractures in adults. Cochrane Database Syst Rev. CDO08471.

Chalidis B Sachinis N Assiotis A et al. 2011 Stimulation of bone formation and fracture healing with pulsed electromagnetic fields: biologic responses and clinical implications. Int J Immunopathol Pharmacol. 24(1 Suppl. 2):17020.

Zhong C Zhao TF Xu ZJ et al. 2012 Effects of electromagnetic fields on bone regeneration in experimental and clinical studies: a review of the literature. Chin Med J. 125:367–72.

Resonance and frequency specificity are key topics for exploring a wide range of phenomena:

- Various energy medicine technologies that apply frequency to the body.
- Consciousness-based therapies.
- Subtle energetic techniques, such as QiGong, Therapeutic Touch, Reiki, Healing Touch, Polarity Therapy, BodyTalk, and many others, that can have profound healing effects with or without direct physical contact.
- The significance of intention.
- Prayer and distant healing.
- Electromagnetic sensitivity, a growing health problem in which people appear to have allergic reactions to low levels of electromagnetic radiation, as from cell towers or cell phones.

We shall therefore examine the physics of resonance from several perspectives to develop explanations for these important phenomena.

Resonance is the process by which a field of a particular frequency or wavelength can transfer vibrational energy from one object to another. Clinical applications of electromagnetic resonance have the advantage that they can act at a distance using tiny fields that excite or energize specific natural processes taking place deep within the body. Electromagnetic resonance can be used to influence processes taking place in areas that are difficult to reach with drugs, such as the interior of the brain, which is protected by the blood–brain barrier, or the interior of pockets of inflammation that are separated from the general circulation by an inflammatory barricade, as will be discussed in Chapter 17. Resonance is based on simple and understandable biophysics that clearly explains why specific frequencies and not others are therapeutically effective and why there are few if any side effects.

In physics, resonance is defined as the tendency of any object to oscillate or vibrate at maximum amplitude at certain frequencies, known as the system's resonant or natural frequencies. At these frequencies, even a tiny rhythmic driving force can build up in the system to produce strong vibrations because the system accumulates or stores each applied pulse of energy.

A familiar example of resonance is pushing a child on a swing (Figure 3.1). When applied at the appropriate intervals, the pushes cause the child to swing higher and higher. Physicists refer to this arrangement as a pendulum. Anyone who has pushed a child on a swing knows how important it is to apply the push at the correct time so that the swinging will go higher and higher.

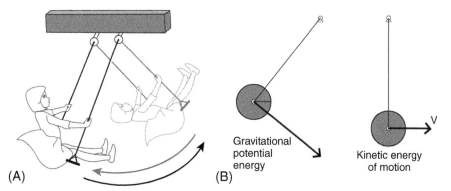

Figure 3.1 A child on a swing (A) provides a good example of an oscillating system in which energy shifts between two forms. Physicists refer to this arrangement as a pendulum (B). At the top of the swing, all of the energy is in the form of gravitational potential energy, i.e., the energy available to the object as a result of its position in relation to the gravity field. At the bottom of the swing, all of the energy is in the form of kinetic energy, or the energy of motion. The energy in the system oscillates back and forth between these two different forms.

A push at the wrong time will take energy away from the pendulum and slow the swinging. There are equations available to calculate the period or frequency of a pendulum as a function of the length of the wire and the acceleration due to gravity. The weight of the swinging object is not a factor in the equations.

The example shown in Figure 3.1 is instructive because it illustrates resonant interactions between two objects, the pusher and the child on the swing. It also illustrates energy being converted from one form to another. Physicists refer to the energy of motion as kinetic energy. At the base of the child's swing, all of the energy is kinetic, whereas at the top of the swing there is no kinetic energy – motion ceases for an instant. The physicist describes that moment as an instant when all of the energy is in the form of gravitational potential energy – the energy that will restart the swinging.

Electromagnetism employs similar principles to enable transmission of energy and information over long distances.

Electricity and Magnetism Combined: The Electromagnetic Field

Electromagnetic interactions taking place within the human body, between the body and its environment, and between a therapist and his or her patient are extremely important but have not received adequate attention. Molecules can behave as resonant antennas, meaning that they can radiate and absorb electromagnetic fields. This concept is inescapable. It is based on fundamental laws of physics but is not widely discussed by biomedical researchers. Many alternative therapies involving energy can seem peculiar from superficial observation, but they are easily explained by electromagnetic interactions between molecules and, especially, arrays of molecules within living systems. All of the conceptual pieces are in place, and they are based on substantial physics that will be described next. This section also provides the basis for an understanding of electromagnetic communication and control systems in the living body to be described Chapter 9.

James Clerk Maxwell (1831–1879) was a Scottish theoretical physicist and mathematician (Figure 3.2A). He developed the classical electromagnetic theory that synthesizes Ampère's circuit law and Faraday's law of induction and optics into a consistent theory. His set of equations – Maxwell's equations – demonstrated that electricity, magnetism, and light are all manifestations of the same phenomenon: the electromagnetic field. Maxwell demonstrated that electric and magnetic fields travel through space in the form of waves. Figure 3.2B shows the way the electrical field and magnetic field are thought to move through space as electromagnetic waves. Note that the electric field is perpendicular to the magnetic field.

In 1864 Maxwell wrote *A Dynamical Theory of the Electromagnetic Field*, proposing that light involves undulations in the same medium in which electric and magnetic phenomena take place. His unified model of electromagnetism is regarded as one of the greatest advances in the history of physics. It helped birth the era of modern physics and electronics by providing the foundation for the fields of special relativity and quantum mechanics and the basis for technologies such as radio, television, radar, and cellular telephones.

As Figure 3.2B shows, an oscillating charge alternately produces an electric field and a magnetic field. When the charge is stationary, the field is purely electrical. As the charge accelerates, the electric component declines and the magnetic component increases. When the charge is moving at the maximum velocity, it produces a purely magnetic field and the electric field falls to zero. The way charges can be made to oscillate involves a simple circuit known as an LC or inductance/capacitance circuit (Figure 3.3).

An LC circuit, also called a resonant circuit, tank circuit, or tuned circuit, consists of an inductor, represented by the letter L, and a capacitor, represented by the letter C. When connected together, the coil and the capacitor can act as an electrical resonator, an electrical analog

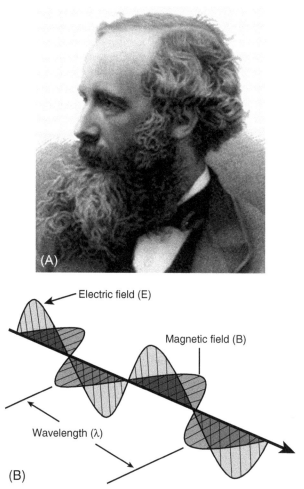

Figure 3.2 (A) James Clerk Maxwell (1831–1879), Scottish theoretical physicist and mathematician who developed the classical electromagnetic theory by synthesizing Ampère's law, Faraday's law of induction and optics into a consistent formulation. (B) According to Maxwell, the electrical field and magnetic field move through space as electromagnetic waves. Note that the electric field is perpendicular to the magnetic field.

of a tuning fork or pendulum, to produce a purely magnetic field; the electrical field has fallen to zero. The way the charges are caused to oscillate involves the LC circuit (Figure 3.3) storing and releasing energy at the circuit's resonant frequency. When L and C are connected, an electric field will create a magnetic field in the inductor and an electric field in the capacitor. Energy alternates between the inductor and the capacitor at the circuit's resonant frequency. The resonant frequency, in turn, is determined by the value of inductance, measured in henrys, and the value of capacitance, measured in farads (see text box). Again, these terms, the henry and the farad, are named for the pioneers of electromagnetism, Joseph Henry and Michael Faraday, as discussed in the previous chapter. Living tissues have both of these properties, inductance and capacitance.

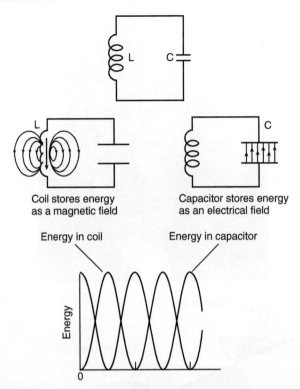

Coil stores energy   Capacitor stores energy
as a magnetic field   as an electrical field

Figure 3.3 Explanation of how an oscillator consisting of a coil (L) and a capacitor (C) produces an oscillating field that can be used to generate an electromagnetic field. Energy is built up in the coil and stored as magnetic energy. The magnetic field then collapses and induces a current flow into the capacitor, which then builds up an electrical field. When the electrical field in the capacitor collapses, current flows back to the coil, etc. Energy oscillates between the coil and capacitor at a frequency that is determined by the inductance and capacitance of the two circuit elements.

LC circuits are used for generating signals at particular frequencies or for picking out a signal at a particular frequency from a more complex signal. They are key components in many applications such as oscillators, filters, and tuners. The living matrix, to be described in detail in Chapters 10 and 11, contains many materials that have inductance and capacitance properties. Figure 3.4 shows a tuned transmitter circuit connected to an antenna and to the ground (the Earth) transmitting a signal to a similarly tuned receiver circuit.

Technical Details: Inductance and Capacitance

The resonant frequency of an LC circuit is determined by the inductance, L, of the coil, measured in henrys, and by the capacitance, C, of the capacitor, measured in farads. A farad is the charge in coulombs a capacitor will accept for the potential across it to change by 1 V. A coulomb, in turn, is the amount of electric charge transported in 1 s by a steady current of one ampere, and is equal to $6.241,509,745 \times 10^{18}$ electrons. The henry is defined in terms of the rate of change of current in a circuit. When the rate of change is $1\,A\,s^{-1}$, and the resulting electromotive force is 1 V, then the inductance of the circuit is 1 H.

Halliday & Resnick (1970)

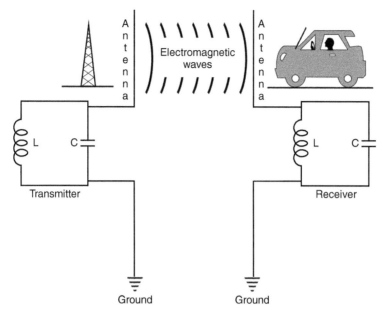

Figure 3.4 A tuned LC circuit on the left provides the basis for a radio transmitter. The tuned circuit on the right, a car radio, is the receiver. When the values of L and C in the two circuits are resonant, an electromagnetic signal will be transmitted from the transmitter to the receiver.

Antennas

Antenna theory may sound like a boring, dry subject, but understanding how an antenna radiates or captures a signal is central to regulatory biology and energy medicine. Antenna theory can help us understand fundamental energetic processes taking place in the human body. Any object that is electrically conductive will have antenna properties. Metallic wires are good antennas, and many molecules, including DNA, are referred to as molecular wires, and are therefore good antennas as well.

At body temperatures, all of the molecules in the body are vibrating. Some of this vibratory energy is converted into electromagnetic fields (radio waves and light) that can travel through space and that can cause vibrations in other resonant molecules a distance away. You don't have to know how an antenna works to understand biology. But understanding a bit about radio and antennas and the mysterious process by which antennas launch energy and information from *Here* to another antenna, *There*, can be very helpful.

As can be seen in Figure 3.5, if you straighten out an ordinary paperclip, you have a 160 m antenna. Obviously the paperclip is not 160 m long. The paperclip is seven octaves below 160 m. When we use a word such as 'octave' we are using musical notation, and this is entirely appropriate for electromagnetics. An orchestra typically uses instruments over eight octaves. Music theory and antenna theory are similar because they deal with harmonics. In both cases dividing the wavelength by 2 increases the resonant frequency by a single octave, and multiplying the wavelength by 2 decreases the resonant frequency by one octave. The human ear tends to hear all of these notes as being essentially 'the same'. Likewise, antennas 'tuned' to different octaves will function similarly. In the Western system of musical notation, notes that are octaves apart are given the same note name. In radio terminology, antennas that are octaves apart are also given the same name. In the Western system of music notation, the name of a note an octave above A is

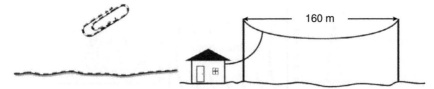

Figure 3.5 Straighten out an ordinary paperclip, and you have a 160 m antenna. 160 m is the wavelength (the length of one wave) corresponding to a frequency of about 2,000,000 cycles per second (abbreviated as Hz). The paperclip is seven octaves below 160 m. An orchestra typically uses instruments over eight octaves.

also A. In music theory, this is called octave equivalency. This process of dividing or multiplying a resonant frequency transposes it into a different octave by doubling or halving its wavelength in an exact and precise manner. An octave-shifted therapeutic resonant frequency will have a precise correlation with the first or primary therapeutic resonant frequency. Again, musical notation applies to this situation. The 160 m paperclip corresponds to a frequency of about 2,000,000 Hz. The abbreviation, Hz, means cycles per second and is named after Heinrich Hertz (1857–1894), a German scientist who was the first to demonstrate the existence of electromagnetic waves by building an apparatus that could both produce and detect radio waves.

For the most efficient energy transfer from one antenna to another, the transmitting and receiving antennas have the same geometry, are a single wavelength long, and are separated by an exact multiple of the wavelength (Figure 3.6). However, efficient energy transfer can also occur if the transmitting and receiving antennas are some fraction or multiple of the wavelength.

Brain Waves

Delta wave: (< 4 Hz)
Theta wave: (4–7 Hz)
Alpha wave: (8–15 Hz)
Mu wave: (8–12 Hz)
Beta wave: (16–31 Hz)
Gamma: (> 32 Hz)

Electroencephalography

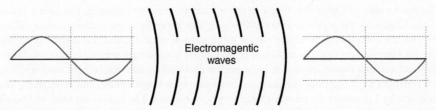

Figure 3.6 For completely efficient energy transfer from one antenna to another, the transmitting and receiving antennas have the same geometry and are a single wavelength long and are separated by an exact multiple of the wavelength.

Occasionally, one hears confusing statements about this. For example, one scientist stated that extremely low frequencies could not possibly interact with living tissues because their wavelength was far too long. For example, an electric power frequency field at 60 Hz has a wavelength of more than 3000 miles – about the distance from Los Angeles to New York! Since the length of the human body is far shorter than this, one might say that such a long wave cannot possibly interact with the human body – but that would be wrong! Living tissues produce frequencies in this range, and external fields will affect those biological rhythms by entraining them. Examples include the electric field of the heart (about 1 Hz if the heart is beating at 60 beats per minute), and brain waves (see text box). The psychoactive correlates of the various brain wave frequencies are well known.

Listening to a favourite public radio station involves adjusting the radio to W282AB Dover at 104.3 MHz (104.3 million hertz). What does this mean, and what does it mean for energy medicine? Every day we use our radios, televisions, and cell phones. These devices use electromagnetic fields of particular frequencies to send information over a distance, from a transmitter to a receiver. All of these devices involve electromagnetic fields of particular frequencies. Setting the dial for 104.3 involves selecting a frequency of 104,300,000 cycles per second. If antennas did not radiate and absorb energy, we would not have radio, television, radar, cell phones, or microwave ovens. If tissues and molecules in the human body did not radiate and absorb energy by the same process, many energy medicine therapies would not exist.

W282AB Dover is an FM station. FM refers to frequency modulation. Other stations are on the AM dial, with AM referring to amplitude modulation. The nature of these two kinds of signals is important for energy medicine, because the human body uses both AM and FM signaling. Figure 3.7 explains the difference between AM and FM. Both types of radio transmission involve a fundamental frequency called the carrier wave. In AM, the amplitude or height of the carrier wave is modulated up and down. The receiver subtracts the carrier wave and retrieves the original information that was used to modulate the carrier. In FM, the frequency instead of the amplitude of the carrier wave is modulated up and down without changes in its amplitude. FM is commonly used for high-fidelity broadcasts of music and speech and television sound.

Figure 3.8 shows some manmade antennas used for television, and cell phone communications. The size and other geometrical characteristics of the antennas determine their resonant frequency.

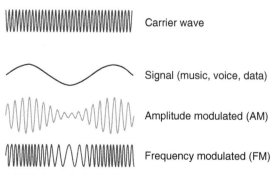

Carrier wave

Signal (music, voice, data)

Amplitude modulated (AM)

Frequency modulated (FM)

Figure 3.7 Both types of radio transmission involve a fundamental frequency called the carrier wave. In AM, the amplitude or height of the carrier wave is modulated up and down. The receiver subtracts the carrier wave and retrieves the original information that was used to modulate the carrier. In FM, the frequency instead of the amplitude of the carrier wave is modulated up and down without changes in its amplitude.

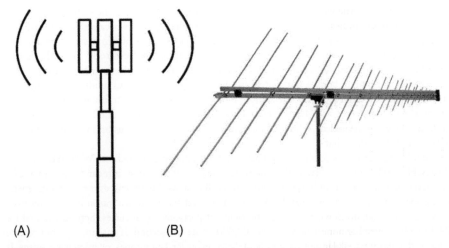

Figure 3.8   Manmade antennas used for television, and cell phone communications.

Biological Antennas

Figure 3.9 shows some biological antennas: an insect antenna, a DNA molecule, and an adenosine triphosphate (ATP) molecule. Each of these natural antennas is the product of millions of years of evolutionary refinement. Study of their properties involves physics, electronics and biophysics. This chapter will explain the basics of how these antennas operate and their biological significance. *There are many phenomena in complementary and alternative medicine that are incomprehensible without the understandings developed in this chapter.*

Studies of the insect antenna have revealed an important aspect of biological resonance. Entomologists had always assumed that the insect antenna was a scent receptor, used by insects of opposite sex to locate each other by following the trail of airborne insect hormones called pheromones. The problem with this idea is that a male moth, for example, can find a female a

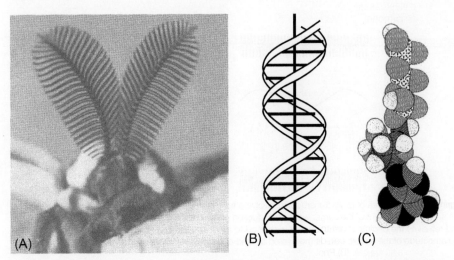

Figure 3.9   Natural antennas. (A) An insect antenna. (B) The DNA molecule. (C) The adenosine triphosphate (ATP) molecule. *(Image (A) courtesy of Philip S. Callahan.)*

mile away even when the wind is blowing the scent molecules away from him instead of toward him. In a series of studies, Phillip Callahan demonstrated that the pheromone molecules are actually molecular antennas that emit radio signals. The male moth looking for the female is not attracted by the scent or smell of the pheromones, but by the radio signals the molecules emit. This research has been summarized by Oschman and Oschman (2004).

Molecular Antennas

Callahan (1975) pioneered the study of the antenna properties of molecules. There is now detailed clinical evidence that molecules can indeed act as transmitting and receiving antennas. More detail will be provided in Chapter 16, where the important subject of allergies is discussed. Previously, it was stated that any electrical conductor can act as an antenna. The DNA molecule is a classic example. DNA is an electronic conductor (e.g., Fink and Schönenberger, 1999; Porath et al., 2000). The movement of charges through DNA is electronic and not ionic. DNA molecules are referred to as quantum wires and can function as antennas.

The usual view of hormone–receptor interactions (Figure 3.10A) involves a secretory cell releasing a hormone into the extracellular fluid, and the molecule diffusing randomly until it chances to bump into a receptor on a distant cell. Many have viewed this type of regulatory phenomenon as highly improbable or even impossible. Certainly it seems far too slow to explain the rapid and subtle ways organisms adapt to their environment. An electromagnetic mechanism (Figure 3.10B) would be much faster.

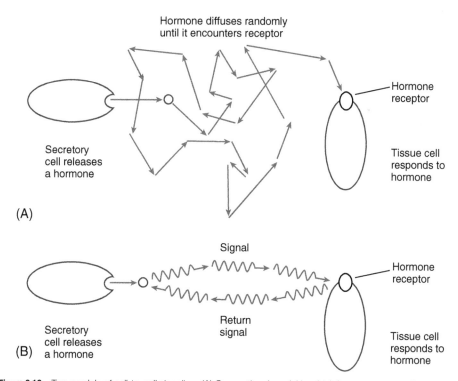

Figure 3.10 Two models of cell-to-cell signaling. (A) Conventional model in which hormone or neurohormone is released from a secretory cell, diffuses randomly through the extracellular fluids, and eventually encounters a receptor on a tissue cell. (B) Photonic model in which the hormone emits an electromagnetic field (photon) that travels through tissue fluids or along surfaces until it activates the receptor, which, in turn, emits a return signal informing the secretory cell that the message has been received.

Studies of interactions between photons and atoms or molecules have long been a corner-stone of quantum physics, quantum chemistry, biochemistry, and pharmacology. Single-molecule spectroscopy was accomplished in the 1990s (Basche et al., 1996). Recent research in Germany has focused on single-photon communications between two identical molecules (Figure 3.11). The efforts are driven by potential technological applications in molecular circuits for computers and other devices. Under some extreme conditions, with very sophisticated techniques, scientists from Switzerland, Germany, and the Netherlands have transmitted streams of single photons between the smallest antennas in the world, i.e., between two molecules (Rezus et al. 2012). The transmitting molecule has to emit photons of exactly the same color as the receiving molecule can absorb – in other words, they need to have matching molecular geometry – they must resonate. One of their goals, which these scientists think they will be able to achieve, is to bounce a photon back and forth several times between two molecules. Such a 'quantum radio' would allow for a return signal. In terms of Figure 3.10B, the secretory cell would be 'notified' that the message was received. The hallmark of an effective cybernetic system is to develop circular, causal chains that move from action to sensing to comparison with desired goal, and again to action (Figure 3.12).

While achievement of such interactions between molecules is very challenging in the labora-tory, it may be much simpler and more effective in the living body. The reason for stating this is that cells and molecules are coated with a special form of water, known as exclusion zone water, or EZ water, that has extraordinary properties (see Figure 13.13). One property is a capacity to

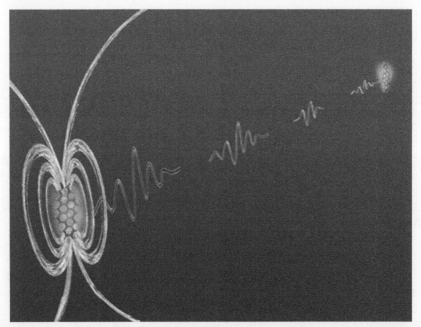

Figure 3.11   Artist's view of a single organic molecule sending a stream of single photons to a second molecule at a distance, in quantum analogy to the communication between two radio stations, shown in the distance. Exciting research from Germany and Switzerland is confirming the idea that molecules can emit photons that interact with molecules a distance away. This fundamental physics research has profound biomedical implications with respect to the physiological regulations discussed in this chapter. A group of scientists at the Max Planck Institute for the Science of Light and Department of Physics, University of Erlangen-Nuremberg in Germany has succeeded in producing single photons from a single organic molecule and measuring its interaction with a second molecule several meters away. The emitter is 1,2:7,8-Dibenzanthanthrene (DBATT). The transmission is extremely efficient. A second group of researchers at the Max Planck Institute for Solid State Research and the University of Stuttgart is doing similar research. See Rezus et al., 2012 and Siyushev et al., 2014. Image modified from the original drawn by Lettow (2012).

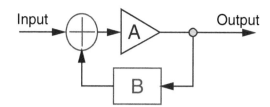

Figure 3.12   The ideal cybernetic feedback model.

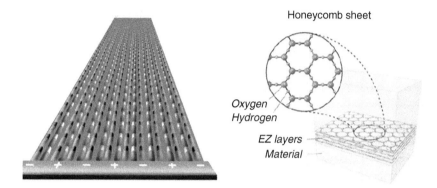

Figure 3.13   The deep exclusion zone (EZ) at the surface of a cell or molecule. *Diagram to the left shows how charges on a surface orient layers of water molecules extending for a considerable distance. Diagram on the right shows how the hexagonally packed water molecules form many layers of honeycomb sheets. (Diagram on the left is from Pollack (2008); diagram on right is from Pollack (2013) page xxiv.)*

exclude solutes from approaching the surfaces of structures such as proteins and cell surfaces. If discovery is confirmed, it adds another dimension of improbability to the scheme shown in Figure 3.10A. If confirmed, it will support the concept of electromagnetic interactions between signal molecules and receptors, with the fields acting through water in the exclusion zone.

Some theoretical and practical aspects of molecular antennas can be found in a United States Patent by Boehm (2007):

> Methods are provided for determining resonant frequencies that can be used therapeutically, for example, for debilitation of specific types of genomic materials, including DNA and/or RNA, genes, and gene sections. The methods can be used in relation to various human and animal diseases and conditions. Therapeutic resonance frequencies are adapted for use with available frequency-emitting devices by shifting frequencies up or down by factors of 2, 4, 6, etc. Boehm (2007), United States Patent 7,280,874.

Boehm, 2007

As an example of her method, Boehm used the pathogen that causes Lyme disease. The pathogen is a spirochete called *Borrelia burgdorferi* (Figure 3.14). This pathogen causes a very serious bacterial infection via a tick bite that affects humans and animals. This little organism has created a worldwide health issue, affecting millions of people. We know the structure of the genome of the B31 strain of this pathogen. Because of its clinical significance, it was the third microbial genome ever sequenced, enabling a determination of the length and resonant frequency of the molecule acting as an antenna. The genome contains 910,725 base pairs and 853 genes. Results of the sequencing project were reported in *Nature* in 1997 (Fraser et al., 1997).

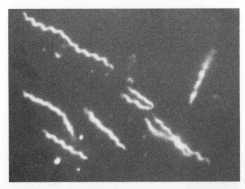

Figure 3.14 An important example of the use of resonant frequencies in medicine is provided by *Borrelia burgdorferi* the spirochete that causes Lyme disease. Infections of this organism have also been linked to non-Hodgkin lymphomas.

Boehm's method can be used more generally to determine therapeutic resonant frequencies that can be used to treat various human and animal diseases and conditions. Specifically, certain frequencies will activate specific enzymes and genes, and other frequencies will inhibit them. When a disorder is caused by a pathogen (bacterium or virus), specific frequencies can have precise effects:

- Inhibition of the processes carried out by DNA and/or RNA, genes, and pieces of genes.
- Inhibition of metabolic pathways that slow or stop reproduction of the pathogen.
- Stimulation of metabolic pathways within the pathogen causing it to reproduce so rapidly that it consumes its sources of nutrients and can therefore no longer proliferate.
- Stimulation of metabolism in cells of the immune system so that they are better able to remove the pathogens and their metabolic products.

Infections by this organism have also been linked to non-Hodgkin lymphomas (Guidoboni et al., 2006). Technical details of how information on the genome is converted to a therapeutic frequency are described in the box.

Calculating the Resonant Frequency of the Lyme Disease Pathogen: Technical Details

- The length of the molecular antenna is obtained by adding the cumulative lengths of the 910,724 base pairs plus the distances between them, 3.403,846 e^{-10} m, giving a total length of 3.099,96 e^{-4} m (Figure 3.13B). This enabled Boehm (2007) to estimate the resonant frequency of the genome of the pathogen as 3.415,150,16 e^{11} Hz. e^{-10} m.
- The resonant frequency must be determined in relation to the velocity of electromagnetic radiation *in vivo*. The primary resonant frequency is calculated to be 3.415,150,16 e^{11} Hz.
- There has to be appropriate 'impedance matching' between the signal propagating in air and in the aqueous environment within the organism, and the method takes this into consideration.
- This frequency is actually in the infrared range of the electromagnetic spectrum.
- To find a convenient sub-harmonic of the primary resonant frequency that falls in the audio range, the primary resonant frequency is divided by the number 2 as many times as necessary.
- In musical terms these frequencies are known as octaves. In the example of the *B. burgdorferi* genome, a multi-octave shift to audio range is obtained by dividing the primary therapeutic resonant frequency by 2^{29}, which gives a corresponding second therapeutic resonant frequency of 636.12 Hz, which is in the audio range.

Boehm (2007)

In some cases, no devices are readily available to emit the primary resonant frequency. In these examples, frequencies that are harmonics (exact multiples) or sub-harmonics (exact fractions) of the primary frequency are effective. The situation is comparable to that described in the discussion of antenna theory: the best match is between antennas of identical geometry, but antennas of ½ wave, ¼ wave, and so on will also resonate. For Lyme disease, caused by *B. burgdorferi*, the following *in vivo* therapeutic resonant frequencies have been determined the audio range:

- 636.12 Hz
- 1272.24 Hz
- 2544.5 Hz
- 5088.9 Hz

The first of these frequencies, 636.12 Hz, is very close to a frequency (640 Hz) that has been used in the past for treating Lyme disease (Boehm, 2007).

Oscillations, Vibrations, and Energy Transfers

Vibrations underlie virtually every aspect of nature. The vibrations of atoms create sound and heat. Light arises from the vibrations of electrons in an object. When we say something is blue, what is really happening is that light has made the electrons within the object vibrate in a way that causes the emission of blue light (see Weisskopf's 1968 article on how light interacts with matter). At a basic level, all life depends upon molecules interacting through vibrating or oscillating energy fields. Virtually all that we know about living systems is based on the analysis of vibrations.

In the living body, each electron, atom, chemical bond, molecule, cell, tissue, organ (and the body as a whole) has its own vibratory character. Since living structure and function are orderly, biological oscillations are organized in meaningful ways, and they contribute information to a dynamic vibratory network that extends throughout the body and into the space around it. 'Energy medicines' and 'vibrational medicines' seek to understand this continuous energetic matrix, and to interact with it to facilitate healing (Gerber, 1988).

Vibrations are a fundamental part of physics. There is a wide spectrum of electromagnetic vibratory frequencies, covering some 90 octaves. Any therapeutic interaction, whether it uses sound, heat, laser beams, herbs, aromas, or movements, involves one or more portions of this energy spectrum.

The science of vibrations applies to all clinical methods. Regardless of the philosophy of the technique being used, intricate energetic interactions occur between nearby individuals, even if they are not in physical contact. Seeing and talking with another person are energetic interactions, involving light and sound vibrations. Information can be transferred from one organism to another via energy fields, and living systems are very sensitive to them. Add therapeutic intention and touch to the equation, and whole new dimensions of subtle but measurable exchanges are brought into play.

Skeptics lump vibrational medicines together as mystical, supernatural, occult, pseudoscience, flaky, twilight zone, new-age gobbledygook, or, simply, unbelievable (e.g., Barrett and Jarvis, 1993; Raso, 1995). The dynamic energy systems of the body are dismissed as involving 'subtle energies that are alien to physics'.

These critiques are out of date, because modern researchers have confirmed that living organisms do, indeed, comprise dynamic energy systems involving the same sorts of field phenomena that physicists have been studying for a long time. For example, clinical medicine is beginning to employ oscillating magnetic fields to 'jump start' healing. Vibrational therapies are not magic or superstition: they are based on biology, chemistry, and physics.

Modern physics … pictures matter not at all as passive and inert, but as being in a continuous dancing and vibrating motion whose rhythmic patterns are determined by the molecular, atomic, and nuclear structures. This is also the way the Eastern mystics see the material world. They all emphasize that the universe has to be grasped dynamically, as it moves, vibrates, and dances: that nature is not a static, but a dynamic equilibrium.

CAPRA (1975)

All objects in the universe are in constant motion. Stillness does not exist. Movements can be linear (in a straight line), rhythmic, vibratory, or orbital. Some objects move from one position to another and then back again. A simple example is a weight hanging from a spring as shown in Figure 3.15A. Put in motion, the weight will move up and down – it will oscillate. The mathematical description of this kind of motion is called a sine wave or sinusoid (Figure 3.15B). It is a pattern that occurs often in nature, including ocean waves, sound waves, light and radio waves and electrical currents. The human ear can recognize single sine waves as a pure clear tone because sine waves are representations of a single frequency with no harmonics; some other wave shapes are also important in energy medicine and are shown in Figure 3.16.

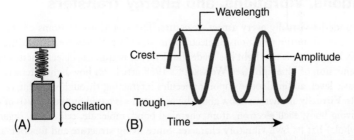

Figure 3.15   (A) The weight is attached to a spring. Put in motion, the weight will move up and down – it will oscillate. The mathematical description of this motion is called a sine wave (B).

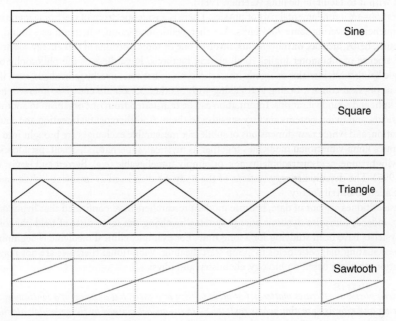

Figure 3.16   Various wave shapes. They all have the same frequency, but their different shapes will produce different effects in living systems.

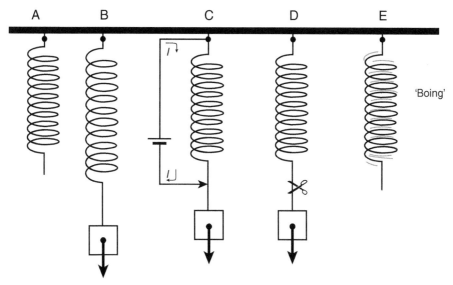

Figure 3.17   Transformation of energy from one form to another. A wire spring is suspended from a solid support such as a ceiling (A). A weight is attached to the spring (B). The spring is stretched as the gravitational potential energy of the weight is converted to the kinetic energy of motion and to elastic energy in the spring. A battery is connected to the two ends of the spring, causing an electric field to flow through the spring (C). The electricity generates magnetic fields around the wire and the magnetic fields attract the loops of the spring toward each other so that the weight is lifted. By lifting the weight, the spring has converted electricity to magnetism to gravitational potential energy. The attachment of the weight is cut (D) so the weight drops to the floor (gravitational potential energy is converted to kinetic energy of motion). The spring, suddenly released from the tension of the weight (E), recoils (elastic is converted to kinetic energy of motion) and 'boings' (elastic energy is converted to sound).

Waves have important characteristics that are crucial to our understanding of energy medicine and the effects of energy therapies on the human body. The most important characteristics of waves are their amplitude, wavelength, frequency, and wave shape. Some other kinds of waves will be discussed later in Chapter 16.

Earlier in this chapter the child on a swing, otherwise known as a pendulum, was given as an example of a system that rhythmically converts energy from one form to another. Another example involves a weight on a spring, as shown in Figure 3.17. In Figure 3.17 we bring in some other forms of energy. Hanging a weight on the spring causes it to stretch, converting gravitational potential energy of the weight into elastic energy that is stored in the spring (Figure 3.17B). Applying a voltage between the top and bottom of the spring creates magnetic fields around the wire and these fields attract the loops of the spring toward each other so that the weight is lifted (Figure 3.17C). By lifting the weight, the spring has converted electricity to magnetism to gravitational potential energy. The attachment of the weight is cut (D) so the weight drops to the floor (gravitational potential energy is converted to kinetic energy of motion). The spring, suddenly released from the tension of the weight (E), recoils (elastic energy is converted to kinetic energy of motion) and 'boings' (elastic energy is converted to sound). When the weight hits the floor, another sound is produced – the kinetic energy of motion is converted into acoustic energy.

Conclusions

Physics and biophysics are the foundation of the discipline of energy medicine. Without these basic concepts other vital phenomena such as resonance and energy fields remain mysterious. Likewise, many of the seemingly baffling results with complementary and alternative therapies make no sense unless they are viewed from the perspectives described in this chapter. Many therapists and many physicians have never had a course in physics, so this part of the subject can be challenging. The aim of this and the previous chapter is to present the basics in an accurate yet understandable manner.

On the centennial of Maxwell's birthday, Albert Einstein described Maxwell's work as the *most profound and the most fruitful that physics has experienced since the time of Newton* (McFall, 2006). Einstein kept a photograph of Maxwell on his study wall, alongside pictures of Michael Faraday and Isaac Newton (Arianrhod, 2003).

References

Arianrhod, R., 2003. Einstein's heroes: imagining the world through the language of mathematics. The Sydney Morning Herald, Sydney, Australia, 10 November.

Barrett, S., Jarvis, W.T., 1993. The Health Robbers: A Close Look at Quackery in America. Prometheus Books, Buffalo, NY.

Basche, T., Moerner, W.E., Orrit, M., Wild, U.P., 1996. Single-Molecule Optical Detection, Imaging and Spectroscopy. VCH Weinheim, Germany.

Boehm, C.A., 2007. Methods for determining therapeutic resonant frequencies. United States Patent 7,280,874, issued October 9, 2007.

Callahan, P.S., 1975. Tuning into Nature. The DDevin Adair Co., Greenwich, CT.

Capra, F., 1975. The Tao of Physics. Shambala, Berkeley, CA. Electroencephalography: http://en.wikipedia.org/wiki/Electroencephalography.

Fink, H.W., Schönenberger, C. 1999. Electrical conduction through DNA molecules. Nature 398 (6726), 407–410.

Fraser, C.M., Casjens, S., Huang, W.M., Sutton, G.G., et al., 1997. Genomic sequence of a Lyme disease spirochaete, *Borrelia burgdorferi*. Nature 390 (6660), 580–586.

Gerber, R., 1988. Vibrational Medicine. Bear, Santa Fe, NM.

Guidoboni, M., Ferreri, A.J., Ponzoni, M., Doglioni, C., Dolcetti, R., (2006). Infectious agents in mucosa-associated lymphoid tissue-type lymphomas: pathogenic role and therapeutic perspectives. Clin. Lymphoma Myeloma 6 (4), 289–300.

Halliday, D., Resnick, R., 1970. Fundamentals of Physics. John Wiley & Sons, Inc., New York, Chapter 34.

Lettow, R., 2012. http://www.rdmag.com/news/2012/02/two-molecules-communicate-single-photons.

Maxwell, J.C., 1865. A dynamical theory of the electromagnetic field. Philos. Trans. R. Soc. Lond. 155, 459–512.

McFall, P., 2006. Brainy young James wasn't so daft after all. The Sunday Post, 23 April.

NASA, 2009. http://nssdc.gsfc.nasa.gov/nmc/spacecraftDisplay.do?id=1972-012A, accessed 15 August 2009.

Oschman, J.L., Oschman, N.H., 2004. Electromagnetic communication and olfaction in insects. Commemorating the research of Phillip S. Callahan, Ph.D. Frontier Perspect. 13 (1), 8–15.

Pall, M.L., 2013. Electromagnetic fields act via activation of voltage-gated calcium channels to produce beneficial or adverse effects. J. Cell. Mol. Med. 17 (8), 958–965.

Pollack, G., 2008. Water, energy, and life: fresh views from the water's edge. 32nd Annual Faculty Lecture, University of Washington. http://www.youtube.com/watch?v=XVBEwn6iWOo.

Pollack, G.H., 2013. The Fourth Phasr of Water. Beyond Solid, Liquid, and Vapor. Ebner & Sons Publishers, Seattle WA.

Porath, D., Bezryadin, A., de Vries, S., Dekker, C., 2000. Direct measurement of electrical transport through DNA molecules. Nature 403, 635–638.

Raso, J., 1995. Mystical medical alternativism. Skeptical Inquirer. 19 (5), 33–37.

Rezus, Y.L., Walt, S.G., Lettow, R., Zumofen, G., Renn, A., Götzinger, S., Sandoghdar, V., 2012. Single-photon spectroscopy of a single molecule. Phys. Rev. Lett. 108, 093601.

Siyushev, P., Guilherme, G., Wrachtrup, J., Gerhardt, I., 2014. Molecular photons interfaced with alkali atoms. Nature 509, 66–70.

Weisskopf, V.F., 1968. How light interacts with matter: the everyday objects around us are white, colored or black, opaque or transparent, depending on how the electrons in their atoms or molecules respond to the driving force of electromagnetic radiation. Sci. Am. 219, 60–71.

CHAPTER 4

Historical Origins of Energy Medicine

*In every culture and in every medical tradition before ours,
healing was accomplished by moving energy.*
Albert Szent-Györgyi (1960)

Chapter Summary

The quotation raises important and fascinating historical questions. Why has modern medicine neglected most of the fundamental principles of the medicines from virtually all of the other cultures and traditions from around the world? Where can we find information about these medicines, some of which have been used successfully by hundreds of millions of people in the most populous regions of the world for many centuries? Why does Western scientific medicine avoid all but superficial consideration of the ways energy moves within living things and discount the medical significance of discoveries made in other parts of the world and in other eras? In this chapter, we point the reader toward rich sources of medical knowledge, wisdom, and philosophy that have enlightened people through the ages and that are incorporated in various schools and technologies encompassed by the term *energy medicine*. The techniques that have incorporated this wisdom are offering much promise toward resolving our modern healthcare dilemmas. Moreover, we see in retrospect that a number of individuals who were regarded as charlatans by their contemporaries were in fact responsible for some of the most important discoveries in the history of medicine. Ancient and new technologies and ideas, which currently focus mainly on biochemistry, molecular biology, pharmacology, and sophisticated high-tech devices, are enriching our definition of life and health. An important perspective is the interaction between discoveries made by sensitive individuals and the evolution of devices.

Discoveries, Ideas, Enlightenments, and 'Golden Ages'

The term *Golden Age* (Χρυσόν Γένος) comes from Greek mythology and refers to legendary periods characterized with such words as *perfect and primordial peace, justice, innocence, goodness, virtue, harmony, stability, abundance, bliss, beauty, happiness, health, ease*, and *prosperity* – in other words, a paradise, a civilized life free of vices, hatred, vanity, evil, disease, sorrow, and fear (Figure 4.1). Whether such times actually existed, much is written about the possibility of past and future utopian societies without war or crime, devoted to culture, learning, peace, and prosperity (e.g., Heinberg, 1989; Hesse, 1970). Many ancient cultures have believed that history is cyclical, composed of alternating Dark and Golden Ages. Indeed, every human culture has 'Adam and Eve' myths of a 'fall' from an original golden age of peace and prosperity to evil, death, and disease. The British poet Percy Bysshe Shelley (1792–1822) hailed the promise of the return of romantic and

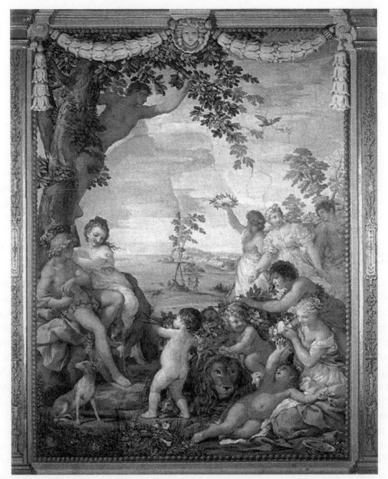

Figure 4.1 'The Golden Age' by Pietro da Cortona.

revolutionary eras, foretelling the dissolution of empires and the advent of a new and truly peaceful religion and world society (see Shelley, 1822). A yearning for the return of such an archetypal period of 'paradise' exists in the hearts of many. Albert Szent-Györgyi offered an actual physical mechanism for such a transformation in his classic and controversial article entitled 'Syntropy – the Drive in Nature to Perfect Itself' (Szent-Györgyi, 1977).

Enlightenments

In a fascinating essay entitled 'The Third Enlightenment', Yasuhiko Genku Kimura has discussed the topic in the context of the history of enlightenment, with references to three main periods:

- *The spiritual enlightenment of the ancient masters*
- *The scientific enlightenment of the industrial revolution*
- *The convergence of the spiritual and scientific enlightenments that is taking place today*

The modern 'age of enlightenment' of the seventeenth and eighteenth centuries, sparked by philosophers Baruch Spinoza (1632–1677), John Locke (1632–1704), and Pierre Bayle

(1647–1706), and by mathematician Isaac Newton (1643–1727), was viewed by Immanuel Kant (1724–1804) as 'mankind's final coming of age, the emancipation of the human consciousness from an immature state of ignorance and error' (Kant, 1784). Bertrand Russell (1872–1970) did not agree, stating that the Age of Enlightenment of Kant was actually the latest phase in a progressive development that began in antiquity. Yasuhiko Kimura expanded on this perspective on the basis of his extensive studies of the evolution of knowledge and consciousness: The first enlightenment permeates world history, as expressed in language, art, and music, and was referred to by Aldous Huxley as 'the perennial philosophy', by Ken Wilber as 'deep spirituality', and by Herbert Günther as 'originary awarenes'.

To appreciate these ideas we need to know more about the spiritual enlightenment of the ancient masters. What were their teachings, what kind of medicine did they have, where can we learn about it, and can this have meaning for us today?

Ayurveda, Vedic, or Yogic medicines are probably the oldest systems, having developed over thousands, perhaps tens of thousands of years, or even longer. These medicines have survived as collections of poetic Sanskrit verses that can be memorized, sung, or chanted. Vedic medicine probably synthesized insights from all over Asia and the Middle East, and perhaps parts of Europe, with Sanskrit serving as the language of the early sciences. Our present medicine arose from Vedic medicine, since it is the direct descendant of Greek, Islamic, and subsequently European medical traditions, all of which can be traced back to Ayurvedic roots. Various miraculous healings are described in early texts from around the world and in the Bible (Figure 4.2).

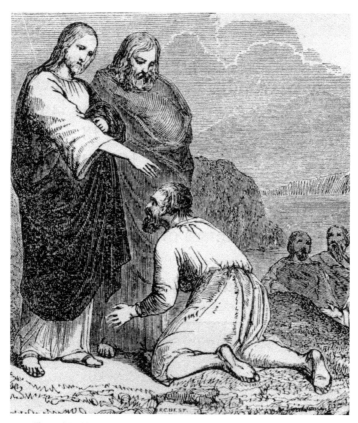

Figure 4.2 Woodcut from an old bible, showing Jesus healing a leper.

A number of scholarly texts assert that Jesus spent some years in India and was inspired by the Buddhist religion. Books such as *The Gnostic Gospels* (1979) and *Beyond Belief: the Secret Gospel of Thomas* (2003) by Princeton Professor Elaine Pagels and *The Original Jesus: The Buddhist Sources of Christianity* by Gruber and Kersten (1995) discuss these theories.

According to Tibetan Buddhism, Dzogchen is the natural or primordial condition of the mind, and the teachings and practises leading to an experience of that condition. Dzogchen or "Great Perfection" is regarded as the highest and most definitive path to enlightenment. Dzogchen teaches that the ultimate nature of all sentient beings is pure, all-encompassing, primordial awareness or naturally occurring timeless awareness. One's nature is like a mirror which reflects with complete openness but is not affected by the reflections, or like a crystal ball that takes on the color of the surface on which it is placed without itself being changed.

Keown (2003), Rinpoche (2008), Shikpo (2011) and Third Dzogchen Rinpoche (2008)

The 'laying on of hands' healings practised by Jesus of Nazareth (Figure 4.2) continues today in some churches and cathedrals around the world. There are many similarities between this method and some of the techniques of more recent approaches such as Reiki, Therapeutic Touch, Healing Touch, Aura Balancing, and Polarity Therapy.

The Bible discusses the healings performed by Jesus:

Jesus went throughout Galilee, teaching in their synagogues, preaching the good news of the kingdom, and healing every disease and sickness among the people. News about Him spread all over Syria, and people brought to Him all who were ill with various diseases, those suffering severe pain, the demon possessed, those having seizures, and the paralyzed, and He healed them.

MATTHEW 4:23–24

Herbert V. Günther

One source of the ancient knowledge can be found in the works of Professor Herbert V. Günther (1917–2006), who was one of the leading Buddhist scholars of our times. While living in India, he encountered many prominent Tibetan and Mongolian lamas and teachers, including His Holiness the Dalai Lama. He hand-copied many important Tibetan texts written by the great teachers and was one of the first translators of the RDzogs-Chen teachings into English. He published many books and articles with translations and interpretations of the teachings of the great lamas (e.g., Günther, 1976, 2001; Günther and Trungpa, 2001). These and many related texts focus on the nature of consciousness and meditative practises that enhance one's personal and interpersonal awareness, skills similar to those that are now being taught in many schools of energy medicine that are transforming healthcare.

Later in this chapter, we will discuss examples of exciting modern energy medicine approaches that are soundly based on the ancient traditional philosophies and wisdom combined with modern discoveries in fields such as quantum physics. The method called BodyTalk provides a brilliant example (Veltheim, 2012; Veltheim and Muiznieks, 2011).

Early Use of Energy in Medicine

The earliest recorded use of electricity for healing dates from 2750 BC, when sick people were exposed to the shocks produced by electric eels (Kellaway, 1946). Around 400 BC, Thales rubbed amber and obtained static electricity, which also appeared to be therapeutic. Different forms of magnet healing may be even older. An African mine over 100,000 years old was a source of red iron ore, called bloodstone or ocher, that was used since ancient times for healing and ceremonial purposes. Magnetite or lodestone was used for healing by the ancient Egyptians, the Chinese, and, later, by the Greeks (Payne, 1990).

Acupuncture has a recorded history of about 2000 years, but probably goes back much further. Some believe that acupuncture began during the Stone Age when stone knives or sharp-edged tools were used to puncture and drain abscesses. Another theory is that solders injured in battle discovered that puncture wounds in certain areas on their skin resolved long-standing digestive or other chronic problems. A scholarly summary of the origins of healing methods is *The Healing Hand. Man and Wound in the Ancient World*, by Harvard Professor Guido Majno (1975).

Franz Anton Mesmer

In 1766 Franz Anton Mesmer (1734–1815) published his doctoral dissertation with the Latin title *De planetarum influxu in corpus humanum* (*On the Influence of the Planets on the Human Body*), which discussed the influence of the sun, moon, and planets on the human body and on disease. This was not astrology because it relied largely on Newton's theory of the tides.

In 1773, Mesmer (Figure 4.3A) began using magnets for healing. His patients frequently felt 'unusual currents' coursing through their bodies prior to the onset of a 'healing crisis' that led to a cure. Soon Mesmer discovered that he could produce the same phenomenon without the magnets, simply by passing his hands above the patient's body (Figure 4.3B). After some careful experimentation, in 1779 Mesmer published his *Memoir on the Discovery of Animal Magnetism* (Mesmer, 1948). Mesmer felt a sort of attraction and repulsion phenomenon around the body, similar to the sensations one has when handling iron magnets. Mesmer found an influential

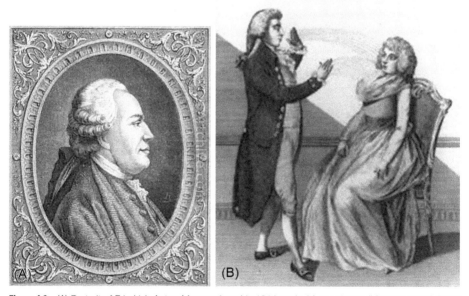

Figure 4.3   (A) Portrait of Friedrich Anton Mesmer from his 1814 work, *Mesmerismus* (Mesmer, 1966) *(From YOONIQ Co., LTD.)*. (B) The common Mesmeric posture (*Dupotet, C., 1862. L'art du magnetiseur, A. Réné, Paris*) with the 'magnetizer' moving his hand closely over his patient.

physician, Charles d'Eslon, who became a disciple. According to d'Eslon, Mesmer understood health as the free flow of the 'process of life' through thousands of channels in the human. Illness was caused by obstacles to this flow. Overcoming these obstacles and restoring flow restored health. When Nature failed to do this spontaneously, contact with a conductor of 'animal magnetism' was the best remedy. These concepts are virtually identical to those of acupuncture and many other energy therapies.

Mesmer invited scientists to witness his very popular work with 'incurable' cases, but the scientific and medical communities responded mainly with ridicule, animosity, malicious rumours, slander, and fear. It must be said, however, that Mesmer's scientific reputation was not always enhanced by his personal demeanour: 'Clothed in a robe embroidered with Rosicrucian alchemical symbols, he stalked the darkened rooms to the accompaniment of a glass harmonica and actively encouraged his clients to luxuriate in their convulsive crises' (Miller, 1995). Three scientific French Royal Commissions investigated Mesmer's methods and found his successes to be the result of his patients' imaginations and not from any real magnetic effect. Benjamin Franklin and Antoine Lavoisier were members of the last Commission, which was set up by Louis XVI in 1784. The Commission agreed that some healings had taken place, but they considered the idea of magnetic emanations 'philosophically unacceptable', although at the same time Franklin was convinced that electricity was a 'weightless fluid', and Lavoisier assumed that heat was also. Of course, Mesmer's studies preceded our modern understanding of magnetism and electricity by about 50 years. Franklin and Lavoisier were great scientific pioneers (Lavoisier is considered the father of modern chemistry) and were widely respected at the time they evaluated Mesmer's work, but they could not know what we know now: Movements of magnets near a person's body will, indeed, induce the flow of microcurrents within tissues and some patients can feel these flows. We will also see that such microcurrents can be profoundly therapeutic, and that the mechanisms involved have been carefully researched using the tools of modern physiology and biophysics (Chapters 2, 9, 15).

Mesmer's method resembled the laying on of hands used by Jesus and other religious figures, as well as the more modern methods mentioned above. Clinical trials are demonstrating the efficacy of these methods, and, as we shall soon see, research has begun to explain how these techniques work.

Mesmer is also credited with the discovery of hypnotism. The process was originally called *Mesmerism* and was subsequently termed *hypnotism* by a physician, James Braid.

An Emotional Controversy

Since ancient times, people have had a deep fear of the powerful and invisible forces of nature. Shamans and other religious figures derived authority and power from their ability to 'explain' the unknown, predict celestial events, calm or frighten the people, and perform 'healings' (Calvin, 1991). In many respects, science is another way of 'seeing' and explaining that which is normally hidden from our view. For biologists, the relationship between energy fields and life has been a subject of bitter and continuous controversy for over 400 years. The battle concerns a fundamental disagreement about the nature of life. Competing philosophies have generated much emotion and dogma. One argument is referred to as mechanism versus vitalism.

Mechanism Versus Vitalism

Mechanists hold that life obeys the laws of chemistry and physics and will ultimately be totally explained by those laws. This philosophy supports reductionism and the belief that the body is like a machine, composed of parts that can be studied individually and, if necessary, replaced. In contrast, vitalists have historically held to the belief that life will never be explained by normal science, that there is some kind of mysterious 'life force' separate from the known laws of nature and that distinguishes living from non-living matter. This concept is ancient and universal, appearing in some form or another in many different cultures and religions.

With the discovery of electricity in 1771 by Luigi Galvani, some vitalists began to associate electrical fields with a life force (for an excellent and detailed account of the history of this subject, see Becker and Marino, 1982). We defined 'healing energy' and "life force" in scientific terms in Chapter 1. We will also see, in Chapter 16, that there are subtle energetic relationships that go deeper than electricity and magnetism and that are opening new avenues for scientific exploration. These include the fundamental quantum processes taking place at the very small scale of the quantum plenum.

Samuel Hahnemann and Homeopathy

In 1790, Samuel Hahnemann (1755–1843) (Figure 4.4) began experimenting with natural remedies. Hahnemann was fascinated with a species of South American tree-bark (cinchona) that was being used at the time to treat the fever induced by malaria. One of the compounds that can be isolated from this natural source is quinine. Hahnemann ingested the bark and found that it caused symptoms similar to malaria. He continued researching various 'cures' and developed the idea of 'similar suffering'. *Similia similibus curentur* is the Latin phrase meaning 'let likes be cured by likes'. This is the primary principle of homeopathy. A homeopathic physician searches for a substance that produces in a healthy person those same symptoms a patient experiences. The substance is diluted and administered to the patient at an extremely low dose to trigger a 'healing crisis'. The symptoms may worsen briefly, followed by rapid healing.

The healing crisis is an important principle of natural medicines. Conventional Western medical thinking and patients seek immediate gratification: Just make the symptom go away. The elimination of the symptom is equated with the elimination of the disease or disorder. However, illnesses do not occur without causes, and symptoms are not causes. They are signals from the body that something is out of balance. They are signs that the body is attempting to heal itself. When the symptoms are treated, the patient feels better in the short term, but the underlying causes remain, and the patient may later develop a more serious condition. Hence the greatest harm from drug treatment is not so much the toxicity or side effects as it is the suppression effect. For example, a symptom such as itchy skin indicates that the body is responding to a deeper problem. If the itch is treated, it may go away, but then another problem arises, such as chronic diarrhoea. If the diarrhoea is then suppressed, the next step may be liver disease. This is the unrecognized and high price patients pay for the quick fix, for the shot or pill that seems to make the problem go away quickly.

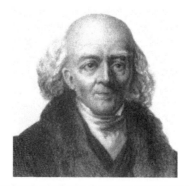

Figure 4.4 Samuel Hahnemann (1755–1843) who developed homeopathy. *(Courtesy of Wellcome Trust.)*

Homeopathy recognizes that this is a frequent problem with conventional medicine and views the healing crisis as a positive sign. The healing crisis is also known as the Herxheimer reaction. Adolf Jarisch (1850–1902), an Austrian dermatologist, and Karl Herxheimer (1861–1942), a German dermatologist, are credited with the discovery of the Herxheimer reaction. It occurs when the body is detoxifying too rapidly and toxins are being released faster than the body can eliminate them. A healing crisis can actually result from *any* holistic/natural therapy such as homeopathy, naturopathy, bodywork, movement therapies, acupuncture, and so on. Holistic practitioners learn to recognize the reaction and support the patient by having him or her drink water, rest, and perhaps take nutritional supplements that support the immune and lymphatic systems. Homeopathy also recognizes that it is often necessary to revisit each illness or trauma the body has been through that brought it to its current condition. This 'reversal process' is also common with a variety of holistic therapies. When it occurs in bodywork, it is sometimes referred to as 'unwinding'.

Homeopathy grew rapidly following Hahnemann's original findings, teachings, and writings. In 1784 Hahnemann published his first large-scale work, *Directions for Curing Radically Old Sores and Indolent Ulcers, with an Appendix Containing a More Appropriate Treatment of Fistulas, Caries, Spina Ventosa, Cancer, White Swelling and Pulmonary Consumption*. Published in Leipzig, the book contained many useful observations on the management of the health in general and of old ulcers in particular.

From its earliest days, homeopathy has been able to treat epidemic diseases with a substantial rate of success when compared to conventional treatments. It was these successes that placed the practise of homeopathy so firmly in the consciousness of people worldwide.

Joseph Pulte was one of the earliest homeopaths in Cincinnati. When he began his practise, many people were so angered by a homeopath being in town that they pelted the house with eggs. He was becoming discouraged enough to think of leaving. His wife said, 'Joseph, do you believe in the truth of homeopathy?' He replied in the affirmative. 'Then', she said, 'you will stay in Cincinnati'.

Shortly after, when the cholera epidemic swept through, Pulte was able to boast of not having lost a single patient – and he was accepted into the community. In the epidemic of 1849, people crowded to his door and stood in the street because the waiting room was full.

Moritz Muller founded the first homeopathic Journal, *Archiv fur der Homoopathischen Heilkunst*, in 1822. Other students of Hahnemann founded the first homeopathic medical school in the United States in the late 1800s. Homeopathy became important because of its success in treating the many epidemics that were rampant at the time – scarlet fever, typhoid, cholera, and yellow fever. According to Ernst and Kaptchuk, (1996), by 1900 8% of American medical practitioners were homeopathic doctors. At that time, there were 22 homeopathic medical schools, 100 homeopathic hospitals, over 1000 homeopathic pharmacies, and 31 homeopathic medical journals in the United States alone. Boston University, Stanford University, and New York Medical College were teaching homeopathy. This widely successful and popular form of medicine was nearly eliminated in the 1920s as a result of the Flexner report (see below) and the reorganization of medical education that followed. At the same time, interest in homeopathy was growing steadily in Europe and Asia. Today homeopathy has a particularly strong following in Russia, India, Switzerland, Mexico, Germany, the Netherlands, Italy, the UK, and South America. Homeopathy is also returning in the United States. This resurgence has been documented by the National Center for Homeopathy in Virginia.

Our understanding of the physiological, electronic, and quantum basis for homeopathic effects has been greatly advanced through the work of Cyril Smith. This will be detailed in Chapter 16.

Andrew Taylor Still, the Palmers, William G. Sutherland, and Randolph Stone

Some of the most significant concepts utilized in modern complementary and alternative therapies appear to be traceable to Andrew Taylor Still (1828–1917) (Figure 4.5), who founded osteopathy. Still had a strong spiritual background and was possibly influenced by Native American healers during a period when he was one of the first white men living in the state of Kansas. He had an intense dislike of drugs, which raised many problems for him. People could not understand his manipulations and the remarkable results they produced. A woman asked him if it was hypnotism, and he replied, 'Yes, madam, I set seventeen hips in one day'.

Whatever works, works!

RANDOLPH STONE

We can trace the influence of Still's teachings through his associates, students, and their students. Prominent figures in this lineage include William Garner Sutherland, who was a student of A.T. Still (circa 1900). Sutherland accepted his mentor's suggestion to 'dig deeper' and was responsible for extending osteopathic principles to the cranium, which led to his discovery of what has been termed the *primary respiratory mechanism*. Sutherland wrote a classic book, *Osteopathy in the Cranial Field*. The Palmers were instrumental in establishing the chiropractic profession. Randolph Stone developed Polarity Therapy. He was an avid student and became a Doctor of Osteopathy, a Doctor of Chiropractic, and a Naturopathic Doctor. He travelled extensively around the world in search of medical insights from other cultures. His motto was, 'Whatever works, works!'

These creative and visionary individuals – Still, Sutherland, the Palmers, and Stone – all had profound insights and experiences in the area of energetics, and their discoveries are having major influences on healthcare worldwide (Figure 4.6).

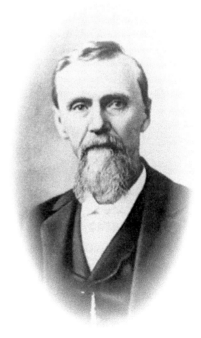

Figure 4.5 Andrew Taylor Still (1828–1917), founder of osteopathy. *(Courtesy of Wellcome Trust.)*

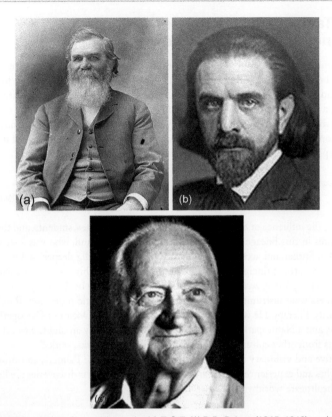

Figure 4.6   Associates and students of the work of A.T. Still, (A) D.D. Palmer (1845–1913), and (B) B.J. Palmer (1881–1961), founders of the chiropractic profession, and (C) Randolph Stone (1890–1981) who developed Polarity Therapy.

The Beginnings of Reiki

It was during this period that Dr. Mikao Usui founded the Usui System of Reiki in Japan. The actual origins of the process are the subject of discussion, but most authorities agree that Dr. Usui (1865–1926) (Figure 4.7) founded the system that was later brought to the United States. Reiki has spread rapidly in the West. It is now practised throughout North and South America, Europe, New Zealand, Australia, and other parts of the world. There are now millions of Reiki Masters throughout the world.

Albert Abrams

At the beginning of the nineteenth century, Albert Abrams (1863–1924) was operating a clinic in San Francisco and laying down the foundations for what would later become known as 'radionics'. Abrams claimed that he could detect energies or vibrations that are emitted from healthy and diseased tissues. He invented devices that he said could measure these energies and systematically interpret them as signs of health or disease (Figure 4.8). This is not a radical idea, in view of Einthoven's important discovery that diseases of the heart are revealed by distortions in the heart's electrical field, as mentioned in Chapter 5. However, Abrams is still considered by some to be

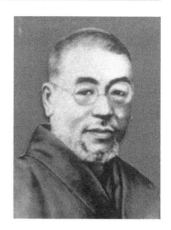

Figure 4.7 Dr. Mikao Usui (1865–1926) founded the Usui System of Reiki in Japan.

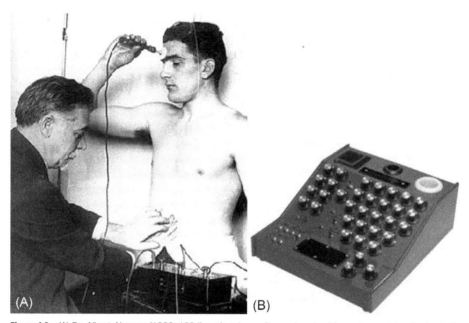

Figure 4.8 (A) Dr. Albert Abrams (1863–1924) performing a diagnosis using his controversial radionics technology. (B) One of his devices used for diagnosis and treatment is viewed by many to have no plausible mechanism of operation.

'the Dean of 20th Century Charlatans' because of widespread disbelief in his methods. Radionic devices continue to provide skeptics with a lot of good material, although there are many patients who report successes.

The operation of the Abrams device is said to contradict known principles of biology and physics, and there is allegedly no scientifically plausible mechanism of function. It is frequently stated that no radionic device has been found effective in the diagnosis or treatment of any disease, and the U.S. Food and Drug Administration does not recognize any legitimate medical application. Most physicians dismiss radionics as complete quackery. It must be remembered, however, that such judgments have been levelled against some of the greatest scientists and clinicians in history. Indeed, history has shown that rejection by 'the establishment' has often been a sign that an important discovery has been made.

A discovery must be, by definition, at variance with existing knowledge.

SZENT-GYÖRGYI (1972)

Franz Anton Mesmer discovered 'animal magnetism' and is still considered a charlatan by many. Yet we now know that he was correct – animals have biomagnetic fields around them (Chapter 9), and mesmerism or hypnosis is still widely applied. Were Abrams and Mesmer charlatans, fakes, and quacks, or were they ahead of their time?

The famous author, Upton Sinclair (1878–1968) heard glowing reports about the work that Abrams was doing in letters from his close friend, the famous California poet George Sterling (1869–1926). 'I should never again be afraid of getting any disease; Abrams would cure it in a week or two. He has utterly revolutionized medicine, and henceforth nine operations out of ten will be unnecessary … his diagnoses are 100 percent correct'. Sinclair found these statements to be extreme and did not take them seriously. However, after listening to this praise of Abrams for some 10–12 years, Sinclair decided to go to San Francisco to investigate. He expected to spend a day or two, but what he found captivated him for several weeks; he would have stayed longer if urgent matters had not called him home. Sinclair was so impressed with the work of Abrams that he wrote a fascinating essay that was published in *Pearson's Magazine* in June 1922. He concluded:

> … *one thing quickly becomes clear to you. The hypothesis of fraud must be excluded … You talk with the physicians who sit watching [Abrams work]. 'Why did you come here?' you ask, and the answer is, 'I sent Abrams some blood specimens, and found his diagnoses were right every time'. You ask another, and get the same response. You ask a third and he says, 'He diagnosed my cancer while I was in Illinois, and cured it, so I came to learn about it'. Half the physicians here have been cured of something, you find, and several are in the process of cure.*

Sinclair was obviously deeply moved by the work of Abrams, by his gentle nature and his scientific rigour. He came to call the Abrams clinic 'The House of Wonder' because of the miracles he saw taking place there. Eventually, the physicians in San Francisco began to refer to Abrams as crazy. Sinclair noted that the same thing had happened to Harvey, who is credited with the discovery of the circulation of the blood, and to Lister, who discovered antisepsis.

In spite of the criticisms, skepticism, and disbelief, the methods originated by Abrams have been refined by a number of investigators and appear to yield reproducible results. The equipment utilizes subtle energies that are not yet fully understood, and the energies involved are very small, as in homeopathy. This does not mean that the concepts should be rejected, for the history of medicine teaches us that what is heresy for one generation can become a dominant paradigm in the next. Valid explanations for the results obtained with these technologies may emerge from quantum physics (see Chapters 9, 11 and 13).

The most tragic case of skepticism, actually causing many deaths, is the story of Semmelweis in Vienna in the mid-1800s. Semmelweis attempted to introduce a completely radical medical concept, hand washing, to protect patients from an invisible force, bacteria (see box below).

If it were not for the pioneers and their struggles at the frontiers of human intellect and accomplishment, most of what we now value in science, medicine, and many other areas would never have become available to us. Science and biomedicine would progress at a much faster pace if the people involved were willing to consider rather than react to new ideas.

When Semmelweis proposed that obstetricians wash their hands before delivering babies, the idea was considered preposterous. He was in effect introducing a new and invisible factor at work in healing, which today we call infection. At the time, however, the theory of an infectious disease did not exist. So Semmelweis did a simple experiment to prove his point. For a year the midwives on one obstetrical ward washed their hands, and the obstetricians on another ward did not. On the hand washing ward mortality from childbirth fever declined by 1000%. But, alas, the data made no difference. Skeptical physicians still could not accept the conclusion that there was a lethal factor lurking on the hospital wards that they were helping spread and that could be controlled by washing one's hands. Semmelweis was regarded as a troublemaker and was vilified. He fled Vienna for Budapest and eventually committed suicide as a result of the emotional strain he experienced.

Garrison (1929)

In this context, recall that in 1633 Galileo was condemned by the Church for supporting the notion that the Earth revolves around the sun, counter to Church teachings at the time. The cardinals refused to look into Galileo's telescope because dogma had it that the moon's surface had to be perfect. More than 350 years later, in 1992, Pope John Paul II declared that the seventeenth century denunciation of Galileo was an error. Scientific politics and judgments are always problematic, but Galileo's case shows that when religion enters into an argument, things can become even more complicated. We now appropriately view the actions of the Church as totally unscientific, although similar behaviour persists in the conventional scientific establishment when confronted with new data or concepts. Many who made important new discoveries have been unable to obtain research grants, get their articles published, or receive academic promotion. The justification: peer review, the process by which new discoveries are evaluated in relationship to the currently held paradigm.

Many of the greatest problems in biology are unsolved, if not untouched. We should not shy away from admitting our ignorance. The first step toward new knowledge is to recognize ignorance.
SZENT-GYÖRGYI (1977)

Flexner Report

The total absence of standards for medical education, clinical practise, and therapeutic devices in the United States led to the passage of the Federal Pure Food and Drugs Act of 1906 and to the publication in 1910 of the Flexner report. These two events changed the course of medicine, and the effects, both positive and negative, are still felt today. The Flexner report is regarded as the defining document for modern medicine because it standardized medical education, supposedly on the basis of scientific principles and demonstrable facts. The Flexner study was funded by the Carnegie Foundation, and it established science as the basis for all medicine and clinical education. Medical schools were completely overhauled. Abraham Flexner (Figure 4.9) had a strong bias against homeopathy and naturopathy, and colleges were gradually forced to eliminate such programmes. Electrotherapy was declared scientifically unsupportable (although no actual research was done to back up this statement) and was legally excluded from clinical practise. Many doctors had equipment removed from their offices and taken to 'museums of quackery'. They were told that if they wanted to continue using electrotherapies, they would be doing it in prison! Dr. Hammond's pills were no longer sold through the Sears catalogue (Chapter 5). The Pure Food and Drug Act and Flexner's work laid the foundation for a century of dominance of pharmaceutical medicine.

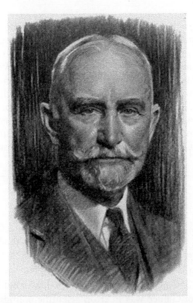

Figure 4.9 Abraham Flexner, author of the Flexner report (1910) funded by the Carnegie Foundation. The report established science as the basis for all medicine and clinical education. Medical schools were completely overhauled.

References

Becker, R.O., Marino, A.A., 1982. Electromagnetism and Life. State University of New York Press, Albany, NY.

Calvin, W.H., 1991. How the Shaman Stole the Moon: In Search of Ancient Prophet-Scientists from Stonehenge to the Grand Canyon. Bantam Books, New York, NY.

Dupotet, C., 1862. L'art du magnetiseur, A. Réné, Paris.

Ernst, E., Kaptchuk, T., 1996. Homeopathy revisited. Arch. Intern. Med. 156, 2162–2164.

Flexner, A., 1910. Medical Education in the United States and Canada: A Report to the Carnegie Foundation for the Advancement of Teaching. Bulletin No. 4. The Carnegie Foundation for the Advancement of Teaching; New York.

Gruber, E.R., Kersten, H., 1995. The Original Jesus: The Buddhist Sources of Christianity Element Books. HarperCollins, London, UK.

Garrison, F.H., 1929. An Introduction to the History of Medicine, 4th edition. W.B. Saunders, Philadelphia, PA, pp. 232–233.

Günther, H.V., 1976. Kindly Bent to Ease Us. Part Two: Meditation. Dharma Publishing, Berkeley, CA.

Günther, H.V., 2001. Matrix of Mystery: Scientific and Humanistic Aspects of rDzogs-chen Thought. Shambhala, Boston, MA.

Günther, H.V., Trungpa, C., 2001. The Dawn of Tantra. Shambhala, Boston, MA.

Heinberg, R., 1989. Memories and Visions of Paradise: Exploring the Universal Myth of a Lost Golden Age. Tarcher, Los Angeles, CA, 282 pp.

Hesse, H., 1970. Magister Ludi. Bantam Books, New York, NY.

Kant, I., 1784. Answering the question: What is Enlightenment?: Beantwortung der Frage: Was ist Aufklärung? In: Gedike, F., Biester, J.E. (Eds.), Berlinische Monatsschrift (Berlin Monthly), Berlin. An English translation can be found at, https://web.cn.edu/kwheeler/documents/What_is_Enlightenment.pdf, accessed July 17, 2014.

Kellaway, P., 1946. The part played by electric fish in the early history of bioelectricity and electrotherapy. Bull. Hist. Med. 20, 112–132.

Keown, D., 2003. A Dictionary of Buddhism. Oxford University Press p. 82.

Majno, G., 1975. The Healing Hand. Man and Wound in the Ancient World. Harvard University Press, Cambridge, MA.

Mesmer, A., 1948. Mesmerism: With an Introduction by Gilbert Frankau. Macdonald, London (This is Mesmer's Memoir of 1779.).

Mesmer, F.A., 1966. Mesmerismus: oder System der Wechselwirkungen, Theorie and Anwendung des thierischen Magnetismus als die allgemeine Heilkunde zur Erhaltung des Menschen. Translated by Karl Christian Wolfart. E.J Bonset, Amsterdam [Mesmer's work was first published in 1814].

Miller, J., 1995. Going unconscious. In: Silvers, R.B. (Ed.), Hidden Histories of Science. Granta Books, London, pp. 1–35.

Pagels, E., 1979. The Gnostic Gospels. Vintage Books, New York, NY.

Pagels, E., 2003. Beyond Belief: The Secret Gospel of Thomas. Vintage Books, New York, NY.

Payne, B., 1990. The Body Magnetic. Privately published, Santa Cruz, CA.

Rinpoche, D., 2008. Great Perfection: Outer and Inner Preliminaries. Snow Lion Publications (Shambhala), Boston, MA.

Shelley, P.B., 1822. Hellas. Charles and James Ollier, London, UK.

Shikpo, R., 2011. Longchen, Longchenpa and the Dzogchen Lineage. A Heart of the Buddha Teaching. DVD recorded December at Friends Meeting House, Oxford Longchen Foundation, Oxford.

Szent-Györgyi, A., 1977. Drive in living matter to perfect itself. Synthesis 1 (1), 14–26.

Szent-Györgyi, A., 1972. Dionysians and Apollonians. Science 176, 966.

Veltheim, J., 2012. Quantum BodyTalk. International BodyTalk Association, Sarasota, FL.

Veltheim, J., Muiznieks, S., 2011. BodyTalk Fundamentals. International BodyTalk Association, Sarasota, FL.

Winter, A., 1998. Mesmerized: Powers of Mind in Victorian Britain. University of Chicago Press, Chicago, IL, Fig. 1, p. 2.

CHAPTER 5

Electrobiology and Electrophysiology

Chapter Summary

Electricity is one of the most significant forces of nature and has had a long history of involvement in biomedicine. As early as 46 CE, the Roman physician Scribonium Largus used electric rays, genus *Torpedo*, to cure the pain of gout and headaches. For headache, the live ray was placed against the painful spot. For gout, the patient's feet are placed on a live black *Torpedo* while standing on the moist shore washed by the sea. From what we now know about electrons and inflammation, this treatment may not be as surprising as it seems (see Preface, Introduction and Chapter 17).

It was not until the late sixteenth century that a true science of bioelectricity was born, suddenly, with an electric spark. This was the discovery of 'animal electricity' by Luigi Galvani, a physician and surgeon in Bologna, Italy. Galvani (it may actually have been his wife, Lucia, who saw it first; Figure 5.1) noticed that recently dissected frog legs twitched vigorously when a nearby electric generator emitted a spark. The phenomenon was so interesting that Galvani made a career of studying the twitches and how, for example, an 'electric fluid' in a nerve could be conducted via a metallic wire to a muscle, which would contract.

Soon one of the most interesting arguments in the history of science began between Galvani and his friend, Alessandro Volta, in nearby Pavia. Volta's invention of the electric battery (the Voltaic pile) was a huge accomplishment, and the unit of measure of electricity, the volt, was named after him. Galvani's name was attached to the early devices for measuring electricity, galvanometers. This is the instrument that Einthoven in Holland used a century later to measure the electricity of the heart and record the electrocardiogram, an energy medicine diagnostic tool now used in virtually every hospital in the world.

Electrophysiology After Galvani

In the centuries since the discovery of animal electricity, much has been learned about how electricity is involved in the activities of all cells and tissues and organs throughout the body. It is remarkable how the research of one man and his wife can lead to entire disciplines such as electrophysiology and neurophysiology, occupying the attention of literally thousands of scientists around the world. In tracing the path from Galvani to the present, we meet remarkable individuals who faced serious questions. For example, the discovery was made that nerves conduct some sort of 'electrical fluid' at a velocity of dozens of meters per second, while electric fields in metal wires move at the speed of light. How could the nerve impulse be electrical in nature if it moved so slowly? This question was resolved with a remarkable experiment done by Bernstein (1868), showing that an electrical 'negative variation' propagated along the nerve at a speed corresponding to that of the nerve signal. This negative variation proved to be the action potential, a phenomenon that was explained in exquisite detail beginning almost exactly 200 years after Galvani's birth by Alan Hodgkin and Andrew Huxley for which they were awarded the Nobel Prize in Physiology or Medicine in 1963.

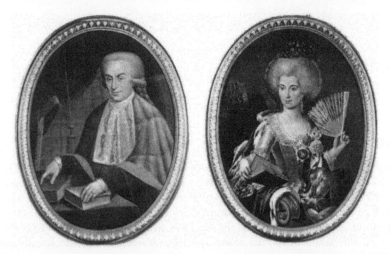

Figure 5.1 Contemporary portraits of Luigi Galvani and his wife Lucia Galeazzi. Notes in Galvani's experimental log of the spark experiment contain a passage alluding to his wife's collaboration in his historic discovery. *(From Piccolino M: Luigi Galvani and animal electricity: two centuries after the foundation of electrophysiology, Trends Neurosci 1997 Oct;20(10):443–448.)*

The Beginnings of Electrobiology and Electrophysiology

And still we could never suppose that fortune were to be so friend to us, such as to allow us to be perhaps the first in handling, as it were, the electricity concealed in nerves, in extracting it from nerves, and, in some way, in putting it under everyone's eyes.

GALVANI (1791)

From his studies of 'animal electricity' in frogs, Luigi Galvani, the scientist from Bologna, demonstrated that there was some sort of 'animating force' that flows from nerves to muscles to trigger movements. The discovery began when he noticed that recently dissected frog legs would twitch when the nerve going to them was touched with a metal implement, but only when a spark jumped from a nearby electric generator. This was a surprise, and he followed up with a series of experiments to find out more details. One experiment involved directly connecting the sciatic nerve of a freshly dissected frog to the exposed leg muscle with a wire (Figure 5.2), causing the

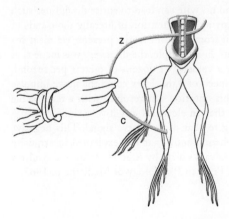

Figure 5.2   Galvani's frog leg experiment.

muscles to contract. Eventually he demonstrated that this effect was due to 'intrinsic electricity' that is involved in fundamental physiological processes. He also showed that this electricity was the same as the atmospheric electricity Benjamin Franklin had demonstrated with his famous 1752 experiment in which he showed that lightning is electricity by flying a kite in a storm and nearly electrocuting himself. Galvani did an experiment in which he attached the nerve that supplies the frog's leg to a wire that was connected to a metal spike at the top of his house. The legs twitched vigorously when lightning flashed during a storm.

Galvani's research laid the foundation for the fields of bioelectricity or medical electricity. The research that followed virtually eliminated from life sciences mysterious fluids and elusive entities like 'humours' and 'animal spirits' and led to the foundation of the new sciences of electrobiology and electrophysiology. Two centuries of research have confirmed Galvani's conception of animal electricity.

Galvani opened the way for the studies of physicist Alessandro Giuseppe Antonio Anastasio Volta at the University of Pavia, culminating in 1800 with the invention of the electric battery. Volta disagreed with Galvani about 'animal electricity'. His view was that frogs, although capable of reacting to external electricity like sensitive electroscopes (Figure 5.3) did not have intrinsic electricity. According to Volta, the electricity originated from the dissimilar metals Galvani had used to connect the frog nerve to his lightning rod – the iron wire from the rod and the brass hooks he had attached to the nerves.

The ensuing controversy between Galvani and Volta is regarded as one of the most important scientific debates in the history of science. It led both scientists to carry out fundamental experiments to support their respective hypotheses. Volta's experiments led to the invention of the electrical battery, the famous Voltaic pile, which led to the subsequent development of electrochemistry, electromagnetism, and related phenomena. Galvani's studies laid the foundations for modern electrophysiology and neuroscience. In retrospect, the development of electrophysiology in the nineteenth century depended critically on the work of both of these scientists.

Volta correctly pointed out that contacts between metals and living tissues were capable of acting as 'motors' of electricity. He stated that *E' la differenza de' metalli che fa* ('It is the difference of metals which does it') (Volta, 1918). This is, in fact, the basis for 'electrode reactions' that occur when a recording electrode touches living tissues. Unless appropriate precautions are taken, measurements of electric fields from living tissues can, in part, be due to voltages set up at the tissue-electrode boundary.

The scientific controversy between Galvani and Volta was followed by two centuries of electrophysiological studies leading to the modern understanding of electrical excitability in nerve and muscle. Here we are referring to the work of scientists such as Nobili, Matteucci, du Bois-Reymond, von Helmholtz, Bernstein, Hermann, Lucas, Adrian, Hodgkin, Huxley, and Katz, some of the most prominent.

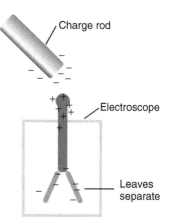

Figure 5.3 The electroscope used to detect static electricity.

In 1791 Galvani published his main work (the famous *De Viribus Electricitatis in Motu Musculari Commentarius – A Commentary on the Effects of Electricity on the Motion of Muscles*) summarizing more than 10 years of research on the effects of electricity on animal preparations (mostly frogs). This publication had an impact on the scientific community comparable to the social and political impact of the French revolution that took place at about the same time (du Bois-Reymond, 1848). Wherever frogs were available, both scientists and laymen set about reproducing Galvani's experiments by inducing contractions in the leg muscles of recently dead animals. One result was a shortage of frogs. The effects of electricity were also studied in other species, including humans. In 1803 in London, Galvani's nephew, Giovanni Aldini (1762–1834), applied electricity to the head of an executed criminal, with dramatic effects that inspired Mary Shelley's famous character, Frankenstein.

Because of his prestige from the development of the voltaic pile or battery, and due to his charismatic and dynamic speaking abilities, Volta's arguments eclipsed the work of the more retiring Galvani. Hence the hypothesis of 'animal electricity' was abandoned for many years. However, although successful with the invention of the electrical battery, Volta was mistaken in many of his conclusions on animal electricity, and this fact emerged over the following century.

About three decades after Galvani, in 1828, Leopoldo Nobili (1784–1835) was able to actually measure what he called *corrente di rana* or *corrente propria* ('frog current' or 'intrinsic current') with an improved galvanometer that corrected for the influence of the Earth's magnetic field on the magnetic needle in the device. Due to the continuing influence of Volta, Nobili incorrectly attributed the measured current to a thermoelectric effect due to the unequal cooling of nerve and muscle.

In 1838, Carlo Matteucci repeated the Nobili experiment and made the correct interpretation that the measured current was truly of biological origin. He then performed a convincing and unequivocal demonstration of the biological source of the muscle current with the ingenious preparation of a group of sectioned frog thighs arranged in series (Figure 5.4). The deflection of the galvanometer needle increased in proportion to the number of elements in the 'biological pile', excluding the possibility that the measured current was due to the contact of the muscular tissue with the metal of the electrodes (Matteucci, 1844). This experiment was also one of the first demonstrations of the injury potential, as will be discussed in the next chapter.

Emile du Bois-Reymond confirmed Matteucci's findings and went on to make the first instrumental recording of what would soon be called the 'action current' or 'action potential' (du Bois-Reymond, 1848). The electrical phenomenon he measured accompanying the excitation of

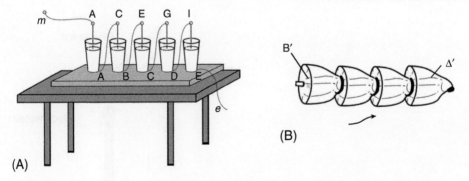

Figure 5.4   (A) The 'cascade battery' of Franklin, essentially a set of Leyden jars in series. (B) Matteucci's 1844 experiment demonstrating that Galvani's 'animal electricity' is of biological origin. A group of sectioned frog thighs was arranged in series. The deflection of the galvanometer needle increased in proportion to the number of the elements in the 'biological pile.' *((A) From Tyndall (1876).)*

muscle and nerve, using a sensitive galvanometer, was referred to by du Bois-Reymond as to the 'negative Schwankung' (the 'negative variation').

Meanwhile, in Berlin the great physiologist Johannes Müller (1845) stated that the nerve signal probably travelled at the speed of light and probably would never be measured. An idea that electricity travels very fast had already been obtained from a striking demonstration by the Abbé Nollet. In 1746, he had 200 of his monks form a circle about a mile in circumference, with each monk connected to the next by holding iron rods between their hands. The Abbé connected the ends of the circle to a bank of Leyden jars, devices that store static electricity. The jar discharged and sent a shock wave through the circle that caused the monks to jump virtually simultaneously. It was clear that electricity travels very fast (Stack, 1753).

It was not long after Müller's statement that it would be impossible to measure the speed of nerve conduction that his brilliant student Hermann von Helmholtz created a simple experimental arrangement that enabled him to measure the time required for the nerve signal to propagate a short distance. He calculated the conduction speed to be a few dozen meters per second. Helmholtz went on to use a rotating smoked drum (Figure 5.5) to graphically record muscle contractions.

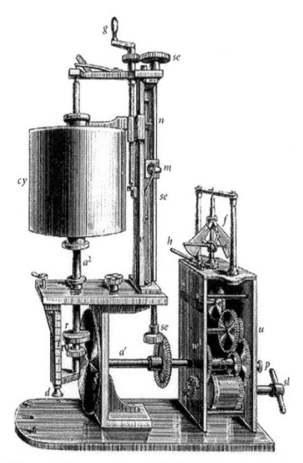

Figure 5.5 Rotating smoked drum apparatus used by Helmholtz to record muscle contractions.

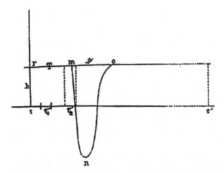

Figure 5.6 The first published recording of the time course of the action current, negative variation, now known as the action potential in a nerve. (*From Bernstein (1868).*)

The measurements of the velocity of nerve conduction raised an important question. Electric fields propagate in metallic wires at close to the speed of light, so how could the nerve impulse be electrical in nature if it moved so slowly? This question was resolved by showing that an electrical 'negative variation' propagated along the nerve had a speed corresponding to that of the nerve signal. This was accomplished by Julius Bernstein, a student of both von Helmholtz and du Bois-Reymond. Bernstein (1868) invented a remarkable device called a 'differential rheotome' that showed the time course of the action current or negative variation in the nerve (Figure 5.6). He also demonstrated that the speed of propagation of the negative variation and of the nerve signal closely corresponded to each other. This was strong evidence the two events were identical.

The unequivocal evidence that the nervous signal is fundamentally an electrical event, as Galvani had supposed at the end of the eighteenth century, had to await for the most modern epoch of electrophysiology (i.e., the period of studies of nerve physiology carried out by Hodgkin and his collaborators in Cambridge), which led to a widely accepted mechanism underlying the generation and propagation of the nerve signal.

Early Electrotherapy

It did not take very long for Galvani's discoveries to be applied in medicine. One early discovery that has endured to this day is the use of electricity to stimulate the healing of bone fractures that have failed to heal. In 1812, Dr. John Birch in London healed a nonunion of the tibia with electric currents passed through needles surgically implanted in the fracture region. By the mid-1800s, this had become the preferred method for treating slow-healing bone fractures. A modern version of this treatment, widely preferred and used by orthopedic surgeons, is an implantable electrical stimulation device (Figure 5.7).

Medical electricity had its golden era between the late 1700s and the early 1900s. During that period, a variety of electrical healing devices were developed and were widely used by physicians for treating a range of ailments.

(REVIEWED BY GEDDES, 1984)

Clinical electrotherapy was thriving at the same time that vitalism was being rejected by mainstream science. A serious effort was made by the founder of the Methodist Church, John Wesley (Figure 5.8), who published *Desideratum or Electricity Made Plain and Useful*, in which he recorded many successful treatments with mild electrotherapies (Wesley, 1871). His noble goal was to bring electrotherapy to the poor of London. Interestingly, he wrote, 'From a thousand experiments, it appears that there is a fluid far more subtle than air, which is everywhere diffused through all space, which surrounds the earth and pervades every part of it.' Could he have anticipated the quantum vacuum? (see Chapter 9).

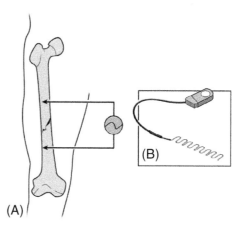

Figure 5.7 Modern method of stimulating bone growth in patients with delayed union of fracture (improper healing within 6 months) or fracture nonunion (failure of union after 6 months).

(A)

(B)

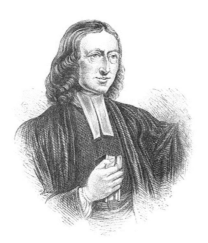

Figure 5.8 John Wesley.

By 1884 it was estimated that 10,000 physicians in the United States were using electricity every day for therapeutic purposes, totally without the blessing of science. Figure 5.9 shows an electromagnetic healing device patented by Elias Smith in 1869, and Figure 5.10 shows a French version (d'Arsonval, 1894).

The popularity of these early electrical devices was compromised by some eighteenth century proponents of electrical therapies, some with noble goals and others with entrepreneurial ambitions. Some were showmen who created spectacular displays of electrical phenomena and made outrageous health claims, many of which were probably nonsense. This period in the history of energy medicine is told entertainingly by Frances Ashcroft (2012) in *The Spark of Life: Electricity in the Human Body*.

Far less noble was the flamboyant work of the notorious 'Dr.' James Graham, who advertised that electricity could remedy all physical defects. His Temple of Health in the elegant Royal Adelphi Terrace only lasted from 1779 to 1782 because it created a mixture of fascination and

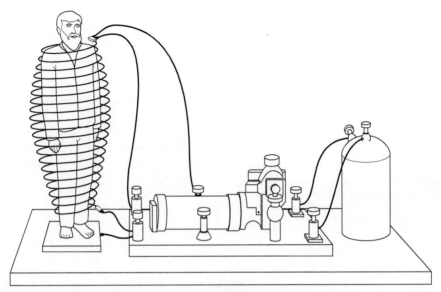

Figure 5.9   Healing device patented by E. Smith on October 19, 1869, US Patent No. 96,044. For convenience the coil is in two parts so the patient can step into the lower one and have the upper one placed over the head. Current flowing through the coil creates a magnetic field around and through the body. This is augmented by passing another current through the body from the head to the feet.

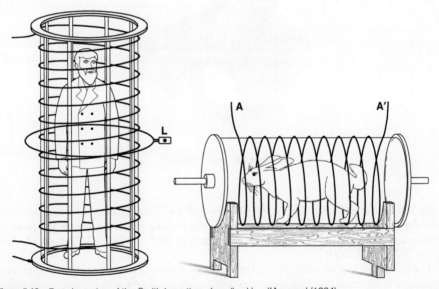

Figure 5.10   French version of the Smith invention, described by d'Arsonval (1894).

outrage. A plethora of electrical machines were promoted in the Victorian age; they produced both outstanding testimonials and suspicion in the medical community.

A popular approach was the 'electric hand' shown in Figure 5.11. The patient sat on a stool with his or her bare feet on a metal plate connected to an induction coil. An electrode attached to the other terminal of the coil was held in one hand by the therapist. The therapist's other hand—the 'electric hand'—was used to stroke or massage various parts of the patient's body

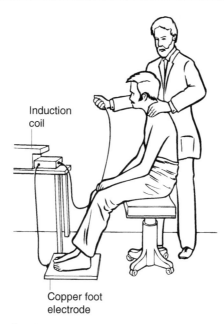

Induction
coil

Copper foot
electrode

Figure 5.11 The 'electric hand' method widely used in the late 1800s. The therapist and patient are connected in series to an induction coil that generates electricity. Here the therapist is shown massaging and 'faradizing' the patient's shoulder with his left hand.

(Ziemssen, 1864). Hence the electricity was passing through both the doctor and the patient. For many, a 'general faradization' of the whole body produced an ecstatic experience. 'Localized faradization' of specific regions was used to treat a variety of medical problems. In some cases, special electrodes were used to stimulate particular parts of the body. It was claimed that nearly all diseases could be cured by electricity, provided it could be passed through the blood. A possible explanation for these effects is that the flow of electricity through the patient's body delivered electrons to sites of chronic inflammation, which modern research recognizes as the cause of many chronic disorders, as mentioned in the Preface and further discussed in Chapter 17.

Four different forms of electricity were described:

- Static, or Franklinic electricity
- Direct, or galvanic current
- Induction-coil, or faradic current
- High-frequency, or d'Arsonval current

One discovery made using the electric hand was that stimulation of specific points on the body surface causes the underlying muscles to contract. In 1864, Ziemssen charted the locations of these points, which are now called 'muscle points' or 'motor points' (Basmajian, 1979). Using fresh cadavers, Ziemssen marked many of the motor points, dissected the underlying tissue, and found they were the places where the nerves entered the muscles. Subsequently, in 1867, Duchenne (1959) published his classic studies of the muscle points (Figure 5.12) that gave rise to the modern field of medical electromyography. The extent of nerve damage, for example, can be determined by making electrical recordings at the motor points to establish whether a muscle is properly innervated. One of the primary uses of electromyography is to determine the degree of injury a person has sustained for legal and insurance purposes.

The discoveries of the cellular and molecular basis of life, the bacterial origin of infectious diseases, Darwin's theory of evolution, and the electrical aspects of nerve conduction were all

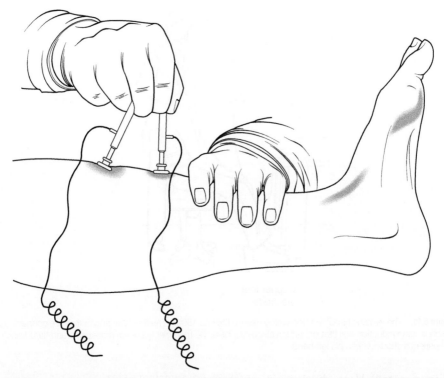

Figure 5.12   Duchenne's (1867) illustration of electrical stimulation of muscles (Duchenne 1959). His research founded the modern medical field of electromyography.

taken by the scientific establishment as the final blows to the vitalist position. All of life, from its beginnings in the primordial sea to its present level of complexity, could be explained scientifically. Organisms, like machines, could be broken down into their components and studied piece by piece until all mysteries were solved. It was just a matter of time and hard work before everything about life and disease could be understood. For the vitalist position, fundamental discoveries in biology caused a steady retreat, but the basic mystery of the driving force for nature remained. We will soon see that there was another mystery that persists to this day: What and where is the blueprint for life, the map or plan that determines how the various components of the organism are assembled into living structures?

Electrotherapy at the Turn of the Twentieth Century

By 1900, a wide variety of electrical and magnetic healing devices were on the market, claiming cures for virtually every disease and problem. Figure 5.13 illustrates some items listed in the 1902 catalogue from Sears Roebuck in Chicago, Illinois. Many claims were made about the miraculous healing powers of these products. Electric belts, bands, chains, plasters, and garters were 'capable of providing a quick cure of all nervous and organic disorders arising from any cause', and Dr. Hammond's Nerve and Brain Pills were 'positively guaranteed to cure any disease'. We shall see that these extravagant claims provided the impetus for strong regulatory actions against energy therapies that continue to this day. Note that it cannot be said that these products were ineffective, but only that there simply was no scientific evidence one way or the other. This was long before the modern era of basic research and clinical trials.

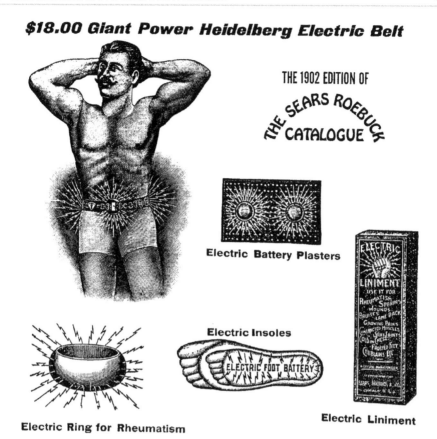

Figure 5.13 Electrical healing devices listed in the 1902 Catalogue of the Sears Roebuck Company, Chicago, Illinois.

Electrobiology, Electrophysiology, Neurophysiology

While medical research and medical school education were shifting toward pharmacology, rapid progress began to take place in electrobiology and electrophysiology – the study of the electrical properties of living systems. Various useful diagnostic tools were developed that involved recording the electrical fields produced by organs such as the heart, the other muscles, the eyes, and the brain (some of this was mentioned in Chapter 1 and is further explored in Chapter 3).

With progress in electrobiology and electrophysiology, electricity gradually lost its mystery and became less attractive as the elusive force the vitalists were searching for. This does not mean that vitalism is dead, nor does it mean we fully understand all of the energies and forces of nature, including electricity and magnetism, and their roles in living systems.

The emotional and dogmatic fervour of the past persists. There continues to be a strong academic bias against any suggestion that the electrical and magnetic fields generated by tissues and organs might have any important biological purpose – they are widely thought to be mere by-products of cellular activities, useful for diagnosis only. We shall see, though, that this view is being replaced. Biological fields are not just by-products of physiological processes; they are part of the mechanism by which the body regulates and communicates with itself. Research on this topic is underway in medical and academic research centers around the world. 'Electromagnetic medicine' is beginning to revive, but with a far more sophisticated scientific base to support it.

In the climate produced by the Flexner report (see Chapter 4), some prominent scientists, seeking to explore the possible role of electricity and magnetism in the control of growth and development and medicine, realized they were entering politically hazardous territory. To avoid problems, some researchers wisely obtained academic tenure by doing mainstream research before they began investigating energy fields. In this way they could be free to explore the role of energetics in living processes without the danger of being fired from their university positions.

HAROLD SAXTON BURR

One such pioneer was Harold Saxton Burr (Figures 5.14 and 5.15), who obtained his PhD at Yale in 1915 and became a full professor at Yale School of Medicine in 1929. He was appointed

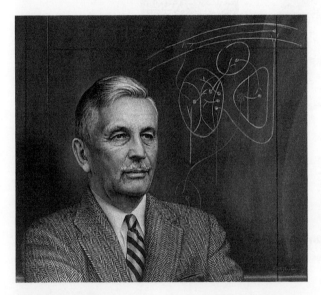

Figure 5.14 Harold Saxton Burr. From a painting by Artzybasheff presented to the Yale University School of Medicine on December 6, 1957 by the Burr Portrait Committee on behalf of Dr. Burr's colleagues and former students.

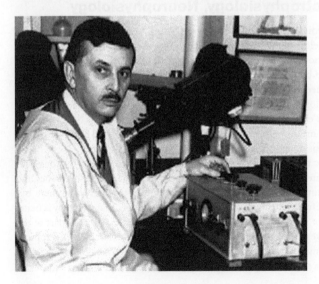

Figure 5.15 Harold Saxton Burr at work in his laboratory at Yale School of Medicine.

E. K. Hunt Professor of Anatomy in 1933 and remained in the post for 40 years. His early work was on the development of the nervous system, and he published nearly 20 papers on this subject between 1916 and 1935.

In 1932, Burr began a series of important and controversial studies of the role of electricity in development and disease. From his work on the development of the nervous system, Burr realized how little was actually known about the control of form in animals. Molecular genetics was revealing how the parts of the body are manufactured, but there was little understanding of the 'blueprint' that directs their assembly into the whole organism. While there continues to be widespread enthusiasm about the discoveries being made in molecular biology and especially in the human genome project, the mystery of the 'blueprint' continues to this day. This is not a trivial issue. All healing must reference the blueprint of the body so that the repair process recreates as closely as possible the form that was present before an injury or disease. We are taught that DNA is the blueprint for the body, but this is a great simplification. DNA is the code for the assembly of the amino acids into proteins, but it remains a mystery how the parts are then assembled into human form. This is one of many examples of a situation where it is widely believed that a problem has been solved when actually it has not.

Burr had many students and collaborators, some of whom were, or became, leading figures in American science. As an example, in 1949 he published a report in collaboration with Alexander Mauro (who later became a Professor at Rockefeller University) describing the electrostatic field of a frog sciatic nerve. The preparation and results are shown in Figure 5.16.

In all, Burr published some 93 papers and stimulated his colleagues in the production of about 100 more. He also wrote a book about his conclusions entitled *Blueprint for Immortality: The Electric Patterns of Life* (Burr, 1972), which was also published under the title *The Fields of Life. Our Links with the Universe* (Burr, 1973).

Burr took advantage of the invention of the vacuum tube voltmeter, a device for measuring the low voltages found in living tissues without drawing current from the sources. The vacuum tube was part of a circuit that amplified the current required to operate the meter. In this way the required energy is supplied by an amplifier and power supply instead of by the biological circuit being studied.

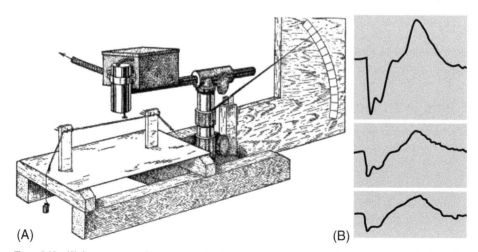

(A)   (B)

Figure 5.16 (A) Apparatus used to measure the electrostatic component of the nerve action potential in the air near the nerve. (B) The measured electrostatic field of the nerve at a distance of 1, 4, and 6 mm from the nerve. *(From Burr, H.S., Mauro, A., 1949. Electrostatic fields of the sciatic nerve in the frog. Yale J. Biol. Med. 21 (6), 455–462.)*

Burr's work on energy fields from 1932 to 1956 was out of step with the mainstream medicine and biology of the time. This was a period of explosive growth in pharmaceutical medicine and in the use of X-rays for diagnosis. Antibiotics were winning the war against disease, and the thrust of medical research and public policy was toward 'a pill for every problem'. The public was dazzled by the seemingly continuous and accelerating rate of scientific and medical progress. There was a very successful concept of bioenergetics, but it was entirely confined to the study of biochemical reactions and the ways molecules such as adenosine triphosphate (ATP) store and release metabolic energy. Few biochemists are aware that the standard textbook models of energy metabolism are far from complete and that many basic questions remain unsolved and even unstudied.

In the 1950s, a visitor to Burr's ancestral home, Mansewood, in Lyme, Connecticut, would discover various kinds of trees connected to recording voltmeters: Burr was convinced that all living things, from mice to humans, from seeds to trees, are formed and controlled by fields that can be measured with standard detectors. He published a series of articles on how the electric fields of trees change in advance of weather patterns and other atmospheric phenomena. Burr was convinced that the 'fields of life' are the basic blueprints for all living things; the fields reflect physical and mental conditions and are therefore useful for diagnostic purposes.

During the period when Burr was researching energy fields, most biologists and physicians were certain that all notions of energy therapy and 'life force' were complete nonsense. The experiences of energy therapies by energy practitioners and their patients were dismissed, either by ignoring them or by stating that the patients were victims of deception, illusion, trickery, fakery, quackery, hallucination, or the placebo effect. Scientists could say with certainty that any energy field around an organism would be far too weak to be detected. If such a field existed, it surely had no biological significance. Healing with energy fields was fantasy, and any notion that light could be emitted by the body was certainly quite foolish. This is a subject that will be discussed again in Chapter 9.

As a student of the history of medicine, Burr was well aware that work published ahead of its time remains in the libraries and is available to future generations when its moment arrives. Such a period is upon us, and Burr's articles are highly recommended, both for the serious student of energetic bodywork and/or movement therapies and for biomedical researchers exploring the role of energy fields in health and disease. A complete listing of Burr's articles can be found in the *Yale Journal of Biology and Medicine* (Burr, 1957) and at the end of Burr's own book (Burr, 1972).

In retrospect, the research of Burr and his many distinguished scientific colleagues anticipated many of the breakthroughs that are being made around the world at the present time. His published work and that of Robert O. Becker (Becker, 1990; Becker and Selden, 1985) are excellent introductions to the subject. The remainder of this book will summarize modern scientific definitions and perspectives on the 'life force' and 'healing energy'.

Fields in Diagnosis

The use of fields for diagnosis is based on the premise that every physiological process in the body has an electrical counterpart. Burr reiterated a position taken years earlier by the physiologist A. P. Mathews:

> *Every excess of action, every change in the physical state of the protoplasm of any organ, or any area in the embryo or in the egg, produces, it is believed, an electrical disturbance.*
>
> MATHEWS (1903)

As we shall soon see, modern research has confirmed the observations of Mathews and Burr. Not only does every event in the body, either normal or pathological, produce electrical changes, it also produces alterations of the biomagnetic fields in the spaces around the body. Again, this is a foundational principle of modern electrocardiography and electroencephalography. Recent research describes how this comes about; valuable summaries updating Burr's early research on cancer have been published by Brewitt (1996, 2002).

OVULATION AS AN EXAMPLE

In 1935, Burr described the detection of ovulation by monitoring the substantial voltage changes during the ovulation cycle. Others attempted to repeat Burr's work, but their results were not consistent. Burr continued to refine his approach and reported in 1936 and 1938 that the timing of ovulation in women could be determined by daily measurements of the electric field between the fingers of each hand. This was confirmed by another scientist in 1939, but others continued to have inconsistent results. Burr persisted in his investigations, publishing his last paper on the subject in 1953.

By 1974 the causes of variation in the ovulation potentials had been determined, and a fertility control system based on Burr's work was awarded a US patent (Friedenberg et al., 1975). The patent is interesting reading because it documents the reason for the inconsistency of previous studies. The ovulation cycle is but one of many bodily rhythms that produce oscillating electric fields. Detection of the ovulation cycle requires careful filtering to eliminate interference from other electrical rhythms generated by the other organs in the body, such as the heart and brain (Figure 5.17). Once the electrical rhythms from other organs have been removed by filtration, the monthly rhythm of the ovary can be recorded (Figure 5.18).

EARLY CANCER DETECTION

Another controversial area of investigation concerned the detection of cancer. Burr was convinced that diseases would alter the energy field before symptoms of pathology, such as tumors. His theory was that if the disturbed energy field could be detected and restored to normal, the pathology could be prevented. This is obviously a concept with profound medical significance. It is also

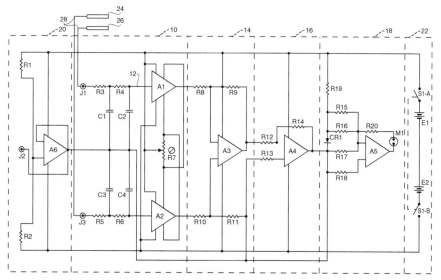

Figure 5.17   The circuit patented by Friedenberg, Reese & Reading (1975) to separate the monthly electrical rhythm of the ovary from the rhythms of other organs in the body. The patent describes this as 'the combined circuitry for milli-volt measurement including the critical means of high impedance and high common mode rejection combined with sufficient isolation and filtration of the essential circuit to reliably indicate and measure the low D.C. ovulation potential'. (From US Patent 3,924,609).

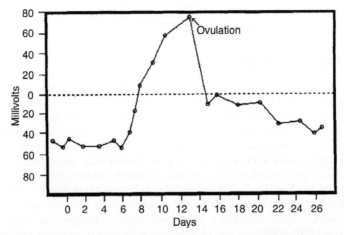

Figure 5.18 The electrical rhythm of the ovulation cycle in the human female recorded between a finger of each hand. Before and after ovulation the potentials are negative. About 5-6 days before ovulation the potential begins to rise and increases above zero a few days before ovulation. Afterwards there is a rapid decline to below zero, at which time the body is free of a fertilizable ovum until the next cycle. (Graph from US Patent 3,924,609).

a fundamental principle of acupuncture and Oriental medicine: that maintenance of energetic balance prevents disease.

In 1936, Burr and his colleagues began a series of studies on the relation between electrical fields and cancer, beginning with spontaneous or induced mammary tumors in mice. Large voltage changes were detected with electrodes attached to the chest from 10 days to 2 weeks before the tumors appeared. In 1945, British researchers attempted to repeat Burr's experiments, but without success. Burr continued to work on the problem and published his last cancer paper in 1949. The following year, critiques of Burr's work were summarized by Crane (1950).

Confirmation of Burr's Cancer Research

In 1996, Brewitt re-analyzed some of Burr's original mouse cancer data using modern statistical methods. The resulting plot of the changes in the electric field at the skin surface during the progression of the cancer is shown in Figure 5.19. There is no question that Burr was correct: The very early stages of disease can be detected by measuring changes in the electrical properties of tissues, making possible early diagnosis and treatments.

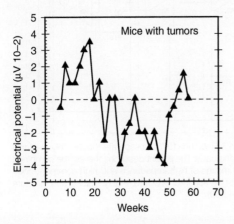

Figure 5.19 In 1936, Burr and colleagues began a series of studies on the relation between electrical fields and cancer, beginning with spontaneous or induced mammary tumors in mice. Large voltage changes were detected with electrodes attached to the chest from 10 days to 2 weeks before the tumors appeared. In 1996, Brewitt re-analyzed some of Burr's original mouse cancer data using modern statistical methods. The resulting plot of the changes in the electric field at the skin surface during the progression of the cancer is shown here.

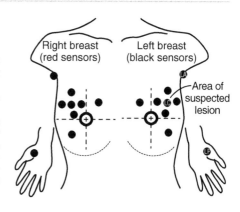

Figure 5.20 In 1998, Cuzick and colleagues reported clinical trials of a method for detecting breast cancer using skin electropotential measurements. The altered membrane potentials extend from the cancerous area to the skin surface above the lesion. These studies confirmed Burr's early conclusions (Figure 5.19) and achieved Burr's original goal of a noninvasive and risk-free test for the presence of breast cancer. *(From Cuzick J, Holland R, Barth V, et al: Electropotential measurements as a new diagnostic modality for breast cancer, Lancet 1998 Aug 1;352(9125):359–363.)*

In 1994, Weiss et al. confirmed Burr's finding that skin surface electrical potentials can be used for the differential diagnosis of breast lesions. The electrical changes arise because rapidly proliferating and transformed cells have lower membrane potentials compared with normal cells (Binggeli and Weinstein, 1986). This has been demonstrated for tumor cells from both breast (Marino et al., 1994) and colon (Davies et al., 1987; Goller et al., 1986). The altered membrane potentials extend from the cancerous area to the skin surface above the lesion. The correlation between cell membrane potentials and cell proliferation had already been detailed in a classic paper by Cone (1970). Cuzick (1998) and Cuzick et al. (1998) reported clinical trials of a method for detecting breast cancer using skin electropotential measurements (Figure 5.20). This noninvasive method is important because it offers the opportunity to resolve the uncertainty of lump detection, whether by self-palpation or by mammograms. In most cases, lumps are benign, but the methods needed to prove this in individual cases are invasive. Burr's goal of a noninvasive and risk-free test for the presence of cancer can be realized.

In 1985, Sullivan and colleagues reported that patients with lung disease (confirmed by chest X-rays) had 30% lower electrical conductances between points along the lung meridian. Other research, summarized by Brewitt (1996, 2002), showed the cellular basis for these effects. Specifically, viral and bacterial infections, as well as cancer, affect the ionic and water content and pH of the extracellular fluids and thereby affect the cell membrane potentials and tissue conductances.

Modern use of electrical fields in diagnosis and therapeutics will be discussed in the next chapter.

Conclusions

This chapter has traced the uses of energy in medicine from early times to the present. Two aspects stand out. First, in retrospect, the early observations of Mesmer and Burr, ridiculed or ignored by their contemporaries, respectively, have been shown to be correct. For example, the existence of 'animal magnetism' introduced by Mesmer has been confirmed (see Chapter 8). Modern devices based on Burr's early discoveries are proving valuable in clinical diagnosis of conditions such as cancer, but they have been very slow to gain acceptance by a medical community whose primary treatment modality is pharmacology. This chapter mentions a few devices; others will be introduced in Chapter 6.

References

Ashcroft, F., 2012. The Spark of Life: Electricity in the Human Body. W.W. Norton & Company, New York, NY.

Basmajian, J.V., 1979. Muscles Alive: Their Functions Revealed by Electromyography. Williams & Wilkins, Baltimore, MD.

Becker, R.O., 1990. Cross Currents: The Perils of Electropollution, the Promise of Electromedicine. Jeremy P. Tarcher, Los Angeles, CA.

Becker, R.O., Selden, G., 1985. The Body Electric: Electromagnetism and the Foundation of Life. William and Morrow Company, New York, NY, p. 172.

Bernstein, J., 1868. Ueber den zeitlichen Verlauf der negativen Schwankung des Nervenstroms. Pflüger's Arch. f. d. ges. Physiol. 1, 173–207.

Binggeli, R., Weinstein, R.C., 1986. Membrane potentials and sodium channels: hypotheses for growth regulation and cancer formation based on changes in sodium channels and gap junctions. J. Theoret. Biol. 123, 377–401.

Brewitt, B., 1996. Quantitative analysis of electrical skin conductance in diagnosis: historical and current views of bioelectric medicine. J. Naturopath. Med. 6 (1), 66–75.

Brewitt, B., 2002. Electromagnetic medicine and HIV/AIDS treatment: clinical data and hypothesis for mechanism of action. In: Standish, L.J., Calabrese, C., Galatino, M.L. (Eds.), AIDS and Alternative Medicine: The Current State of the Science. Harcourt Brace, New York, NY.

Burr, H.S., 1957. Harold Saxton Burr. Yale J. Biol. Med. 30 (3), 161–167.

Burr, H.S., 1972. Blueprint for Immortality. CW Daniel, Saffron Walden, UK.

Burr, H.S., 1973. The Fields of Life. Our Links with the Universe. Ballantine Books, New York, NY.

Burr, H.S., Mauro, A., 1949. Electrostatic fields of the sciatic nerve in the frog. Yale J. Biol. Med. 21 (6), 455–462.

Cone, C.D., 1970. Variation of the transmembrane potential level as a basic mechanism of mitosis control. Oncology 24, 438–470.

Crane, E. E., 1950. Bioelectric potentials, their maintenance and function. Prog. Biophys. Mol. Biol. 1, 85–136.

Cuzick, J., 1998. Continuation of the international breast cancer intervention study (IBIS). Eur. J. Cancer 34 (11), 1647–1648.

Cuzick, J.R., Holland, V., Barth, R., et al., 1998. Electropotential measurements as a new diagnostic modality for breast cancer. Lancet 352, 359–363.

d'Arsonval, J.-A., 1894. Action de l'electricite sur les etres vivants. Cours d'Appel, Paris.

du Bois-Reymond, E., 1848. Untersuchungen über thierische elektricität, 2 voll. G Reimer, Berlin.

Davies, R., Joseph, R., Kaplan, D., Juncosa, R.D., Pempinello, C., Asbun, H., Sedwitz, M.M., 1987. Epithelial impedance analysis in experimentally induced colon cancer. Biophys. J. 52(5), 783–790.

Duchenne, G.B.A., 1959. Physiologie des mouvements. W. B. Saunders, Philadelphia, PA, Translated by EB Kaplan 1949 from 1st edn 1867.

Friedenberg, R., Reese, W., Reading, W.H., 1975. Detector device and process for detecting ovulation. United States Patent 3,924.609, December 9, 1975.

Galvani, L., 1791. De viribus electricitatis in motu musculari commentarius. Bon. Sci. Art. Inst. Acad. Comm. 7, 363–418.

Geddes, L.A., 1984. A short history of the electrical stimulation of excitable tissue including electrotherapeutic applications. Physiologist 27 (1), S1–S47.

Goller, D.A., Weidema, W.F., Davies, R.J., 1986. Transmural electrical potential difference as an early marker in colon cancer. Arch. Surg. 121, 345–350.

Marino, A.A., Ilev, I.G., Schwalke, M.A., et al., 1994. Association between cell membrane potential and breast cancer. Tumor Biology 15, 82–89.

Mathews, A.P., 1903. Electric polarity in hydroids. Am. J. Physiol. 8, 294–299.

Matteucci, C., 1844. Traité des phénomènes électro-physiologiques des animaux suivi d'études anatomiques sur le systhème nerveux et sur l'organe électrique de la torpille par Paul Savi. Fortin, Masson et C.ie, Paris.

Müller, J., 1845. Manuel de physiologie. Baillière, Paris.

Stack, T., 1753. Extract of the observations made in Italy, by the Abbe Nollet, F. R. S. on the Grotta de Cani. Translated from the French by Tho. Stack, MD FRS, Phil. Trans. 47, 48–61.

Sullivan, S.G., Eggleston, W.W., Martinoff, J.T., Kroenig, R.I., 1985. Evoked electrical conductivity on the lung acupuncture points in healthy individuals and confirmed lung cancer patients. Am. J. Acupunc. 13 (3), 261–266.

Tyndall, J., 1876. Lessons in electricity IV. Popular Science Monthly 9, July Issue.

Volta, A., 1918. Le opere di Alessandro Volta (edizione nazionale), vol. I. Hoepli, Milano.

Wesley, J., 1871. The Desideratum: Or, Electricity made Plain and Useful (1871). Baillière, Tindall & Cox, London.

Ziemssen, H., 1864. Die Electricitat in der Medicin, second ed. Von August Hirschwald, Berlin.

CHAPTER 6

Electricity and Magnetism in Diagnosis and Therapeutics

Chapter Summary

During the centuries since Galvani made his historic discovery of animal electricity, scientists from many different disciplines have studied the electrical aspects of life. Much of this has been basic research – studies designed to simply find out the role of electricity in various biological processes such as nerve conduction, muscle contraction, secretion, and reproduction. Applied research on bioelectricity has been aimed at understanding the possible roles of electrical fields in wound healing and defence against disease. For example, it has been discovered that an injury potential arises when the skin is broken or when an organ is injured. This potential flows as a wave away from the site of trauma. It is thought that the injury potential sets in action the various cellular and tissue responses that are necessary for restoration of the tissue to its normal state. This is a remarkable phenomenon because to repair an injury, the body must reference the original blueprint for the design of the cell and tissue components that have been damaged. Artificial enhancement of the injury potential increases the rate of wound closure and the extent of regeneration. This has important clinical applications such as stimulating the healing of chronic wounds.

As we understood more and more about the roles of electricity in healthy functioning and in injury repair, a wide variety of therapeutic devices were created. Some of these devices appeared to be very successful, as judged from the testimonials of those who used them. However, testimonials are not science. The reorganization of medical education that followed the Flexner report led to a medicine that was focused on pharmaceuticals, and the economic and regulatory atmosphere put major emphasis on the development of new drugs while discouraging energetic approaches. For approximately half a century after the Flexner report, the use of electricity, magnetism, and light for healing purposes was essentially illegal. The situation began to change in 1979 when the U.S. Food and Drug Administration (FDA) approved the use of pulsing electric, magnetic, and electromagnetic fields to stimulate bone healing. These methods followed from the work of Birch in London who used electricity to stimulate healing of bone fractures, as mentioned in Chapter 5. The regulatory process involved in getting FDA certification for energy medicine technologies is described in Appendix II. A number of medical electrical devices have been allowed by the FDA, often after a long and expensive approval process. Some of these devices will be described in this chapter, without attempting an exhaustive listing. A thorough discussion of all of these technologies would require a book much larger than this one. Key technologies include various diagnostic systems and therapeutic devices such as transcutaneous electrical nerve stimulation (TENS) for treating intractable pain; frequency-specific microcurrent (FSM), which seems to have a wide variety of applications; various feedback systems; and electro acupuncture.

The Injury Potential

The injury potential, also called the demarcation potential, is the difference in electrical potential between the injured and uninjured parts of a nerve, muscle, skin, or other tissue. It is an energetic phenomenon with important roles in wound healing – the intricate process in which the skin or another tissue or organ repairs itself after injury (Huttenlocher and Horwitz, 2007; Nguyen et al., 2009; Zaho et al., 2006). Carlo Matteucci (1811–1868) was a pioneer in the study of bioelectricity. Using a sensitive galvanometer that had been developed by Leopoldo Nobili in 1825 (Figure 6.1), Matteucci showed that injured excitable biological tissues generate direct electrical currents and that they can be summed by adding elements in series, as was shown in Figure 5.4 in Chapter 5. He identified an injury potential resulting from current flowing between a site of injury and an intact region of muscle (Matteucci, 1844). Emil Heinrich du Bois-Reymond (1865) confirmed this and found a similar potential arising in injured nerves. This places the discovery of the injury potential historically before the discovery of the nerve resting and action potentials (Davson, 1970). Du Bois-Reymond (1848–1884) also discovered that currents are produced by small epidermal wounds in human fingers immersed in saline. This was confirmed by Herlitzka (1910). In 1980, Illingworth and Barker reported that currents are produced by the stumps of accidentally amputated human fingers immersed in saline. Research has shown that artificial enhancement of the injury potential increases the rate of wound closure and the extent of regeneration. This means that a wide range of energy therapies, ranging from medical devices to hands-on treatments to acupuncture, can facilitate the healing of chronic wounds.

The most thorough research on the injury potential has been done on the skin and cornea of the eye. When the skin is cut or punctured, there begins a sequence of electrical, electronic, and probably photonic processes that activate the healing process. An understanding of the injury potential provides a basis for a number of energy medicine technologies.

Many chronic wounds heal very slowly, do not heal, or worsen despite the best efforts to promote tissue repair. An intervention commonly used to treat such difficult chronic wounds, especially by nurses and physical therapists, is electrical stimulation. The method is based on the fact that the human body has endogenous bioelectric systems that enhance healing of bone fractures and soft-tissue injuries. When the body's endogenous bioelectric system does not produce normal wound repair, therapeutic electrical currents may be delivered into the 'repair field' from an external source. The applied current may serve to mimic the failed natural bioelectric currents, thereby promoting wound healing.

One mechanism for the success of this method is that electric fields can attract cells into the repair field. The surfaces of neutrophils, macrophages, fibroblasts, and epidermal cells involved in wound repair are electrically charged (see Figure 6.2). An applied electric field can facilitate galvanotaxic[1] migrations of these cells into the repair field and thereby accelerate healing. Another effect of electric fields is the enhancement of ATP production in the cells involved in the repair process. This is important because energy from ATP is needed to power cell migrations and the synthesis of new proteins and other molecules that must be replaced. This was demonstrated by Cheng et al. (1982), who found that currents of 10–1000 µA produced a three- to five-fold increase in ATP levels. Higher current levels, into the milliampere range, decreased protein synthesis. This has important clinical applications, such as stimulating the healing of chronic wounds (Kloth and McCulloch, 1996; Messerli and Graham, 2011). Interestingly, electrical stimulation also enhances ATP production in chloroplasts of green plants (Vinkler and Korenstein, 1982).

In 2007, English researchers Clegg and Guest studied the cost effectiveness of electric stimulation therapy compared to standard care in elderly patients with chronic, non-healing wounds of over 6 months' duration. They found that use of the bioelectric stimulation led 33% of these intractable wounds to heal within 16 weeks, reduced the need for clinician visits from 4.7 to 2.3 per week, and reduced costs by 16%. Most clinical trials have reported a significant increase in the rate of healing from 13 to 50% (Nuccitelli, 2003).

---

[1]Galvanotaxis or electrotaxis is the directional movement of motile cells in response to an electric field. By detecting and orienting themselves in an electric field, cells are able to direct their movement toward a wound to begin the repair process. Such directed movements may also contribute to directional growth of cells and tissues during development and regeneration. This idea is based on (1) measurements of electric fields that naturally occur during wound healing (current of injury), development, and regeneration; and (2) the fact that cells in cultures respond to applied electric fields by directional cell migration.

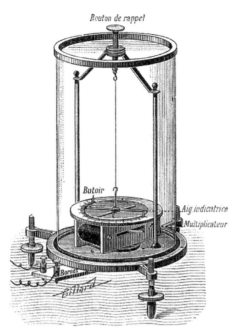

Figure 6.1 The astatic galvanometer developed by Nobili (1825) and used by Matteucci to measure the injury potential.

Zhao Forrester & McCaig, 1999 studied corneal epithelial cells in culture and found that the orientation of cell division is directed by small, applied electric fields. The field strength used was 150 mV/mm, which is within the range of those measured in many developing and regenerating systems (Nuccitelli, 1988). There are many instances in which cell divisions *in vivo* occur in the presence of direct-current electrical fields, for example, during embryonic morphogenesis, neuronal and epithelial differentiation, wound healing, or tumor formation. Endogenous physiological electrical fields may play important roles in some or all of these processes by regulating the axis of cell division and, hence, the positioning of daughter cells. Recent researches have provided significant insights into how naturally occurring electrical fields may participate in the control of tissue repair and regeneration. Applied electrical fields equivalent to the size of fields measured *in vivo* direct cell migration, cell proliferation, and nerve sprouting at wounds (reviewed by Wang and Zago, 2010).

In 1982, Barker Jaffe and Vanable reported a detailed electrophysiological study of the properties of the skin of the guinea pig and human. The guinea pig was studied because it has regions (the glabrous or hairless epidermis) that are free of hair and glands. Guinea pig skin has a battery that is comparable in power to that of the frog skin. In frogs the skin is an osmoregulatory organ, absorbing salts from the surrounding pond water. In mammals the skin battery is thought to function mainly in epidermal wound healing.

The 1982, study by Barker and colleagues indicated that the skin battery is located in the deeper living layer of the epidermis, the stratum germinativum, rather than in the superficial dead layers, the stratum corneum. The resting potential of the skin varies from place to place and is in the range of 20–200 mV with the inside positive.

Barker and colleagues suggested that the fields in the skin help guide the movements of cells that close the wound, a process known as re-epithelialization, which restores the epithelial barrier function. That such cellular migrations take place has been known for a long time (Peters, 1885) and dynamic aspects of these movements were beautifully documented in amphibian skin by Lash (1955), who injected individual skin cells with carmine granules. The injected cells remain viable and visible. Using a microscope, Lash was able to follow the migrations of injected cells during wound closure. He found that there was a wave of mobilization of epidermal cells, which detach from the underlying basement lamina and form a sheet that migrates toward the center of the wound. This migration ceases when the wound is closed.

Much is now known about the cellular mechanisms involving the migration of epidermal and other cell types (Masopust and Schenkel, 2013; Stossel, 1994; Krawczyk, 1971). Cell crawling is achieved by reversible changes in the gel state of the cytoskeleton and reversible attachments to the underlying substrate.

Lash found the wave of activation of epidermal cells begins near the wound border and spreads into the surrounding tissue at a rate of about 0.4 mm/h. Barker and colleagues suggested that the cells migrate in response to the steady lateral fields set up by the skin battery in the region around the wound. These fields decline in strength by about three-fold for each 0.3 mm from the wound edge. Hinkle et al. (1981) showed that various kinds of mammalian cells will migrate toward the negative pole at field strengths considerably smaller than those present near wounds.

The polarization of the skin battery, with the inside positive, and the current that flows inward at the site of an injury are shown in Figure 6.2. The injury potential is thought to trigger the migration of epidermal cells, fibroblasts, leukocytes, nerve growth, and the extension of new blood vessels (angiogenesis) toward the site of injury. For a detailed description of the cell migrations in other activities taking place during wound healing, see Majno (1975).

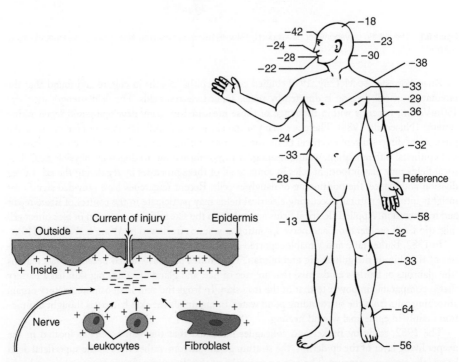

Figure 6.2 The skin battery is thought to activate wound healing. To the left, the inward flow of anions at the site of a puncture or scratch. The resulting electrical field is thought to trigger the migration of epidermal cells, fibroblasts, leukocytes, and nerve growth toward the site of injury. To the right is a map of the transcutaneous voltages in the calm and conscious human. The figure on the right is based on the work of Barker Jaffe and Venable, 1982. The glabrous epidermis of cavies contains a powerful battery. American Journal of Physiology 242, R358–366. *(Modified from Barker AT, Jaffe LF, Venable JW Jr.: The glabrous epidermis of cavies contains a powerful battery, Am J Physiol 1982 Mar;242(3):R358–R366.)*

Also shown in Figure 6.2 is a map of transcutaneous voltages. Note that the voltage varies from place to place on the skin. Because the skin battery is important for activating wound healing, regional variations in its strength may explain why in some areas it's easier to trigger wound healing responses than in others.

In 1971, Lykken reported studies of the impedance properties of skin in relation to wound healing. The method involves applying square-wave pulses to the skin and observing the current waveforms with an oscilloscope (Lykken, 1971). The skin's electronic properties during healing changed little during the first 3–4 days, then the skin potential recovered suddenly. Leakage or shunt resistance, thought to be a property of the superficial layers, may not be entirely restored until 1–2 weeks after injury.

The final step in wound healing is contraction. The wound is made smaller by the action of myofibroblasts, which grip the wound edges and contract themselves using a mechanism similar to that in smooth muscle cells. When the cells' roles are close to complete, unneeded cells undergo apoptosis (Midwood et al., 2004).

TENS and MENS

TENS has been an accepted mode of electrotherapy for many years and is well characterized (Kahn, 1987) (Figure 6.3). Microcurrent electrotherapy, sometimes abbreviated as 'MENS' (microcurrent electrical neuromuscular stimulation), is becoming a more widely accepted clinical practise for decreasing or eliminating pain and stimulating the healing process. MENS is typically used for pain relief and, more typically, for tissue healing by affecting the injured tissue at the cellular level. Tissues that respond to MENS include muscle, tendon, bone, nerve, and skin. The effectiveness and use of microcurrent electrotherapy has also been well documented (Kahn, 1987; Snyder-Mackler and Robinson, 2007). MENS devices deliver a much smaller current than TENS devices (typically 20–600 μA). The waveforms used are typically a positive direct current (DC), negative DC, or a combination of these in which the polarity is switched at an adjustable rate (usually 0.3–30 Hz using a 50% duty cycle[2] waveform). The use of microamperes of electrical current in MENS therapy,

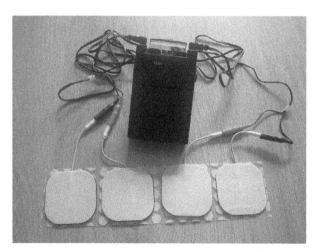

Figure 6.3 A typical battery-operated transcutaneous electrical nerve stimulation (TENS) unit with four leads. The operator can adjust pulse width, frequency, and intensity. Generally, TENS is applied at high frequency (> 50 Hz) with an intensity below motor contraction (sensory intensity) or low frequency (< 10 Hz) with an intensity that produces muscle contraction.

---

[2]Duty cycle refers to the percent of time that current is flowing, as a fraction of the total time. In an electrical device, a 60% duty cycle means the power is on 60% of the time and off 40% of the time.

as opposed to TENS therapy, results in little or no patient discomfort or even sensation during application. As with TENS, electrodes must be manually placed over the tissue that is to receive the stimulation. Electrode pads are placed to follow an electrical pathway within the body, e.g., from the origin to the insertion of a muscle following muscular electrical flow, down the pathway of radiating nerve pain, through acupuncture or trigger points, or medial/lateral through a swollen joint. Sometimes electrodes are implanted into the tissue. Microcurrent and interferential therapy devices are regulated by the FDA as Class II devices, with more than 50 instruments receiving 510(k) approval. Common user controls include amplitude (intensity), polarity, and frequency.

Treating pain by reducing inflammation is supported by the vast amount of research on the role of inflammation in chronic disease and by the hypothesis presented in a paper by Sota Omoigui (2007) entitled 'The biochemical origin of pain – proposing a new law of pain: The origin of all pain is inflammation and the inflammatory response. Part 1 of 3 – A unifying law of pain.' Omoigui proposed that all pain is caused by inflammation. This is a reasonable hypothesis given the abundance of research connecting inflammation with virtually every chronic disease.

Frequency-Specific Microcurrent

FSM is an emerging technique for treating diverse health conditions. Pairs of frequencies of microampere-level electrical stimulation are applied to particular places on the skin of a patient via combinations of conductive graphite gloves, moistened towels, or gel electrode patches. The current range is much lower than that used in TENS, i.e., microamperes (millionths of an Ampere) instead of milliamperes (thousandths of an Ampere). These currents are similar in strength to those the body uses to communicate with itself.

A consistent finding with FSM is a profound and palpable tissue softening and warming within seconds of applying frequencies at the correct places appropriate for treating particular conditions. Similar phenomena are often observed with other energy-based techniques.

Specific changes include:

- The tissue rapidly and profoundly softens within seconds.
- Usually tissue all over the body softens when a beneficial frequency combination is applied anywhere on the body for any condition – likely a change in system-wide muscle tone.
- Sometimes there are unresponsive regions that stand out amidst the softened tissue, apparently due to localized muscle tension. These areas can be addressed with additional frequency choices and locations of the conductors.
- Muscle tissue that is hard, tough, scarred, firm, rigid, 'gnarly', or stiff begins to soften and within minutes feels 'smooshy', like pudding in a plastic sack.
- The tissue becomes warm. This can be felt through the conductive gloves. Some sensitive practitioners can feel the warming with their hand several inches away from the skin.
- The patient may become somewhat dreamy or 'spaced out'.

There are two contrasting perspectives on tissue softening with FSM. One is that it is a 'side effect' of the application of therapeutic frequencies and has no physiological significance. Another is that injuries, physical or emotional traumas, or other pathological conditions can increase body-wide muscle tone or local muscle tension and that tissue softening indicates that the pathophysiology is being addressed. On the basis of the work of Irvin Korr and others to be described below, it was suggested that patients often have some degree of elevated muscle tone or tension stemming from the trauma, disease, injury, or other condition that brought them to the physician's office and that tissue softening indicates that treatment is progressing.

In the 1970s, neuroscientist and osteopathic researcher Irvin Korr developed a 'gamma loop hypothesis' to explain the persistence of increased systemic muscle tone associated with various somatic dysfunctions (Korr, 1978). Physiologists, neuroscientists, osteopaths, chiropractors, and fascial researchers have expanded on Korr's ideas by exploring various mechanisms by which injury or disease increase local muscle tension or systemic muscle tone (e.g., Knutson, 2000; Matre et al., 1998; Mense, 1997). Following on Korr's hypothesis, it was suggested that most patients actually present with elevated muscle tone or tense areas due to prior traumas or other disorders and that tissue softening indicates that FSM or other methods are affecting the cause of their pathophysiology.

For example, psychological factors have been associated with primary fibromyalgia syndrome: Antes et al. (1984) and Mines (2003) suggest that most people are 'in shock' from old traumatic experiences.

Recent publications summarize the origins, possible mechanisms, applications, and practical details of FSM (McMakin, 2003, 2011a,b). The technique is based on pairs of frequencies, low-level microamperage currents, and the principles of biological resonance. Clinical experience using graphite gloves as the 'electrodes' has revealed that specific microcurrent frequencies applied to appropriate places on the body are highly effective at reducing pain and inflammation in a wide variety of conditions. As with many microcurrent devices, a dual channel system was used. The frequencies can be varied from 0.1 to 999 Hz. The two channels, termed channel A and channel B, can be set at different frequencies. A long series of trial and error tests involving hundreds of patients revealed certain pairs of frequencies to be effective for specific conditions. A consistent finding was that channel A set at 40 Hz was effective with channel B adjusted until the optimal effect was obtained. Because an interferential effect takes place between the two graphite gloves, a complex of frequencies was created in the body that included each frequency by itself as well as the sum of the two frequencies and their difference.

The publications describe protocols for treating various health complaints; multicenter clinical case reports documenting successful applications; and review condition pathophysiology, differential diagnosis, and current research. An article on the use of FSM for delayed onset muscle soreness (DOMS) summarizes the history of FSM, including the history of the discovery of effective frequencies and frequency combinations (Curtis et al., 2010).

FSM practitioners consistently observe a profound and easily palpable change in tissue texture within seconds of applying frequencies appropriate for a particular disorder. This 'state change' can usually be detected anywhere on the body when one has found the correct frequencies and placements of the conductors (conductive graphite gloves, gloves wrapped in moist cloth, or gel electrode patches – Figures 6.4 and 6.5), provided the patient is hydrated. The softening is not superficial, as in the epidermal layer, but is in the deeper skeletal muscles. Tissue softening

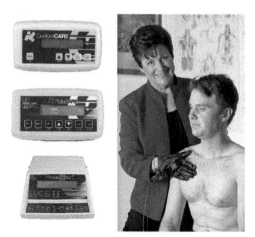

Figure 6.4 Frequency-specific microcurrent developed by Carol McMakin is applied with graphite gloves or electrode patches attached to a signal generator.

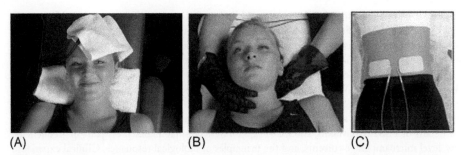

(A)   (B)   (C)

Figure 6.5 Examples of frequency-specific microcurrent methods for delivering microcurrents to the body. (A) Conductive gloves are placed in warm wet hand towels or face cloths placed on the neck and forehead for treatment of shingles affecting the opthalmic branch of cranial nerve V or for treating sinus conditions. One frequency arrangement is effective for both shingles and oral and genital herpes, 230 Hz on channel A and 430 Hz on channel B, although positions of leads depend on which nerve root is involved. (B) Treatment of the upper back, shoulder, and posterior part of the neck using conductive graphite gloves to restore biomechanics and relieve pain. The fingers sense change rather than force it. The frequencies and currents do the work. A latex or nitrile glove is worn under the graphite glove to prevent current conduction to the practitioner. (C) Gel electrode pads used to treat lumbar ligaments without nerve involvement. Another pair of electrode pads is placed on corresponding points on the abdomen (not shown). Electrode polarities are arranged to produce an interferential field so that the current and the frequencies pass diagonally through the area to be treated like an 'X' in three dimensions. For details and other treatment techniques, see McMakin (2011a).

provides rapid feedback when one is optimizing a protocol for a condition not previously treated with FSM. Since so many variables are involved – two separate frequencies, signal intensities and waveforms, positioning of the conductive materials, and the patient's condition – tissue softening facilitates the determination of the best therapeutic combinations. It has been suggested that the reason for the tissue softening is that most patients actually present with tension due to prior traumas or disorders, and that tissue softening indicates that FSM or other methods are affecting the cause of their pathophysiology (McMakin and Oschman, 2012).

Methods that accomplish relief of pain and inflammation may be based on the physical process of delivering antioxidant electrons to the site of an injury. The anti-inflammatory effects of FSM using a mouse ear model have been described in a study by Reilly et al. (2004).

Pulsing Electromagnetic Field Therapy

Pulsing electromagnetic field frequency therapy (PEMF) was in use well over 100 years ago, but competition from pharmaceutical approaches in the West led to a rapid eclipse of virtually all electrotherapy techniques (http://masmagnetics.com/pemf-frequency-therapy/). However, in the former Soviet Union, the use of electrotherapy continued to flourish and was regarded as complementary to pharmacology. During the Soviet space explorations, pulsing electromagnetic field therapy (PEMF) was used by the cosmonauts to help reduce the loss of bone density that occurs when they are removed from the Earth's gravitational and magnetic fields. Back on Earth, this form of therapy was embraced by Soviet medical doctors, who wanted to use the technology on their patients. Eventually, it was used in hospitals throughout the Soviet Union and in Eastern Europe, in particular East Germany, Hungary, and the Czech Republic. When these countries gained their independence, their scientific medical research and electronic devices became available to the Western world via nearby German-speaking countries: Germany, Switzerland, and Austria. These countries incorporated the technology into their healthcare systems, and it became available in hospitals, medical clinics, health spas, and to the general consumer. Hundreds of studies from Eastern Europe and decades of experience in Western Europe have led to detailed understanding of how various frequencies and waveforms work best with each other for specific conditions.

In the meantime, the American space program operated by the National Aeronautical and Space Administration (NASA) recognized a critical need to develop effective prevention and treatments for bone loss and muscle atrophy to enable future human space exploration to the moon, Mars, and beyond. Progressive muscle atrophy leads to weakness, fatigue, and the inability efficiently perform tasks, including emergency procedures. Bone loss causes increased risk of bone fracture and kidney stones, which can also compromise astronaut health and mission objectives. Consequently, NASA mobilized its resources to develop methods that can enhance bone retention, prevent or alleviate muscle atrophy, and augment natural healing/regeneration processes in a space environment with little access to conventional treatments. On Earth, this device was found useful in the treatment of various muscle diseases, age- and cancer-related muscle atrophy, osteoporosis, and other bone diseases. By the time NASA began research in this area, it had been accepted that weak, non-ionizing electromagnetic fields can exert effects on biological targets without heating them. Moreover, the use of pulsing electromagnetic fields for stimulating healing in fracture nonunions had become an established orthopedic practise and had been approved by the FDA in 1979.

Research by NASA identified which PEMF frequencies are most effective in producing biological responses in bone and muscle cells. Studies were undertaken at the molecular and cellular levels to define the alterations induced by micro gravity and the ability of PEMF to reverse these effects. The long-term goal was to produce garments incorporating PEMF devices that could be worn by astronauts. Eventually NASA contractors patented systems for this purpose. The patent claims that the apparatus is for enhancing tissue repair in mammals. The apparatus includes a sleeve, an electrically conductive coil, a sleeve support, and an electrical circuit that supplies the coil with a square wave time-varying electrical current sufficient to create ~0.05–0.5 gauss magnetic field. When in use, the time-varying electromagnetic field is from ~0.05 to 0.5 gauss and is used long enough to produce tissue regeneration at a rate that is faster than what would take place without the use of the device. Figure 6.6 shows one such device for use on a limb. The illustration is from the NASA patent.

In 1952, at the Technical University of Munich in Germany, Professor Winfried Schumann mathematically predicted that the Earth had a pulse, a resonant frequency of around 10 pulses per

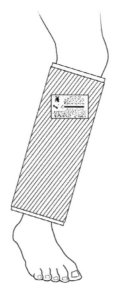

Figure 6.6 Pulsating electromagnetic field therapy (PEMF) device patented by NASA contractors, U.S. Patent Number 7,601,114 dated October 13, 2009.

second. His theory stated that this pulse should arise from the resonance taking place between the surface of the Earth and the charged layer called the ionosphere, some hundreds of miles above the Earth. As we shall see in Chapter 15, Schumann's theory was confirmed. This frequency corresponded to some of the measured frequencies taking place within the brain, the so-called brain waves, as measured with the electroencephalogram. Subsequent research on test subjects in Germany showed that if the Earth's natural magnetic resonant field was removed, health would deteriorate. In an attempt to reverse that process, a frequency generator was utilized to introduce artificial magnetic fields into a test chamber, and it was discovered that 7.83 Hz was the ideal artificial frequency to support life. That frequency, 7.83 Hz, is now known as the Schumann Resonance. This discovery, virtually ignored by Western medicine, was embraced by the Soviet Union. It was decided to develop a healthcare system based upon an earlier form of electrotherapy that now utilized frequencies for electric acupuncture and electromagnets. Like NASA, the Soviet space program provided its citizens with many medical breakthroughs that were used to keep the cosmonauts healthy in space.

A resurgence of interest occurred in the United States and Japan in the 1950s and 1960s. The validity of DC stimulation of bone healing was confirmed in animal studies (Bassett et al., 1964; Yasuda, 1953). Subsequently, an ever-broadening search for mechanisms of action began at the cellular level. NASA patented two chambers for studying cellular effects of PEMF signals (Wolf and Goodwin, 2002, 2004) Simultaneously, efforts were launched to bypass the need for surgical implantation of electrodes and to place electric stimulation of fracture repair on a more practical, less risky, and less costly basis. As a result of these parallel but interlinked efforts, great progress was made in the care of fractures that fail to heal and in opening new horizons to the benefits to be gained in other diseases and disorders by inducing purposeful and precise modifications in the electric microenvironments of many different cell types.

In 2009, NASA released its PEMF patents. Two of the patents were for studying the effects of pulsing electromagnetic fields on cells in culture (Wolf and Goodwin, 2002, 2004), and the third was for a system that a person could wear that would enhance tissue repair in mammals (Goodwin and Parker, 2007). In 2011, the FDA approved PEMF for difficult to treat depression. In the same year, Dr. Oz, a popular television show host, introduced PEMF therapy to millions of his loyal viewers who were asked to help 'spread the word'. The North American medical community is now starting to examine this form of frequency therapy as a method for pain management, cell rejuvenation, and the treatment of a wide variety of neurological disorders. An example of one of these devices is shown in Figure 6.7.

Western medicine has now begun to return to its early roots in electrotherapy and has brought frequency therapy into the healthcare system. It was invented for space travel and is now available on Earth. The scientific literature in support of this conclusion is very compelling.

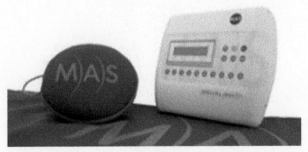

Figure 6.7 MAS (MAgnetic Systems) manufactured in Leibnitz/Austria. The device generates pulsating electromagnetic field therapy (PEMF) signals similar to those developed by the Soviet Space Agency and NASA. *(Courtesy MAS Magnetic Field Systems, New York, NY.)*

Low-Energy Neural Stimulation

ELECTRO INTERSTITIAL SCANNING AND ELECTRICAL IMPEDANCE TOMOGRAPHY

Electrical impedance tomography (EIT) and electro interstitial scanning (EIS) are medical analytical and imaging techniques in which physiological functions are monitored on the basis of the conductivity or permittivity of tissues in the body. The method involves taking electrical measurements at the surface of the body. Conducting electrodes are attached to the skin of the subject, and small (mA) alternating currents are applied. The resulting electrical potentials are measured.

Frederick Gardner Cottrell (1903) developed an equation to describe the change in electric current flowing through a solution when the potential is increased step by step. Over the years Cottrell's equation went through a series of modifications and led to a host of increasingly refined technologies for making noninvasive measurements of the properties of tissues and fluids within the human body. The method evolved into a variety of applications that have been called chronopotentiometry, chronocoulometry, coulometry, voltammetry, electrorheometry, bioelectrical impedance, EIT, impedance cardiography, and electro interstitial scanning (EIS). The basic disciplines are electrochemistry and bioelectrochemistry (Ota et al., 2013). Modern systems can perform noninvasive measurements of a variety of important body systems. Steps in this development can be summarized as follows:

- In the 1950s, Nyboer and associates developed a method for measuring blood volume changes in the arm by using four electrodes. This technique is known as impedance plethysmography.
- In 1962, Thomaset discovered the relation between bioimpedance and the total water body.
- In 1966, Kubicek and colleagues designed the first clinical electrical device that could noninvasively measure the stroke volume of the heart. The system was tested on NASA astronauts.
- In 1970, Nyboer further advanced the theory of bioimpedance by introducing the concept of the resistivity of blood to measure the variation of blood flow.
- In 1978, EIT was developed into a medical imaging system by Henderson and Webster.
- In 1980, Settle and colleagues developed methods for nutritional assessment with measurements of whole body and fluid compartment impedance.
- Extensive mathematical research was required to interpret the results and was accomplished by Alberto P. Calderón (1980), updated by Uhlmann (1999).
- In 1984, the first practical medical system was developed by Barber and Brown.
- The first commercial medical device was introduced in 2011 for monitoring lung function in intensive care patients (Dräger, 2010; Figure 6.8).

A sophisticated system that applies this technology is called the electro interstitial scan (EIS).[3] It uses six electrodes placed on the skin with two on the forehead (one on the left, one on the right), two in contact with the palms of the hands, and two in contact with the soles of the feet (Figure 6.9). Once the EIS programme begins, a sequence of successive measurements is performed on eleven pathways in the body using weak DC current ($200\,\mu A$) and an imposed voltage of $1.28\,V$ between the six electrodes. The software changes the polarity for each pathway, first from anode to cathode and then from cathode to anode. The conductance of each pathway is measured every $32\,ms$ for $1\,s$ for each polarity. In its present state of development, the device can detect five physiological indicators of disease (Maarek, 2012).

This technology is valuable for assessing the physiological balance in a wide range of important organs and systems in a patient. It is also very useful for assessing the effects of particular treatments, including those provided by other energy medicine devices.

---

[3]Electro Interstitial Scan, LD Technology, Miami, FL.

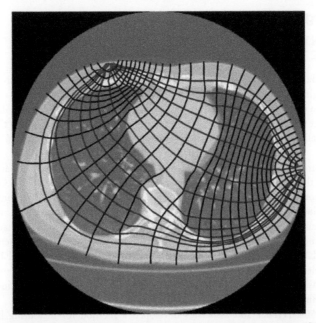

Figure 6.8 A cross section of a human thorax from an X-ray computed tomography (CT) scan showing current flows and equi-potentials from drive electrodes at the surface. Note how lines are bent by the change in conductivity within different organs. *(From Adler (2010).)*

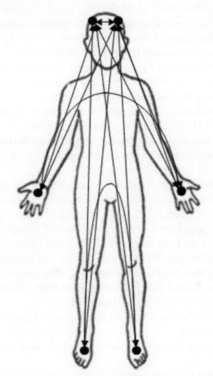

Figure 6.9   Positions for the six electrodes used in electro interstitial scan (EIS).

Electrical Properties of Tumours

The fact that malignant cells have different electrical properties compared to normal cells was first demonstrated by Fricke and Morse (1926). They suggested that reliable diagnosis could be based on such differences. There followed a series of investigations in which various electrical properties were studied: conductance, conductivity, capacitance, resistance, resistivity, impedivity, admittivity, and so on. These different terms have specific technical meanings that need not be detailed here. For example, the term *impedance* usually refers to alternating current (AC) forms of electricity, and the term *resistance* refers to DC.

Differences in conductivity between benign and malignant breast tissue have been thought to be caused by differences in water and electrolyte content related to hormonal changes and to blood supply (angiogenesis), changes in membrane permeability and polarization (Morucci & Rigaud 1996, Morucci & Marsili 1996, Rigaud & Morucci 1996, Valentinuzzi Morucci & Felice 1996, Rigaud Morucci & Chauveau 1996), and changes in orientation and packing density of cells (Foster and Schwan, 1989). An important technique is to pass currents through the tissues at different frequencies. Surowiec et al. (1987) showed that the conductance of tumours is highly frequency dependent. The electrical conductance of breast tumors is seven times higher than that of normal tissues at specific frequencies of 106–108 Hz (Jossinet, 1998; Morimoto et al., 1993; Scholz and Anderson, 2000). Measurements showed 6.0–7.5 times higher conductance in tumors compared to normal tissues (Smith et al., 1986). In later stages of both cancer and AIDS, tissues begin to deteriorate and electrical conductances drop. Haemmerich et al. (2003) found that the electrical differences between tumours and normal tissue correlated with necrosis within the tumours. Others suggested that the differences arose because of the higher water content of tumours (Burdette et al., 1977; Schepps and Foster, 1980; Zywietz and Knoechel, 1986; Figures 6.10 and 6.11).

Low frequency   **High frequency**

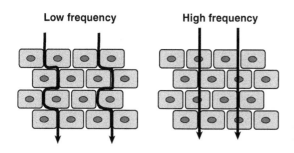

Figure 6.10 At low frequencies the current is mostly extracellular, whereas with higher frequencies intracellular contributions become increasingly significant and the observations more cell-specific.

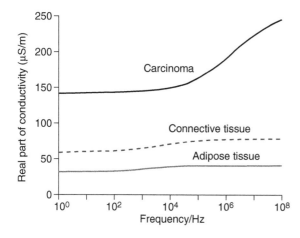

Figure 6.11 Conductivity for different breast tissues, based on Jossinet (1998).

Tabriz for Early Detection of Bladder Cancer

A method developed in Iran focuses on early detection of bladder cancer. The research of Keshtkar and colleagues (2012) used electrical impedance spectroscopy, a minimally invasive screening technique, to separate malignant areas from nonmalignant areas in the urinary bladder. The technique can be used to screen for bladder cancer and abnormalities during cystoscopy (endoscopy of the urinary bladder via the urethra). The results have been compared with histopathological evaluation of urinary bladder lesions. *Ex vivo* studies[4] were carried out in this study by using a total of 30 measured points from malignant and 100 measured points from nonmalignant areas of patient's bladders to determine if their biopsy reports matched the electrical impedance measurements. In all measurements, the impedivity of malignant area of bladder tissue was significantly higher than the impedivity of nonmalignant area this tissue ($P<0.005$).

Electrotherapy Treatments for Cancer

Various energetic therapies for treating cancer have been developed over the past century or so. Extravagant claims for cancer electrotherapy treatments led to the shutdown of virtually all forms of energy medicine following the Pure Food and Drug Act in 1906. Some of the methods were probably successful, but all were declared illegal as the Flexner report aimed to make medicine more scientific. However, there was actually no science to separate out the valid claims from the nonsense, and there was little scientific information on how these devices might work.

An example of an early system was the Lakhovsky multi-wave oscillator (MWO). Information on Georges Lakhovsky is provided in the box.

Lakhovsky's MWO produced a broad range of frequencies from very low all the way to the gigahertz radio waves, with lots of short-wave harmonics. He favoured such a wide bandwidth device so that 'The cell with very weak vibrations, when placed in the field of multiple vibrations, finds its own frequency and starts to oscillate normally through the phenomenon of resonance'.

Other systems were developed by Nikola Tesla, Royal Raymond Rife, and many others. Most of these are controversial and are not approved by the FDA (Vibe Machine, Quantum Pulse, Tesla Energy Lights, Biocharger, Teslastar, Evenstar, Novalite, SEAD Machine, Multiwave Oscillator,

Georges Lakhovsky and the Multiple Wave Oscillator

Georges Lakhovsky was convinced that living cells emit and receive electromagnetic radiations. We now know that this statement was probably accurate (see Chapter 3), although the idea is not part of the scientific mainstream. In 1925 Lakhovsky wrote an article entitled 'Curing Cancer with Ultra Radio Frequencies'. While in France, Lakhovsky worked with the famous French physician, physicist, and inventor of the moving-coil galvanometer, Jacques-Arsène d'Arsonval (1851-1940). Together they developed the Multiple Wave Oscillator (Figure 6.12), which Lakhovsky claimed would revitalize and strengthen the health of cells. The device consisted of two broadband antennae (a sending and a receiving pair) composed of concentric sets of curved open-ended copper pieces suspended/held in place by silk threads, two metal stands to hold the two antennae, Oudin coil(s), and electromagnetic spark/pulse generator. In June 1934 he was awarded U.S. patent 1,962,565 for the device. In 1929, while in France, he wrote 'The Secret of Life: Electricity, Radiation and Your Body' (French) in which he claimed that good or bad health was determined by the relative health of these cellular oscillations, and bacteria, cancers, and other pathogens corrupted them, causing interference with these oscillations. The book was translated into English in 1935. The book contains pictures supposedly taken in a Paris hospital showing cancer patients before, during, and after treatments with his device.

---

[4] *Ex vivo* refers to experiments or measurements done in or on tissue that has been removed from the organism, ideally with a minimum of alteration of natural conditions. *Ex vivo* conditions allow experimentation under more controlled conditions than is possible in *in vivo* experiments (in the intact organism), but at the expense of altering the 'natural' environment.

RIFE machines, Radionics, Zappers, Ionic Footbaths, Gas Plasma, Scalar Energy Devices, Activated Air, Whole Body Vibration, BELS, Violet Ray Device, and so on).

Dr. Royal R. Rife (1888–1971) was a brilliant, passionate scientist who discovered that every virus, bacterium, parasite, and pathogen is sensitive to a specific frequency of sound and can be destroyed by intensifying that frequency until it literally explodes, much like an intense musical note can shatter a crystal wine glass. He called this the mortal oscillatory rate (MOR).

For the past century, medical schools and universities focused their research on pharmacology, and energy medicine was more or less a taboo subject for investigation. This legal status did not deter some inventors from developing new electrical and electromagnetic healing devices. Some were developed in Europe and Russia and imported into the United States. Others were developed by American inventors. With some exceptions, the U.S. FDA has not allowed any of these devices to be used by American doctors. This situation has now changed with the development of some new technologies that show much promise as alternatives to conventional oncology, which uses surgery, radiation, and chemotherapy.

Electrotherapy Treatments for Cancer

On April 8, 2011, the FDA gave a company called Novocure™[5] approval to market a new electrotherapy treatment for patients as an alternative to chemotherapy. The promising new noninvasive system (Figure 6.12) is now available for adult patients with recurring brain tumors (recurrent glioblastoma or GBM). Called NovoTTF™ the device uses specific frequencies called tumor

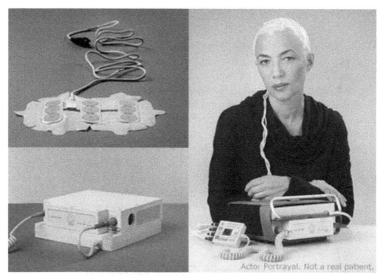

Figure 6.12   Treatment parameters are preset by Novocure™ such that there are no electrical output adjustments available to the patient. All the patient needs to do is change and recharge depleted device batteries and connect to an external power supply overnight. In addition, the transducer arrays need to be replaced once to twice a week and the scalp shaved in order to maintain optimal contact. Patients can carry the device in an over-the-shoulder bag or backpack and receive continuous treatment without changing their daily routine.

---

[5]U.S. Operations, 195 Commerce Way, Portsmouth, NH 03801; Israel Operations, PO Box 15022 Sha'ar HaCarmel, Haifa 31905, Israel.

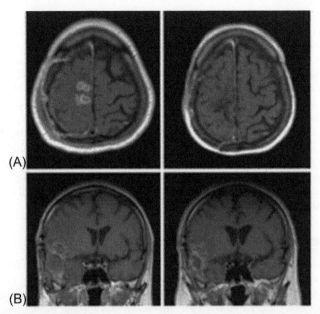

Figure 6.13 Magnetic resonance imaging (MRI) scans of recurrent glioblastoma patients before (A) and after (B) treatment

treating fields to treat cancerous growths. The electric fields are delivered from a portable, wearable device that permits the patient to maintain normal daily activities. Eilon Kirson, M.D., Ph.D., is Novocure's Chief Medical Officer and senior author on two publications validating the method (Kirson et al., 2004, 2007). It is safe and effective in slowing tumor growth *in vitro*, *in vivo*, and in human cancer patients. The device allows for continuous treatment without the side effects that chemotherapies inflict on recurrent GBM patients and indirectly on their families (Figure 6.13).

The portable device, which weighs about 6 pounds (3 kg), is used continuously throughout the day (Figure 6.14). Tests indicate that the devices can slow and reverse tumor growth by inhibiting mitosis, the process by which cancerous cells divide and replicate (Figure 6.15). It has little or no effect on normal brain cells, which replicate slowly if at all. Stupp and colleagues conducted a randomized clinical trial of the device on 237 patients at 28 cancer centers in the United States and Europe. They were treated with either NovoTTF™ or best standard chemotherapy. NovoTTF™ (TTF=tumor treating fields) as a single modality showed a higher response rate and longer time to treatment failure compared to best available chemotherapy.

Electrotherapy for Liver and Other Cancers

An electrical modality for treating tumors with a dramatic reduction in trauma and cost has been described in three reports from an international team of researchers from world-class research centers (Barbault et al., 2009; Costa et al., 2011; Zimmerman et al., 2012; Kuster et al., 2012).

Their earlier studies showed that the intrabuccal administration (sublingual, literally 'under the tongue') of low and safe levels of electromagnetic fields, amplitude-modulated at a frequency of 42.7 Hz by means of a battery-powered portable device, modifies the electroencephalographic activity of healthy subjects (Lebet et al., 1996; Reite et al., 1994), and is associated with subjective

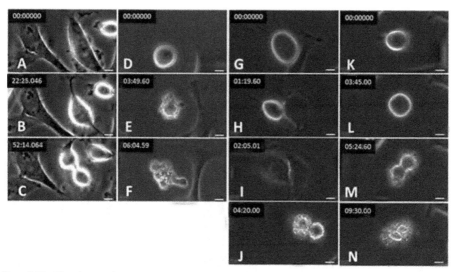

Figure 6.14 Time-lapse video microscopy was used to follow the effects of TTFields on mitotic spindle structures and nuclei in the daughter cells of HeLa cervix adenocarcinoma cells. Control cells (A-C) exhibit normal spindle structure, and cytokinesis occurs after a period of 52 hours and 14 minutes. When cells are exposed to TTFields (D-N) the structure and conformation of the spindle apparatus is completely disrupted and the mitotic process is prolonged. The disruption of the spindle structure leads to mitotic arrest and cell death (D-F) occurring after 6 hours and 5 minutes; disploidy, referring to various kinds of chromosomal rearrangements (G-J) occurring after 4 hours and 20 minutes; or to cell death in cytokinesis (K-M) occurring after 9 hours and 30 minutes. Simultaneous images (not shown) used fluorescent dyes to show that the cells expressed Tubulin-GFP (green fluorescent protein) during exposure to TTFields. Scale bars 10 μ. [microns]. *(Images courtesy of Moshe Giladi, Ph.D, and Novocure Ltd., Haifa, Israel.)*

and objective relaxation effects (Higgs et al., 1994). They also found that sequential administration of four insomnia-specific frequencies, including 42.7 Hz, results in a significant decrease in sleep latency and a significant increase in total sleep time in patients suffering from chronic insomnia (Pasche et al., 1990, 1996). They called this approach low energy emission therapy (LEET). Dosimetric studies have shown that the amount of electromagnetic fields delivered to the brain with this approach is 100–1000 times lower than the amount of electromagnetic fields delivered by handheld cellular phones and does not result in any heating effect within the brain (Pasche and Barbault, 2003). Exposure to these frequencies results in minimal absorption by the human body, which is well below international electromagnetic safety limits (ICNIRP, 1998; IEEE, 2005; Figure 6.16).

The U.S. FDA has determined that such a device is not a significant risk device. A long-term follow-up survey of 807 patients who have received this therapy in the U.S., Europe and Asia revealed that the rate of adverse reactions were low and were not associated with increases in the incidence of malignancy or coronary heart disease (Amato and Pasche, 1994). Their *in vitro* studies on tumor cells suggested that low levels of electromagnetic fields could modify cancer cell growth. They therefore hypothesized that systemic delivery of a combination of tumor-specific frequencies could have a therapeutic effect. They looked for and identified tumor-specific frequencies, and tested the feasibility of administering such frequencies to patients with advanced cancer.

The following frequencies were common to most patients with a diagnosis of breast cancer, hepatocellular carcinoma, prostate cancer, and pancreatic cancer: 1873.477, 2221.323, 6350.333, and 10456.383 Hz (Figure 6.17).

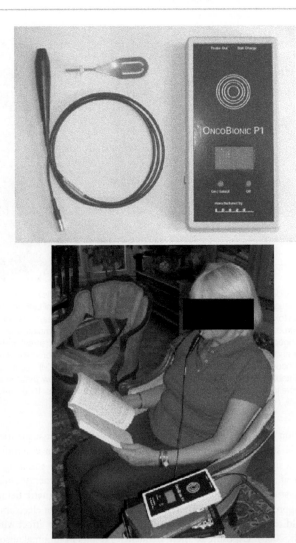

Figure 6.15 (A), battery-driven radio frequency electromagnetic field generator connected to a spoon-shaped mouthpiece that is placed under the tongue. (B), patient receiving a treatment for hepatocellular carcinoma. *(From Costa et al. (2011).)*

Nutri-Energetic Systems and miHealth

A system combining biophysics, quantum physics, and acupuncture theory was developed by Peter Fraser and Harry Massey. Fraser was a visionary Australian scholar of Traditional Chinese Medicine, Homeopathy and Ayurveda. He mapped the complex human biofield, based biophysics and quantum theory. Fraser's studies of information transfer, in collaboration with inventor Harry Massey, led to the development of the miHealth scanner. The device sends information from a map or "blueprint" of the optimal human biofield into the body and reads the response of each physiological system. On the basis of this assessment, practitioners suggest "Infoceuticals" and supplements that restore balance and energetic efficiency. It is the

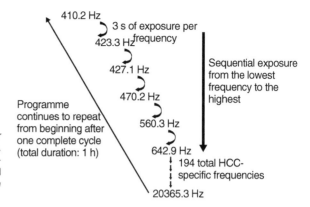

Figure 6.16 Frequency schedule for treating hepatocellular carcinoma. One hundred and ninety-four modulation frequencies were sequenced for 60 min and then repeated. *(From Costa et al. (2011).)*

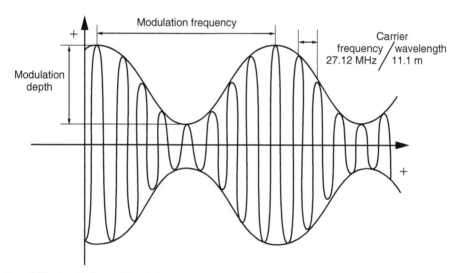

Figure 6.17 Amplitude-modulated electromagnetic field used to treat patients with advanced hepatocellular carcinoma. The carrier frequency is 27.12 MHz, and it is sinusoidally modulated at specific frequencies. *(From Costa et al. (2011).)*

first technology of this kind, and shows how knowledge from quantum physics can be integrated into modern medicine (Fraser & Massey, 2008).

Low Level (cold) Laser Therapy

A variety of low level lasers have demonstrated effectiveness in reducing and eliminating acute and chronic pain from a variety of conditions and surgeries (Figure 6.18). Many patients find this solution a much more effective and an immediate alternative to traditional pain medications. Combined with forms of chiropractic and other hands-on therapies, the lasers can help patients lead a normal, active, and healthy life without debilitating pain. A laser called the Dermalaser targets bacteria responsible for acne. This treatment does not irritate the skin and only attacks the bacteria.

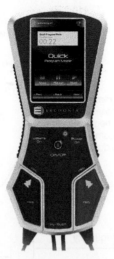

Figure 6.18 The Erchonia low level laser therapy (3LT®) device widely used in physical medicine to treat a number of issues. Erchonia Medical has been an industry leader in conducting randomized clinical trials needed for FDA clearances for conditions including chronic neck and shoulder pain and pain associated with breast augmentation and other surgeries, acne vulgaris-dermatological conditions, non-invasive fat reduction and body contouring, appearance of cellulite, chronic heel pain arising from plantar fasciitis, non-invasive dermatological aesthetic treatment for reduction of circumference of hips, waist, thighs and upper abdomen. *(Courtesy of Erchonia Medical, McKinney, TX.)*

Light and Sound Therapies Combined

Research has shown that pulsing light and/or sound varying in intensity, frequency and color (in the case of light) or tone (in the case of sound) can be both pleasing and therapeutic. Many color therapy systems apply single static colors, sometimes presented in sequences. While these methods have seemed effective, more sophisticated light systems combine color sequences with brainwave photic driving (in which flash frequencies entrain electrical activity recorded over the parieto-occipital regions of the brain). Previous technologies making use of this combination included the Color Receptivity Trainer by Jacob Liberman (1991).

More complex light projections involve the simultaneous presentation of rapid sequences of colors, synchronized with carefully selected sounds. Two award-winning technologies of this kind are the Sensora developed by Canadian physicist Anadi Martel, and the AlphaSphere, invented by Austrian artist and perception researcher, sha (Figure 6.19 and 6.20).

Sensora is a multi-sensorial device that surrounds a person with carefully selected and programmable stimulation sources: a colored light-projection system, a spatially organized sound system and a multi-transducer chair for kinesthetic stimulation in the form of vibrations. The multi-media programs generate a rich experience, with the potential of facilitating various processes such as relaxation and creativity enhancement, as well as more specialized therapies. Martel (1991, 2013) has summarized research on light modulation.

The AlphaSphere developed by sha is a three-dimensional experience room presenting sound, light and movement. It enables people to perceive sound structures and vibrations with their whole bodies. AlphaSpheres have been placed in private lofts, public museums, luxurious spas, therapy practises, offices, and churches. In the Netherlands, AlphaSphere can be found at railway stations, because a few minutes in the device increases a conductor's power of concentration and therefore decreases accident risk. Four studies have been published on the Web: Schiesser (2006), Slunecko (2007), Kriener (2008) and Slunecko (2009).

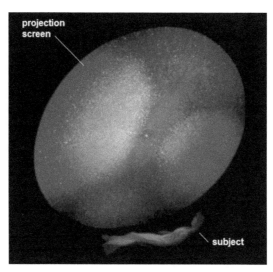

Figure 6.19 Sensora is an award-winning multi-sensorial therapeutic system that provides a rich experience by surrounding a person with carefully programmed patterns of sound and light as well as with vibrations through a multi-transducer chair. It was developed by Canadian physicist, Anadi Martel. *(Courtesy of Sensortech, Inc., Canada.)*

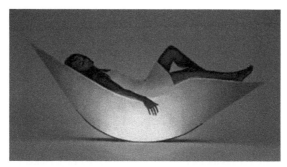

Figure 6.20 The award-winning AlphaSphere was developed by Austrian artist and perception researcher, sha. It is a three-dimensional experience room, presenting sound, light and movement. It gives a person a relaxing and therapeutic whole-body experience. *(Courtesy of Sha-Art, Vienna Australia.)*

Conclusions

This chapter has traced the uses of energy in medicine from antiquity to the present. Two aspects stand out. First, in retrospect, the early observations of Mesmer and Burr, ridiculed or ignored by their contemporaries, respectively, have been shown to be correct. For example, the existence of 'animal magnetism' introduced by Mesmer has been confirmed (see Chapter 8) Second, modern devices based on Burr's early discoveries and those that followed from Cottrell are proving to be valuable in clinical diagnosis of conditions such as cancer, but they have been very slow to gain acceptance by a medical community whose primary treatment modality is pharmacology.

References

Amato, D., Pasche, B., 1994. An evaluation of the safety of low energy emission therapy [published erratum appears in Compr Ther 1994;20(12):681]. Compr Ther 1993 (19), 242–247.

Antes, T.A., Yunus, M.B., Ritey, S.D., Bradley, J.M., Masi, A.T., 1984. Psychological factors associated with primary fibromyalgia syndrome. Arthritis Rheum. 2, 1101–1106.

Barbault, A., Costa, F.P., Bottger, B., Munden, R.F., Bomholt, F., Kuster, N., Pasche, B., 2009. Amplitude-modulated electromagnetic fields for the treatment of cancer: discovery of tumor-specific frequencies and assessment of a novel therapeutic approach. J. Exp. Clin. Cancer Res. 28, 51.

Barber, D.C., Brown, B.H., 1984. Applied potential tomography. J. Phys. E Sci. Instrum. 17 (9), 723–733.

Barker, A.T., Jaffe, L.F., Venable, J.W., 1982. The glaborous epidermis of cavies contains a powerful battery. Am. J. Physiol. 242, R358–R366.

Bassett, L.S., Pawluk, R.J., Becker, R.O., 1964. Effects of electric currents on bone in vivo. Nature (London) 204, 652.

Burdette, E.C., Seals, J., Toler, T.C., Cain, F.L., Magin, R.L., 1977. Preliminary in vivo probe measurements of electrical properties of tumours in mice. In: International Microwave Symposium Digest (San Diego), pp. 344–347.

Calderón, A.P., 1980. "On an inverse boundary value problem", in Seminar on Numerical Analysis and its Applications to Continuum Physics, Rio de Janeiro. Scanned copy of paper. The paper has been reprinted as Calderon, Alberto P. (2006). "On an inverse boundary value problem". Mat. Apl. Comput. 25 (2–3): 133–138.

Cheng, N., et al., 1982. The effect of electric currents on ATP generation, protein synthesis, and membrane transport in rat skin. Clin. Orthop. 171, 264–272.

Clegg, J.P., Guest, J.F., 2007. Modelling the cost-utility of bio-electric stimulation therapy compared to standard care in the treatment of elderly patients with chronic non-healing wounds in the UK. Curr. Med. Res. Opin. 23 (4), 871–883.

Costa, F.P., de Oliveira, A.C., Meirelles, et al., 2011. Treatment of advanced hepatocellular carcinoma with very low levels of amplitude-modulated electromagnetic fields. Br J Cancer 105, 640–648.

Cottrell, F.G., 1903. Application to the Cottrell equation to chronoamperometry. Z. Physik. Chem. 42, 385.

Curtis, D., Fallows, S., Morris, M., McMakin, C., 2010. The efficacy of frequency specific microcurrent therapy on delayed onset muscle soreness. J. Bodyw. Mov. Ther. 14, 272–279.

Dräger, 2010. The Dräger PulmoVista® 500 http://www.draeger.net/media/10/08/96/10089606/rsp_pulmovista_500_pi_9066475_en.pdf (accessed 18.07.2013).

du Bois-Reymond, E., 1848-1884. Untersuchungen uber thierische elektricitat, 2 Reimer, Berlin.

Fraser, P.H., Massey, H., 2008. Decoding the human body-field. The new science of information as medicine. Healing Arts Press, Rochester, VT.

Foster, K.R., Schwan, H.P., 1989. Biomed. Eng. 17, 25–104.

Fricke, H., Morse, S., 1926. The electric capacity of tumours of the breast. J. Cancer Res. 10, 340–376.

Goodwin, T.J., Parker, C.R., 2007. Apparatus for enhancing tissue repair in mammals. US Patent No. 7,179,217.

Haemmerich, D., Staelin, S.T., Tsai, J.Z., Tungjitkusolmun, S., Mahvi, D.M., Webster, J.G., 2003. In vivo electrical conductivity of hepatic tumours. Physiol. Meas. 24, 251–260.

Henderson, R.P., Webster, J.G., 1978. An impedance camera for spatially specific measurements of the thorax. IEEE Trans. Biomed. Eng. 25 (3), 250–254.

Herlitzka, A., 1910. Ein Beitrag zur Physiologie der Regeneration. Wilhelm Roux Arch Entwicklungsmech Org. 10, 126–159.

Higgs, L., Reite, M., Barbault, A., Lebet, J.P., Rossel, C., Amato, D., Dafni, U., Pasche, B., 1994. Subjective and objective relaxation effects of low energy emission therapy. Stress Medicine 10, 5–13.

Hinkle, L., McCaig, C.D., Robinson, K.R., 1981. The direction of growth of differentiating neurons and myoblasts from frog embryos in an applied electric field. J. Physiol. Lond. 314, 121–135.

Huttenlocher, A., Horwitz, A.R., 2007. Wound healing with electric potential. N Engl J Med 356, 303–304.

ICNIRP, 1998. Guidelines for limiting exposure to time-varying electric, magnetic and electromagnetic fields (up to 300 GHz). Health Physics 74, 494–522.

Institute of Electrical and Electronics Engineers: Safety Levels with Respect to Human Exposure to Radio Frequency Electromagnetic Fields, 3 kHz to 300 GHz, IEEE C95.1-2005. New York, Institute of Electrical and Electronics Engineers; 2005.

Illingworth, C.M., Barker, A.T., 1980. Measurement of electrical currents emerging during the regeneration of amputated finger tips in children. Clin. Phys. Physiol. Meas. 1, 87–89.

Jossinet, J., 1998. The impedivity of freshly excised human breast tissue. Physiol. Meas. 19 (1), 61–75.

Kahn, J., 1987. Principles and Practice of Electrotherapy. Churchill Livingstone, New York.

Keshtkar, A., Salehnia, Z., Keshtkar, A., Shokouhi, B., 2012. Bladder cancer detection using electrical imped- ance technique (Tabriz Mark 1). Pathol. Res. Int. 2012, 1–5.

Kirson, E.D., Gurvich, Z., Schneiderman, R., Dekel, E., Itzhaki, A., Wasserman, Y., Schatzberger, R., Palti, Y., 2004. Disruption of cancer cell replication by alternating electric fields. Cancer Res. 64, 3288–3295.

Kirson, E.D., Dbaly, V., Tovarys, F., Vymazal, J., Soustiel, J.F., Aviran Itzhaki, A., Mordechovich, D., Steinberg-Shapira, S., Gurvich, S., Schneiderman, R., Wasserman, Y., Salzberg, M., RyffelB Goldsher, D., Dekel, E., Palti, Y., 2007. Alternating electric fields arrest cell proliferation in animal tumor models and human brain tumors. Proc. Natl. Acad. Sci. U. S. A. 104 (24), 10152–10157.

Kloth, L.C., McCulloch, J.M., 1996. Promotion of wound healing with electrical stimulation. Adv. Wound Care 9 (5), 42–45.

Knutson, G., 2000. The role of the γ-motor system in increasing muscle tone and muscle pain syndromes: a review of the Johansson/Sojka hypothesis. J. Manipulative Physiol. Ther. 23, 564–572.

Korr, I.M., 1978. Sustained sympathicotonia as a factor in disease. In: Korr, I.M. (Ed.), The Neurobiologic Mechanisms in Manipulative Therapy. Plenum Press, New York.

Krawczyk, W.S., 1971. A pattern of epidermal cell migration during wound healing. J. Cell Biol. 49, 247–263.

Kriener, H., 2008. Power Napping and the AlphaSphere as tools to increase efficiency in companies. Master thesis, Faculty of Psychology, University of Vienna. http://www.sha-art.com/content.asp?id=116&id2=238 &id3=266&id4=315&lid=2&eid=4&sid=2&gid=3.

Kuster, N., Costa, F.P., Barbault, A., Pasche, B., 2012. Cancer cell proliferation is inhibited by specific modu- lation frequencies. Br. J. Cancer 106, 307–313.

Lash, J.W., 1955. Studies on wound closure in Urodeles. J. Exp. Zool. 128, 13–28.

Lebet, J.P., Barbault, A., Rossel, C., Tomic, Z., Reite, M., Higgs, L., Dafni, U., Amato, D., Pasche, B., 1996. Electroencephalographic changes following low energy emission therapy. Ann. Biomed. Eng. 24, 424–429.

Liberman, J., 1991. Light, medicine of the future, Edition 1, Bear and Company Publishers, Santa Fe, New Mexico.

Lykken, D.T., 1971. Square-wave analysis of skin impedance. Psychophysiology 7, 262–275.

Maarek, A., 2012. Electro interstitial scan system: assessment of 10 years of research and development. Med. Devices (Auckl) 5, 23–30, 2 March issue.

Majno, G., 1975. The Healing Hand. Man and Wound in the Ancient World. Harvard University Press, Cambridge, MA.

Martel, A., 1991. U.S. Pat. No. 5,070,399 entitled, Light Color and Intensity Modulation System, issued December 3, 1991.

Martel, A., 2013. U.S. Pat. No. 8,579,795, Light modulation device and system, issued November 12, 1913. Schiesser 2006.

Masopust, D., Schenkel, J.M., 2013. The integration of T cell migration, and function. Nat. Rev. Immunol. 13 (5), 309–320.

Matre, D.A., Sinkjaer, T., Svensson, P., Arendt-Nielsen, L., 1998. Experimental muscle pain increases the human stretch reflex. Pain 75, 331–339.

Matteucci, C., 1844. Traité des phénomènes électro-physiologiques des animaux suivi d'études anatomiques sur le système nerveux et sur l'organe électrique de la torpille par Paul Savi. Fortin, Masson et C., Paris.

McMakin, C., 2003. Microcurrent therapy in the treatment of fibromyalgia. In: Chaitow, L. (Ed.), Fibromyalgia Syndrome: A Practitioner's Guide to Treatment. Churchill Livingstone, Edinburgh, pp. 179–206.

McMakin, C., 2011a. Frequency Specific Microcurrent in Pain Management. Churchill Livingstone/Elsevier, Edinburgh.

McMakin, C., 2011b. Qi in chronic fatigue and fibromyalgia. In: Mayor, D., Micozzi, M. (Eds.), Energy Medicine East and West. Churchill Livingstone/Elsevier, Edinburgh, pp. 289–296.

McMakin, C., Oschman, J., 2012. Visceral and somatic disorders: tissue softening with frequency-specific microcurrent. J. Bodyw. Mov. Ther. 19 (2), 170–177.

Mense, S., 1997. Pathophysiologic basis of muscle pain syndromes. Phys. Med. Rehabil. Clinics North Am. 8, 23–53.

Messerli, M.A., Graham, D.M., 2011. Extracellular electrical fields direct wound healing and regeneration. Biol. Bull. 221, 79–92.

Midwood, K.S., Williams, L.V., Schwarzbauer, J.E., 2004. Tissue repair and the dynamics of the extracellular matrix. Int. J. Biochem. Cell Biol. 36 (6), 1031–1037.

Mines, S., 2003. We Are All in Shock. How Overwhelming Experiences Shatter You … and What You Can Do About It. New Page Books, Franklin Lakes, NJ, 256 pp.

Morucci, J.P., Rigaud, B., 1996. Bioelectrical impedance techniques in medicine. Part III: Impedance imaging. Third section: medical applications. Crit Rev Biomed Eng. 24 (4–6), 655–677. Review.

Morucci, J.P., Marsili, P.M., 1996. Bioelectrical impedance techniques in medicine. Part III: Impedance imaging. Second section: reconstruction algorithms. Crit Rev Biomed Eng. 24 (4–6), 599–654. Review.

Nguyen, D.T., Orgill, D.P., Murphy, G.F., 2009. The pathophysiologic basis for wound healing and cutaneous regeneration. In: Biomaterials for Treating Skin Loss. Woodhead Publishing (UK/Europe) & CRC Press (US), Cambridge, UK/Boca Raton, FL, pp. 25–57, Chapter 4.

Nobili, 1825. Astatic Galvanometer. See Greenslade T Instruments for Natural Philosophy—Astatic Galvanometer. http://physics.kenyon.edu/EarlyApparatus/Electrical_Measurements/Astatic_Galvanometer/Astatic_Galvanometer.html (accessed 15.07. 2013).

Nuccitelli, R., 1988. Physiological electric fields can influence cell motility, growth, and polarity. Adv. Cell Biol. 2, 213–233.

Nuccitelli, R., 2003. A role for endogenous electric fields in wound healing. Curr. Top. Dev. Biol. 58, 1–26.

Omoigui, S., 2007. The biochemical origin of pain—proposing a new law of pain: the origin of all pain is inflammation and the inflammatory response. Part 1 of 3—a unifying law of pain. Med. Hypotheses 69, 70–82.

Ota, K.-i., Savinell RF, Kreysa G. (Eds.), 2013. Encyclopedia of Applied Electrochemistry. Springer-Verlag, New York, NY, 4000 pp.

Pasche, B., Barbault, A., 2003. Low-energy emission therapy: current status and future directions. In: Rosch, P.J., Markov, M.S. (Eds.), Bioelectromagnetic Medicine. Marcel Dekker, Inc, New York, pp. 321–327.

Pasche, B., Erman, M., Mitler, M., 1990. Diagnosis and management of insomnia. N Engl J Med 323, 486–487.

Pasche, B., Erman, M., Hayduk, R., Mitler, M., Reite, M., Higgs, L., Dafni, U., Rossel, C., Kuster, N., Barbault, A., Lebet, J.-P., 1996. Effects of Low Energy Emission Therapy in chronic psychophysiological insomnia. Sleep. 19, 327–336.

Peters, C., 1885. Ueber die Regeneration des Epithels der Cornea. Inaug. Diss. Bonn. Cited in Barfurthe D 1991 Zir Regemeratopm der Gewebe. Arch für Mikroskopische Anatomie 37, 406–491.

Reilly, W., Reeve, V.E., Quinn, C., 2004. Anti-inflammatory effects of interferential frequency-specific applied microcurrent. In: Proceedings of the Australian Health and Medical Research Congress, Abstract ID: ABSLN-3TVEH-RYZ99-A78C8.

Reite, M., Higgs, L., Lebet, J.P., Barbault, A., Rossel, C., Kuster, N., Dafni, U., Amato, D., Pasche, B., 1994. Sleep inducing effect of low energy emission therapy. Bioelectromagnetics 15, 67–75.

Rigaud, B., Morucci, J.P., Chauveau, N., 1996. Bioelectrical impedance techniques in medicine. Part I: Bioimpedance measurement. Second section: impedance spectrometry. Crit Rev Biomed Eng. 24 (4–6), 257–351. Review.

Rigaud, B., Morucci, J.P., 1996. Bioelectrical impedance techniques in medicine. Part III: impedance imaging. First section: general concepts and hardware. Crit Rev Biomed Eng. 24 (4–6), 467–597. Review.

Schepps, J.L., Foster, K.R., 1980. The UHF and microwave dielectric properties of normal and tumour tissues: variation in dielectric properties with tissue water content. Phys. Med. Biol. 25, 1149–1159.

Schiesser, I., 2006. Relaxation on the AlphaLounger. A psycho-physiological study. http://www.sha-art.com/upload/downloads/Biofeedback_Messreihe_ENG.pdf.

Settle, R.G., Foster, K.R., Epstein, B.R., Mullen, J.L., 1980. Nutritional assessment: whole body impedance and fluid compartments. Nutr. Cancer 2 (1), 72–80.

Slunecko, T., 2007. Effects and potentials of the AlphaLounger/AlphaSphere. Immersive art as an option for psychotherapy. http://www.sha-art.com/upload/downloads/Psycological_Study_ENG.pdf.

Slunecko, T., 2009. Therapeutic effectiveness of the AlphaSphere. Summary at http://www.sha-art.com/upload/downloads/Researchreport_Shortversion_E.pdf.

Snyder-Mackler, L., Robinson, A., 2007. Clinical Electrophysiology: Electrotherapy and Electrophysiologic Testing. Williams & Wilkins, Baltimore, MD.

Stossel, T.P., 1994. The machinery of cell crawlikng. Sci. Am. 271, 54–63.

Uhlmann, G., 1999. Developments in inverse problems since Calderón's foundational paper. In: Christ, M.E., Kenig, C.E. (Eds.), Harmonic Analysis and Partial Differential Equations: Essays in Honor of Alberto P. Calderón. University of Chicago Press, Chicago, IL.

Valentinuzzi, M.E., Morucci, J.P., Felice, C.J., 1996. Bioelectrical impedance techniques in medicine. Part II: Monitoring of physiological events by impedance. Crit Rev Biomed Eng. 24 (4–6), 353–466. Review.

Vinkler, C., Korenstein, R., 1982. Characterization of external electric field-driven ATP synthesis in chloroplasts. Proc. Natl. Acad. Sci. U. S. A. 79, 3183–3187.

Wang, E.T., Zhao, M., 2010. 2010 Regulation of tissue repair and regeneration by electric fields. Chin. J. Traumatol. 13 (1), 55–61.

Wolf, D.A., Goodwin, T.J., 2002. Growth stimulation of biological cells and tissue by electromagnetic fields and uses thereof. US Patent No. 6,485,963, B1.

Wolf, D.A., Goodwin, T.J., 2004. Growth stimulation of biological cells and tissue by electromagnetic fields and uses thereof. US Patent No. 6,673,597.

Yasuda, I., 1953. The Classic Fundamental Aspects of Fracture Treatment. J. Kyoto Med. Soc. 4, 395.

Zaho, M., Song, B., Pu, J., et al., 2006. Electrical signals control wound healing through phosphatidylinositol-3OH kinase-gamma and PTEN. Nature 442, 457–460.

Zhao, M., Forrester, J.V., McCaig, C.D., 1999. A small, physiological electric field orients cell division. Proc. Natl. Acad. Sci. U. S. A. 96, 4942–4946.

Zimmerman, J.W., Pennison, M.J., Brezovich, I., et al., 2012. Cancer cell proliferation is inhibited by specific modulation frequencies. Br. J. Cancer 106 (2), 307–313.

Zywietz, F., Knoechel, R., 1986. Dielectric properties of Co-χ-irradiated and microwave-heated rat tumour and skin measured in vivo between 0.2 and 2.4 GHz. Phys. Med. Biol. 31, 1021–1029.

CHAPTER 7

Bodywork, Energetic and Movement Therapies

Chapter Summary

During the past century a number of innovators have established therapeutic schools that include training in hands-on and hands-off energy techniques, movement therapies, neuromuscular re-education, and Structural Integration. Many of these innovators were or are medical doctors, scientists, physical therapists, or other kinds of healthcare providers. Each of them had insights into human structure and function that made a huge difference to their students and patients. Driven by a desire to share their skills, each of them established schools that continue their work. Many of these techniques are making an impact in hospitals and other healthcare facilities around the world. Some of these methods relate to the way the body moves in relation to the gravitational field of the Earth. At least two of these pioneers began their training at the Esalen Institute in Big Sur, California, where they found a stimulating and creative atmosphere with a great deal of interest in their work.

Jin Shin Jyutsu®

According to ancient records, the precursors of this method date from before Moses and Gautama Buddha but were dormant for 1200 years. The Knowledge was transmitted by oral tradition until it was written down in the Kojiki (Record of Ancient Things, 712 CE). Around the turn of the century in Japan, Jiro Murai, a young philosopher from a prominent medical family, became terminally ill. He asked his family to leave him at their mountain retreat alone for 7 days and return on the eighth to collect his body. Jiro Murai had read about great sages in the past who had experienced 'miracles' and enlightenment. In the isolation of the wilderness, he utilized the techniques of ancient teachings and experienced a profound healing. From that moment on, he dedicated his life to research to understand his life altering experience. The result was a method that he later called Jin Shin Jyutsu®. In the 1930s, Jiro was summoned to the Royal Palace by the Emperor of Japan. Upon treating the Emperor, he was granted permission to study the sacred information in the Imperial Archives. This enabled him to research this lost art and rediscover it in its totality. After World War II, Jiro sought out a young Japanese American interpreter, Mary Burmeister, to bring this art to America. Mary studied with Jiro for several years and later became a master of Jin Shin Jyutsu®. She wrote the first English language texts on Jin Shin (Burmeister, 1985) and held classes in many countries. In the United States, Pamela Markarian Smith was struggling with an unknown and potentially critical condition when she learned of Mary and Jin Shin Jyutsu® in the early 1960s. She took one of Mary's first classes in Los Angeles. Pamela received treatments from Mary for several months and her symptoms gradually went away. She realized she had found her life's work. After moving to Sonoma County, California, in 1973, Pamela continued her practise and self-help classes. In the late 1970s, Mary Burmeister came to Bodega Bay to give her first class in Northern California. Thereafter, Pamela continued to coordinate annual Jin Shin Jyutsu® seminars for Mary during the next 13 years. In 1992, Pamela founded the Jin Shin Institute as a means to share her understanding of Jin Shin Jyutsu®.

The Alexander Technique

Frederick Matthias Alexander was a Shakespearean orator who developed chronic laryngitis a number of times while he was performing. His voice training had come from experts, and physicians informed him that they could find no physical cause for his problems. To restore his voice, Alexander carefully watched himself in a mirror while he was speaking and noticed that his vocal problem came from undue muscular tension in his neck that extended to his whole body. It took him 8 years to resolve his own problem, and, in the meantime, he observed that many others had similar difficulties. He realized that the pattern of tensing would rotate the head backwards and downwards in relationship to the spine and disrupt efficient overall body alignment. When neck tension is reduced, the head no longer compresses the spine, and the spine is free to lengthen. Alexander restored his own natural capacity for ease by changing the way he thought while initiating all movements. From this work on himself and others during the period 1890–1900, he evolved a hands-on teaching method that encourages all the body's processes to work more efficiently, as an integrated, dynamic whole. The method makes the performance of any movement easier: sitting, standing, walking, using the hands, and speaking. F.M. Alexander trained educators in his technique mainly while living in London, UK, from 1931 until his death in 1955. Proponents believe that the method improves awareness and descriptive ability, ease of movement, balance, and stamina and reduces muscular tension. Some report enhanced clarity in thinking and freedom from self-imposed limitations. The Alexander Technique provides ways to use less effort for movement and thus perform more efficiently, feeling younger and moving gracefully (Alexander, 1932; Jones, 1997, 1999). Training in the method is available worldwide through the Society of Teachers of the Alexander Technique.

Rolfing®/Structural Integration

Ida P. Rolf (Figure 7.1) was a native New Yorker. She graduated from Barnard College in 1916, and in 1920 she earned a PhD in biological chemistry from the College of Physicians and Surgeons of Columbia University. For the next 12 years she worked at the Rockefeller Institute, now the Rockefeller University, first in the Department of Chemotherapy and later in the Department of Organic Chemistry. Eventually, she rose to the rank of Associate, an unusual achievement for a young woman in those times. In 1927, she took a leave of absence from her work to study mathematics and atomic physics at the Swiss Technical University in Zurich. During this time, she also studied homeopathic medicine in Geneva. Returning from Europe, she spent the decade of the 1930s seeking answers to personal and family health problems. Frustrated with the medical treatments available at that time, she explored osteopathy, chiropractic medicine, yoga, the Alexander Technique, and the work of Korzybski (1879–1950) on general semantics and states of consciousness. By the 1940s, Dr. Rolf had developed her own hands-on methods and worked on people with a variety of medical problems in her Manhattan apartment. She was committed to a scientific point of view, yet many breakthroughs came intuitively through the work she did with chronically disabled persons who were unable to find help elsewhere. Her methods eventually became known as Structural Integration or Rolfing®. In the mid-1960s, Dr. Rolf was invited to Esalen Institute in California at the suggestion of Fritz Perls, the founder of Gestalt Therapy. There she began her first training of practitioners and instructors of Structural Integration. In 1967, the first Guild for Structural Integration was formed in Boulder, Colorado. Her methods are still taught there at the Rolf Institute and the Guild for Structural Integration. Aspects of her work have been incorporated into other schools, including Hellerwork (developed in the 1970s by aerospace engineer Joseph Heller), Kinesis Myofascial Integration (developed by Tom Myers, who studied directly with Dr. Ida Rolf, Moshe Feldenkrais, and Buckminster Fuller), and Postural Integration (originally developed in the 1960s by Jack Painter, PhD). Ida Rolf wrote a book about her work (Rolf, 1977), and another fascinating book was compiled by her close associate and companion, Rosemary Feitis (1985).

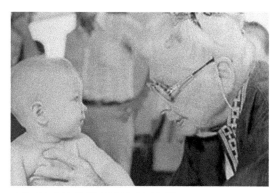

Figure 7.1 Ida P. Rolf, PhD (1896–1979). *(Courtesy of Ron Thompson.)*

The Feldenkrais Method

Dr. Moshé Feldenkrais (1904–1984) was a Ukrainian-born physicist and judo practitioner who moved to Israel. He developed the view that good health means *functioning* well – working well, having satisfying relationships with emotional maturity, being able to access a full range of responses to any situation, in contrast to medically defined health, which is described as not 'sick or disabled'. He asserted that the method of body/mind exploration he evolved leads to improved functioning (health) through individuals becoming more aware and finding improved use of their bodies. His focus on exploration and awareness is typified by his statement, 'What I am after is more flexible minds, not just more flexible bodies'.

The Feldenkrais Method attracts those seeking to improve their movement repertoire (e.g., dancers, musicians, artists), as well as those wishing to reduce pain or limitations in movement and many who want to improve their general well-being and personal development. Because it uses movement as the primary vehicle for gaining awareness, it is directly applicable to disorders that arise from restricted movement, whether due to accident, illness, or genetic challenges. However, practitioners generally don't regard their work as 'treatment' or 'cure' because they are not working from a medical model. Feldenkrais techniques can expand a person's choices and responses to many aspects of life: emotions, relationships, and intellectual tasks; it can be applied at any level, from severe disorder to highly professional performance. The Feldenkrais Method holds that there is no separation between mind and body and that learning to move better can improve one's overall well-being on many levels (Feldenkrais, 1981, 2002). Feldenkrais began teaching his work in Israel and Europe in the early 1970s. His first professional trainings in the United States were done in the early 1980s in San Francisco and Amherst, MA, assisted by his long-time friend and associate, Mia Segal. The work is continued by the Feldenkrais Guild of North America in New York and by an International Feldenkrais Federation that was incorporated in Paris in 1992.

The Trager Approach

The Trager Approach is the discovery of Milton Trager, MD (Figure 7.2), who developed his method somewhat serendipitously at the age of 18. His motivation was to cope with his own congenital spinal deformity and, later, to help his father, who had been suffering from sciatica. His father's chronic complaint cleared up after two sessions from his son. Dr. Trager then spent the next 50 years as a lay practitioner and later as a medical doctor refining and expanding his discovery. Dr. Trager began to teach his work at a late age. He taught others for more than 20 years. Work with people with all kinds of neuromuscular complaints convinced him that he had something to offer the medical profession, and he began to apply to medical schools at the age of 42.

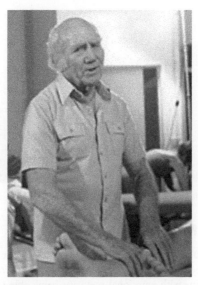

Figure 7.2   Milton Trager, MD (1908–1997).

Because of the results he was getting, he was determined to teach his work to registered physical therapists. After many rejections, he was accepted into the Universidad Autonoma de Guadalajara in Mexico. In 1955, he received his MD. Dr. Trager continued to work with clients within his practise for the next 20 years. An opportunity to teach his work came when he was invited to Esalen Institute in Big Sur, California, to give a demonstration. Betty Fuller (who had also been instrumental in bringing Moshe Feldenkrais to the United States) was teaching at Esalen at the time and having tremendous problems with her neck. Dr. Trager offered to help, and after a few minutes her neck was no longer in pain. Betty was very impressed and went on to co-found the Trager Institute in 1980. Shortly thereafter, a certification program was established to train and certify people in the Trager Approach. There are now thousands of certified Trager practitioners throughout the world. Forty years after his determination to reach the medical profession, holisti-cally minded doctors, nurses, and physical therapists began make use of the Trager Approach in their practices. The Trager training program is now taught throughout the world in many differ-ent languages. For a comprehensive history of Dr. Trager and his life, see Liskin (1996).

CranioSacral Therapy and SomatoEmotional Release

Dr. John Upledger, DO OMM (1932–2012) (Figure 7.3), was an osteopathic physician, clini-cal researcher, and developer of two innovative forms of bodywork, CranioSacral Therapy and SomatoEmotional Release. His unique contribution has been to confirm scientifically the discov-eries of Sutherland and the other early cranial osteopaths and to make a variety of clinical proce-dures available to many people through worldwide training and continuing education programs. Dr. Upledger conducted basic research on the cranial sacral system during the period 1975–1983 when he served as a clinical researcher and Professor of Biomechanics at Michigan State University. With a team of anatomists, physiologists, biophysicists, and bioengineers, Upledger was able to confirm scientifically the movements of the cranial bones and the membranes (dura mater, tentorium cerebelli, and falx cerebri) and cerebrospinal fluid that surround and protect the brain and spinal cord. Dr. Upledger established the Upledger Foundation in 1987 to reach out to those less fortunate and help improve their life experiences. This nonprofit organization

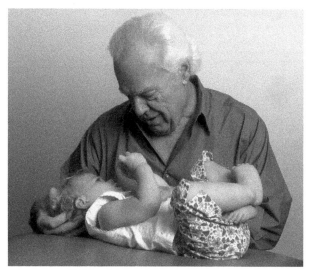

Figure 7.3   John Upledger, DO, OMM. (1932–2012) founder of CranioSacral Therapy. *(Photo courtesy of Upledger Institute International, Inc.)*

is dedicated to ongoing research and development of new therapeutic applications and to the establishment of community-outreach programs that enhance total health. Dr. Upledger has written numerous study guides, research articles, and books (e.g., Upledger and Vredevoogd, 1983; Upledger, 1987, 1997, 2002).

Active Isolated Stretching

Active Isolated Stretching (AIS) was developed by Aaron L. Mattes (Figure 7.4) and is widely used by leading athletes, massage therapists, personal/athletic trainers, and other healthcare professionals. The technique involves individually and systematically stretching virtually every muscle and every myofascial plane in the body and holding each stretch for only 2 s. The result is improved circulation and elasticity of muscles and connective tissue throughout the body. The method facilitates self-repair and enhances peak performance.

AIS was developed over 35 years from the work Aaron Mattes did with thousands of patients, doctors, and health professionals. His stretching book (Mattes, 2000) teaches an individual how to actively stretch him- or herself. Mattes also developed a variety of ingenious tools that can improve flexibility and help alleviate problems associated with many athletic or overuse injuries such as carpel tunnel, tennis elbow, lower back problems, and other ailments resulting from a lack of flexibility. Qualified Active Isolated Stretching practitioners can be found throughout the United States and in other countries. Many of the top athletes in the world attest to the successes they have had in competitions after being treated with AIS.

Therapeutic Touch

Therapeutic Touch (TT) started at Pumpkin Hollow Farm, a family camp and spiritual retreat center of the Theosophical Society in the foothills of the Berkshires in New York State. It was preceded by the work of Dora Kunz, who had a highly developed natural sensitivity to human energy systems. She was able to perceive blockages in a patient's energy field that are not generally accessible with other medical technologies. Dora diagnosed numerous perplexing cases referred

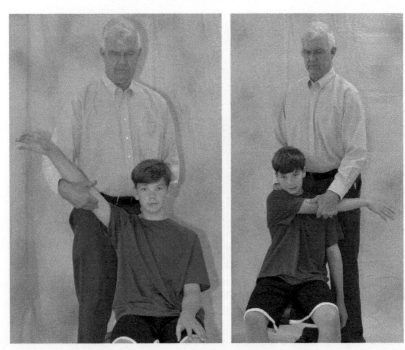

Figure 7.4   Aaron Mattes demonstrating Active Isolated Stretching.

by physicians. In the 1970's, Dora and her long-time student and colleague Dolores Krieger, PhD RN, developed TT (Figure 7.5). Dr. Krieger was Professor of Nursing at New York University.

The practise is based on the assumptions that human beings are complex fields of energy and that the ability to enhance healing in another is a natural potential (Krieger, 1993). Kunz and Krieger developed a program for teaching the procedures and attitudes necessary for TT. Formal

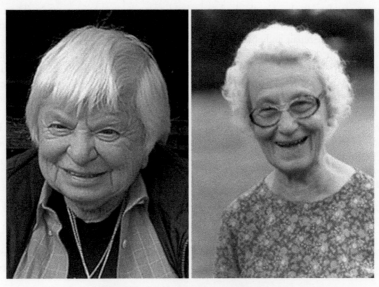

Figure 7.5   Dolores Krieger and Dora Kunz.

classes began at Pumpkin Hollow Farm, where many patients were referred by their physicians. Intensive summer teaching sessions for TT continue at Pumpkin Hollow. In addition, TT is being taught worldwide in universities and workshops for healthcare professionals as well as interested lay people. TT has become a widely accepted form of alternative therapy in hospitals and other health agencies. The method has a substantial base of formal and clinical research. This research has shown that TT is useful in reducing pain, improving wound healing, aiding relaxation, and easing the dying process.

Continuum Movement

Continuum Movement was developed by Emilie Conrad, a professional dancer who was born and raised in New York City. Emilie moved to Haiti in the late 1950s to study primitive dance. She became choreographer and leader of a Haitian dance company. From her experiences in an indigenous society, she questioned how our movements are shaped by our culture. She began developing Continuum Movement in the early 1960s as a way to teach a new view of movement based on the primary motions common to all life forms.

Continuum uses movement, breath, and the resonance of sound to enhance the communication systems within and around the body. In 1963 she moved to Los Angeles where she began teaching at the Actors Studio. Her novel approach to movement enriched performing artists and led to her choreographing and directing plays and other performance works. Her explorations have attracted and inspired an international audience from fields such as Rolfing, Zero Balancing, Hellerwork, craniosacral, osteopathy, physical therapy, dance, psychoneuroimmunology, and physical fitness. She has led workshops throughout the United States, Canada, and Europe. In 1974, Emilie began pioneering work on protocols for spinal cord injury. This remarkable work has helped many 'hopelessly' paralyzed individuals to regain precious movements that conventional medicine regarded to be impossible. From 1974 to 1979, Emilie was part of a research study conducted by Dr. Valerie Hunt at University of California, Los Angeles (UCLA). She has originated a dynamic process that strengthens by incorporating multiple angles in gravity to develop diverse muscular and skeletal relationships. Emilie's most recent contribution is her revolutionary concept of 'The Three Anatomies', which define three distinct tissue structures, the cultural, primordial, and cosmic. The Continuum Studio in Santa Monica offers a wide range of classes, workshops, retreats, and professional programmes. Continuum teachers can be found around the United States and in many other countries around the world. Emilie Conrad published a book describing her work (Conrad, 2007).

Zero Balancing

Zero Balancing is a hands-on system designed by Dr. Fritz Frederick Smith (Figure 7.6), who became a doctor of osteopathic medicine (DO) in 1955 and an MD in 1961. He then studied Rolfing®, yoga, meditation, and Eastern philosophies. He became a licensed acupuncturist in 1972 and later studied with J.R. Worsley at the Chinese College of Acupuncture in England, earning both bachelor's and master's degrees in acupuncture. It was during this time that he also experienced intense personal revelations under the teaching of Swami Muktananda. The Zero Balancing approach emerged in 1975 as an integration of Eastern views of energy with Western views of science. The technique aligns body energy with physical structure. (http://www.zerobalancing.com/fritz_moves.shtml) Throughout the Zero Balancing session, attention is given to the skeleton in particular because it contains the densest matter and the deepest and strongest currents. The process is distinguished by a gentle form of touch known as interface (Hamwee, 2000). The outcome of a Zero Balancing session is relief of physical and mental symptoms; improvements in the ability to deal with life stresses; and improved organization of the body's energy fields to promote a sense of wholeness and well-being.

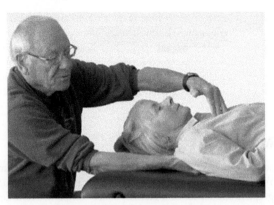

Figure 7.6   Fritz Smith, DO, MD.

It can be useful to think of the structural body as the sail of a boat and the energy body as the wind. At some point the wind meets the sail. When structure and energy are not integrated, you're like a sailor floundering at sea, not "tacked into the winds of life". Life is less satisfying and you're more susceptible to all manner of emotional distress and disease—from simple irritability and headaches to more profound mental or physical symptoms and illnesses.

Zero Balancing has been taught internationally since 1973. The Zero Balancing Health Association was founded in 1991 to promote and support the teaching and practise of Zero Balancing. Dr. Smith has written two books (Smith, 1986, 2005).

Bowen Technique

Tom Bowen developed what is now called the Bowen Technique in Geelong, Australia. Bowen was not formally trained in any medical or alternative therapy discipline. In the late 1950s he developed an interest in healing. He started helping people with 'bad backs' and other ailments and so his life of helping others began. He had a Saturday morning clinic for disabled children who were treated free. Parents would bring their children from many miles away, sometimes travelling 3–4 h. He held a clinic every Saturday evening for athletes who had injured themselves during the day. This was also a free clinic and many people came from near and far. Today Bowen's work is taught at university level in Australia as well as worldwide. Oswald and Elaine Rentsch documented the work and established the Bowen Therapy Academy of Australia in the late 1980s.

The first Bowen seminar in the United States was taught by Ossie Rentsch in 1989. The Bowen Technique uses a series of simple, gentle moves across muscle and connective tissue. It is similar to tuning a stringed instrument that sends harmonic vibrations that balance the body. Because it works in harmony with the body, the Bowen Technique is incredibly effective for any muscular, skeletal, or nerve imbalance. It has also been successful in treating chronic pain due to injury or surgery. The technique is so gentle it can be used on anyone from infants to the elderly. It produces a deep relaxation and can release blocked emotional energy, which can accelerate the healing process. The basic Bowen *move* is precise and light. It targets specific muscles and tendons. Using fingers and thumb, the area is manipulated and the muscle is then challenged and moved in the opposite direction. The patient is left for 2 min, allowing the released energy to travel through the body before the next *move* is performed. This technique is effective for balancing the autonomic nervous system. A book about the Bowen Technique has been written by Wilks (2007).

Healing Touch

Janet Mentgen, BSN, RN (Figure 7.7), founded Healing Touch International, Inc. Janet taught the first official Healing Touch course in 1989. The technique is now taught in more than 20 countries and used by nurses in many hospitals. While all touch can have healing effects, Healing Touch is a very specific program of energy healing that induces deep relaxation and restores the body's natural flow of energy, facilitating self-healing. The method is based on the healing philosophies and methods of well-known healers, such as Alice Bailey, Dr. Brugh Joy, Barbara Brennan, and Rosalyn Bruyere. In 1990, Healing Touch was accepted as a certificate program of the American Holistic Nurses Association (AHNA). The Canadian Holistic Nurses Association has endorsed it as well. In 1996, Healing Touch International, Inc. became the certifying organization for this hands-on energy-based therapy. Healing Touch consists of six levels of training, each requiring hands-on practise to develop skill in Healing Touch (Hover-Kramer, 2000). Healing Touch International probably has the most active research program of any of the complementary and alternative medicine modalities. This has come about because of the diligent efforts of Cynthia Hutchison and, more recently, Diane Wind Wardell, PhD.

Resonance Repatterning

Chloe Faith Wordsworth (Figure 7.8) immigrated to the United States from England in 1964. She is a Phi Beta Kappa Cum Laude graduate of the University of California (UCLA). Following graduation, she began an intensive study of complementary healthcare methods that now form the basis of the Resonance Repatterning system. These include Polarity Therapy, which she studied with its founder, Dr. Randolph Stone in 1972; the five element system of acupuncture, as passed down by Dr. J.R. Worsley; Edu-Kinesiology, which she studied with its founder, Dr. Paul Dennison; and an introduction to Sharry Edwards' method of working with sound frequencies. In the early 1990s Chloe began to explore the use of tuning forks and color frequencies to balance meridian flow. As she discovered that a certain combination of techniques worked effectively on one client and different combinations worked more effectively on other clients, she naturally began to include her knowledge and practise of Jin Shin Jyutsu®, cranial sacral work, harmonic overtones, movement, diet, and breathing patterns to support her clients'

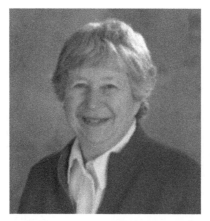

Figure 7.7 Janet Mentgen (1938–2005) founded the Healing Touch Program, the only continuing education program in the field of energy medicine with two national accreditations, American Nurses Credentialing Center (ANCC), and National Commission for Certifying Agencies (NCCA).

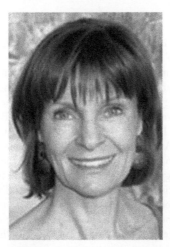

Figure 7.8   Chloe Faith Wordsworth.

self-healing processes. Ultimately, Chloe created a practical system that would give tangible results in every session; a system she could teach so others could apply the method to themselves,
their families, and friends; and that practitioners could learn. In 1990, she began to synthesize
her system of complementary energy healthcare and called it Holographic Repatterning (later
renamed Resonance Repatterning). Chloe has written eleven books that enable practitioners to
access the core frequency patterns that cause dissonance in their lives and relationships and to
transform these patterns. In addition, she has created a Resonance Repatterning training curriculum for students and teachers. The system has caught on by word of mouth and now has practitioners all over the world. The system uses the body's natural biofeedback response to access the
unconscious mind. The most recent book on Resonance Repatterning is *Quantum Change Made
Easy* (Wordsworth and Glanville, 2007).

BodyTalk

Dr. John Veltheim (Figure 7.9) founded the BodyTalk system in 1995 after extensive experience
as a chiropractor, traditional acupuncturist, philosopher, and teacher. John ran a successful acupuncture and chiropractic clinic in Brisbane, Australia, for 15 years and served as the principal of
the Brisbane College of Acupuncture and Natural Therapies for 5 years. His extensive postgrad-
uate studies have included applied kinesiology, bioenergetic psychology, osteopathy, sports
medicine, counselling, comparative philosophy, and theology. The BodyTalk system works by first
identifying the weakened energy circuits within the body. The practitioner relies on the body's
inherent knowledge of itself to locate the energy circuits that need repair by using a form of biofeedback involving a subtle muscle-testing technique. The BodyTalk protocol is straightforward
and requires no diagnoses. The practitioner relies on the guidance of the body's natural wisdom
to not only locate the weakened lines of communication but also to find the proper order in
which they are to be addressed. The result is that the general energy balance of the body is greatly
improved. Because of its simplicity and powerful effects, BodyTalk is one of the fastest growing
approaches to healthcare worldwide. Graduates include medical doctors and specialists, psychologists, psychotherapists, chiropractors, acupuncturists, naturopaths, physical therapists, osteopaths,
nurses, licensed massage therapists, and laypeople. The International BodyTalk Association (IBA)
was formed in Sarasota, Florida, in 2000 and is now a worldwide organization that establishes
practitioner standards, credentialing, training, and scheduling of courses. For further details of the
BodyTalk process, see Veltheim (1999).

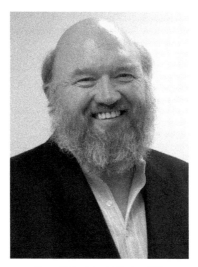

Figure 7.9   John Veltheim, DC.

Many Others

This short survey of the field of energetic, bodywork, and movement therapies has described some of the individuals who have made major contributions and whose students and teachers are scattered throughout the world. It is by no means a complete listing and has not included many established and new schools, each of which is making important practical contributions to healthcare. *The Encyclopedia of Energy Medicine* (Thomas, 2010) is a valuable resource for the field.

Massage has not been mentioned, specifically because there is no single individual we can credit with its invention. Massage has been the wellspring and inspiration for many of the therapies discussed here. The following is a partial listing of some other major contributors and the therapeutic techniques and schools they have established:

- Bonnie Bainbridge Cohen: Body-Mind Centering®
- George Roth: Matrix Repatterning
- John F. Barnes: Myofascial Release
- Herwig Schoen and Eric Pearl: Reconnective Therapy
- Risa Kaparo: Somatic Learning
- Ann and Chris Frederick: Stretch to Win

While this has been a chapter on history, it is by no means complete and up-to-date. Other major contributors will be described in the subsequent chapters. Many of them are inventors of breakthrough therapeutic devices and hands-on therapies.

References

Alexander, F.M., 1932. The Use of Self 1985 Edition. Orion Books Limited, London.

Burmeister, M., 1985. Jin Shin Jyutsu Is: Book 1 (Getting to Know Myself Art of Living), Book 2 (Cosmic Artless Art to Know Myself Physio-Philosophy: Nature – The Effortless).

Conrad, E., 2007. Life on Land: The Story of Continuum, The World-Renowned Self-Discovery and Movement Method. North Atlantic Books, Berkeley, CA.

Feitis, R., 1985. Ida Rolf Talks About Rolfing and Physical Reality. Bookslinger, Indianapolis, IN.

Feldenkrais, M., 1981. The Elusive Obvious. Meta Publications, Cupertino, CA, pp. 7–9.

Feldenkrais, M., 2002. The Potent Self: A Study of Spontaneity and Compulsion. Frog Publications, San Antonio, FL.

Hamwee, J., 2000. Zero Balancing: Touching the Energy of Bone. North Atlantic Books, Berkeley, CA.

Hover-Kramer, D., 2000. Healing Touch: A Guidebook for Practitioners. Delmar Publishers, Clifton Park, NY.

Jones, F.P., 1997. Freedom to Change: The Development and Science of the Alexander Technique. Mouritz, London.

Jones, F.P., 1999. In: Dimon, T., Brown, R. (Eds.), Collected Writings on the Alexander Technique. Alexander Technique Archives, Massachusetts.

Krieger, D., 1993. Accepting Your Power to Heal: The Personal Practice of Therapeutic Touch. Bear & Company, Rochester, VT.

Liskin, J., 1996. Moving Medicine: The Life and Work of Milton Trager, M.D. Station Hill Press, Barrytown, NY.

Mattes, A.L., 2000. Active Isolated Stretching: The Mattes Method. Aaron Mattes Therapy, Sarasota, FL.

Rolf, I.P., 1977. Rolfing: The Integration of Human Structures. Harper and Row Publishers, New York.

Smith, F.F., 1986. Inner Bridges: A Guide to Energy Movement and Body Structure. Humanics Ltd Partners, Internet Archive, San Francisco, California.

Smith, F.F., 2005. The Alchemy of Touch: Moving Towards Mastery Through the Lens of Zero Balancing. Complementary Medicine Press, Taos, NM.

Thomas, L., 2010. The Encyclopedia of Energy Medicine. Fairview Press, Minneapolis, MN.

Upledger, J.E., 1987. CranioSacral Therapy II – Beyond the Dura. Eastland Press, Seattle, WA.

Upledger, J., 1997. Your Inner Physician and You. North Atlantic Books, Berkeley, CA.

Upledger, J., 2002. SomatoEmotional Release. North Atlantic Books, Berkeley, CA.

Upledger, J.E., Vredevoogd, J., 1983. CranioSacral Therapy. Eastland Press, Seattle, WA.

Veltheim, J., 1999. The Body Talk System: The Missing Link to Optimum Health. PaRama, LLC.

Wilks, J., 2007. The Bowen Technique: The Inside Story. Butler & Tanner, Somerset, UK.

Wordsworth, C.F., Glanville, G.N., 2007. Quantum Change Made Easy. Resonance Publishing, Phoenix, AZ.

CHAPTER 8

Measuring the Fields of Life

Something deeply hidden has to be behind things.

Albert Einstein (while playing with a compass his father had given him)

Chapter Summary

In the current era of rapid scientific progress, many of the concepts we were absolutely certain about 20 years ago are no longer true at all. But of all the tales of exploration and discovery that could be told, none is more fascinating and important than the story of the human energy field. In a few decades scientists have gone from a conviction that energy fields in and around the human body are science fiction to an absolute certainty that they exist. Consequently, biomedical researchers are beginning to explore the discoveries of practitioners of energy methods. These are individuals who have felt and manipulated energy fields for healing purposes for centuries but who have usually been disparaged and disregarded by conventional medical practitioners. The synthesis of ancient wisdom and modern research benefits everyone, particularly those who have injuries or diseases that are difficult to treat with conventional techniques but appear to respond well, and quickly, to energetic therapies.

Medical interest has focused on the *magnetic* fields around the body, which are now referred to as *biomagnetic* fields. Interest in biomagnetism has spread widely in the biomedical research community. We know a lot about electricity and magnetism from more than 180 years of research in physics, beginning with famous discoveries of Ørsted (or Oersted), Ampère, and Faraday that were described in Chapters 2 and 3. Einthoven's discovery of the electric field of the heart, and his invention of the electrocardiogram, established the heart as a source of a large electric field. Electric fields from other organs are used for diagnosis. These include the electroencephalogram, the electromyogram, and the electrooculogram. Ørsted and Ampère showed that when an electric current flows, a magnetic field arises in the surrounding space. Hence each of the electrical systems just mentioned has a corresponding magnetic field that is also measurable (the magnetocardiogram, magnetoencephalogram (MEG), and magnetoretinogram, respectively). The roles of other fields, including light, heat, gravity, kinetic energy, and sound will be taken up in later chapters.

Heart Electricity

Our story begins with the investigation of bioelectricity, for it is from electric currents that magnetic fields arise. If you do not understand electricity and magnetism, you have the company of the leading physicists in history. For example, we recognize different forms of energy, such as electricity, magnetism, heat, light, electromagnetism, kinetic energy of motion, sound, gravity, vibration, elastic energy, etc. But there must be some fundamental principle that underlies these different forms of energy. Albert Einstein spent the last decades of his life in an unsuccessful search for a 'common denominator', or the 'something deeply hidden' that has to be behind the various forms of energy: a unifying field. At a fundamental level, we still do not know exactly what electricity and magnetism really are. The electron is a basic unit of matter and has properties such as charge, mass, spin, and gravity, but a deeper explanation of how these properties arise is missing. G. Johnstone Stoney coined the term *electron* in 1894. The name comes from the Greek word for amber, ήλεκτρον. The electron is the unit of charge in electrochemistry. Valuable perspectives on this problem have been published by Day (1989, 1996), Wolff (1993, 1997), and Panvini and Weiler (1998).

About a hundred years ago a Dutch physician, Willem Einthoven, discovered that electricity produced by the heart could be routinely recorded with a very sensitive galvanometer (Einthoven, 1906). Einthoven received a Nobel Prize in 1924 for this discovery. His method has been improved to the point that the electrocardiogram is a standard tool for medical diagnosis. Every physician has prepared and interpreted electrocardiograms.

We now know that each heartbeat begins with a pulse of electricity through the heart muscle. This electricity arises because a large number of charged particles (ions of sodium, potassium, chloride, calcium, and magnesium) flow across the muscle membranes to excite contraction. These currents also spread out into surrounding tissues and to the skin surface, where they can be detected with the appropriate instruments.

Some of the flow of current from the heart is through the circulatory system, which is an excellent conductor of electricity because of its high content of ions that can carry charge. Just as the circulation carries blood to every tissue, the circulatory system carries the heart's electricity everywhere in the body. Hence the electrocardiogram can be picked up anywhere on the skin, even from the toes. Einthoven discovered that if there is a problem in the functioning of part of the heart, the electrocardiogram will be distorted in a characteristic manner. This important discovery has been repeatedly confirmed and is an essential part of cardiology. The enigma is that Einthoven as well as most modern cardiologists was certain that the heart's electrical field is a by-product, almost a waste product, of the heart's activities and has no significant physiological role except as a diagnostic tool. However, there are alternative interpretations that will be discussed in Chapter 15. Specifically, the heart produces a mixture of pulses of electricity, magnetism, sound, heat, vibration, and light that are transmitted to every part of the body via the circulatory system and extracellular fluids and thereby reach every cell in the body (see Figure 15.6). These signals may serve a variety of vital regulatory roles.

Magnetism from Electricity

It is a basic law in physics that when an electric current flows through a conductor, a magnetic field is created in the surrounding space. This profoundly important phenomenon was discovered by accident by Hans Christian Ørsted (Figure 2.4) during a physics lecture he was giving in Copenhagen in 1820. Many of our modern electrical appliances and conveniences, from telephones to elevators, are consequences of Ørsted's discovery.

Heart Magnetism

On the basis of Ørsted's discovery, some scientists predicted that the heart's electricity must create a magnetic field, but it was not until 1963 that anyone was able to detect it. In that year, Baule and McFee (1963), from the electrical engineering department of Syracuse University in New York, used a pair of 2 million-turn coils near the chest to detect the magnetic field produced by the electrical activity of the heart muscle (Figure 8.1). The coils were wound on dumbbell-shaped cores composed of a magnetic material called ferrite. Baule and McFee chose the heart for study because it produces the strongest electrical and magnetic activity of any tissue in the body. Even so, they had to do their initial studies in a cornfield, as far away as possible from sources of electromagnetic noise. The fact that the functioning heart produces a strong pulsating magnetic field, spreading out in front of and behind the body, is important in itself and is discussed in more detail later.

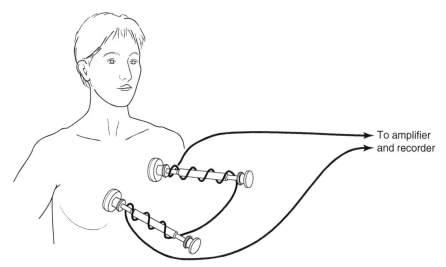

Figure 8.1   Setup used by Baule and McFee (1963) to detect the magnetic field of the heart. The two coils each have 2 million turns of wire wound around dumbbell-shaped cores of a magnetic material called ferrite. The wires go to an amplifier and recording system. The heart's field is about one-millionth that of the Earth's. *(Adapted from Baule, G.M., McFee, R., 1963. Detection of the magnetic field of the heart. Am. Heart J. 66, 95–96.)*

One of the academic questions created by the discovery of the heart's magnetic field is the location of the boundary between the organism and its environment.

The recent results indicating an intimate spatiotemporal relationship of living things to their planetary field have raised to a significance the long-time academic problem concerning the limits of the individual organism, whether at the structural surface of the body or out in the area encompassed by the physical fields generated by the individual. The answer may be very different for the anatomist, on the one hand, and the physiologist, behaviorist and psychologist, on the other. The life of the individual organism cannot be fully described by its organized aggregate of molecules, nor can at this level the powerful tools and concepts of modern physics be brought to bear on it. Rather it must be supplemented by the dynamic fields that are metabolically generated in the organism operating as a bioelectronic entity, and which continuously and mutually interacts with the counterpart fields of its ambient physical surroundings. The organism can only arbitrarily be defined as separate. The organism and the physical environment are mutually invasive.

FRANK A. BROWN, JR, 1980

In the past, we could define an individual as that which lies within the skin, but it is a fact of physics that energy fields are unbounded. The biomagnetic field of the heart extends indefinitely into space. Every heartbeat produces an electromagnetic field that propagates into space at the speed of light, 186,000 miles per second. While its strength diminishes with distance, there is no point at which we can say the field ends. In practice, the field gets weaker and weaker until it becomes undetectable in the noise produced by other fields in the environment; but scientists are constantly developing tricks to make their instruments more sensitive and to separate signals from noise.

A QUANTUM BREAKTHROUGH

Baule and McFee (1963) predicted that the heart should produce magnetic fields, and they went to a lot of trouble to detect those fields. This was a definite breakthrough, but what happened next was even more significant. A discovery in quantum physics led to the development of instruments that can map the energy fields of the human body with unprecedented sensitivity and accuracy. For example, there are devices that can pick up the field of the heart 15 feet away from the body.

In the same year as the article by Baule and McFee was published, a number of scientists (Anderson and Rowell, 1963; Shapiro, 1963) showed that something that seems impossible could actually happen. The seemingly impossible process was the movement of pairs of electrons through a material (called an insulator) that, according to classical physics, the electrons should not be able to penetrate. The phenomenon is called tunnelling and is something that is forbidden in the classical world, the world we are familiar with, but is readily explained in the quantum realm. The reason for this difference is that in the quantum world, classical *particles* such as electrons are at the same time *waves,* and waves can do tricks that solid particles cannot do.

Several kinds of tunnelling can take place, called Josephson effects, named after an English physicist, Brian Josephson, who predicted them in 1962 while he was a graduate student at the University of Cambridge (Josephson, 1962, 1965; Langenberg et al., 1966). In 1973, Josephson received a Nobel Prize for his work, which has had many practical applications and has led to the development of important new technologies.

THE SQUID MAGNETOMETER

If a thin insulating barrier is placed between two superconductors (such as two metals cooled in liquid helium), a supercurrent consisting of pairs of electrons will flow across the barrier. Josephson effects are utilized in electronic devices and ultra-fast computers. But for us the most exciting application is in the SQUID (an acronym for superconducting quantum interference device). A SQUID consists of one or more Josephson junctions immersed in liquid helium. The device was developed by J. E. Zimmerman and his colleagues (Zimmerman, 1972; Zimmerman et al., 1970). Under the appropriate conditions, the properties of the Josephson junction become exceedingly sensitive to ambient magnetic fields. Specifically, the tunnelling current is proportional to the strength of the magnetic field. Figure 8.2 shows the design of a SQUID magnetometer of the kind used to study biomagnetic fields. Figure 8.3 shows that the strength of the magnetic field in the center of the coil is converted into a measurable voltage across the junctions.

SQUIDs and arrays of SQUIDs are now being used in medical research laboratories around the world to map the biomagnetic fields produced by physiological processes inside the human body. A global network of SQUIDs is also being used to monitor moment-to-moment fluctuations in the geomagnetic field of the Earth.

Magnetocardiography

The first biological application of the SQUID took place inside a heavily shielded room at Massachusetts Institute of Technology's (MIT's) Francis Bitter National Magnet Laboratory in Cambridge, Massachusetts. The shielding was essential because the heart's field is one-millionth of the Earth's magnetic field and one-thousandth of the varying background magnetic field in an urban environment.

Cohen and his colleagues (Cohen, 1967; Cohen et al., 1970) described the heart's magnetic field with more clarity and sensitivity than ever before. Their work laid the foundation for a whole new field of diagnostics, magnetocardiography, and marked the beginning of the study of biomagnetism. Figure 8.4 shows a recording of the magnetocardiogram, with a standard electrocardiogram from skin electrodes beside it for comparison. The magnetocardiogram has many advantages compared with the electrocardiogram. It is a noninvasive and noncontact technology.

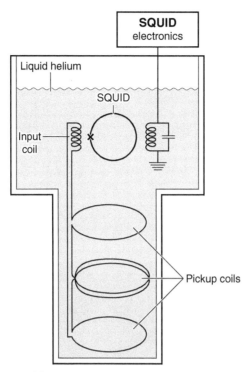

Figure 8.2 Basic design of the SQUID magnetometer used to detect, measure and map biomagnetic fields around the human body. The biomagnetic field induces a current flow in the pickup coils. Design of the pickup coils is such that noise signals from the environment are cancelled. The input coil influences the Josephson junctions in the SQUID proper, and changes in the properties of the junctions are sensed by another circuit that is connected to various amplifiers and filters of the SQUID electronics. The coils and the Josephson junctions are immersed in liquid helium to maintain the superconducting state. *(Adapted from Kaufman, L., Okada, Y., Tripp, J., et al, 1984. Evoked neuromagnetic fields, Ann. NY Acad. Sci. 425:722–742.)* The Josephson junctions are detailed in the next illustration.

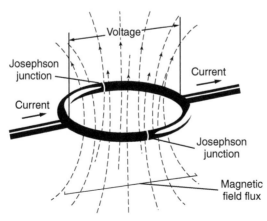

Figure 8.3 Detail of the magnetic sensor using Josephson junctions. The strength of the magnetic field in the center of the coil is converted into a measurable voltage across the junctions.

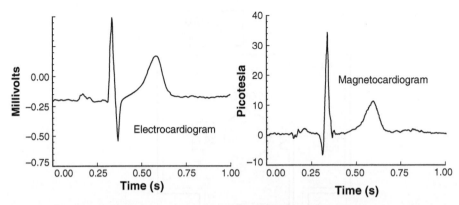

Figure 8.4 Recordings of the heart's electric field or electrocardiogram (left) and the corresponding magnetic field or magnetocardiogram (right). *(After Brockmeier et al., 1995, with kind permission from Dr Konrad Brockmeier and Elsevier Science, IOS Press.)*

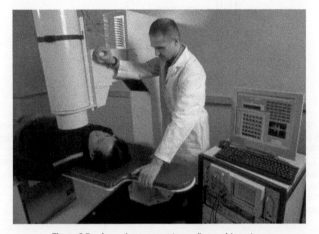

Figure 8.5 A modern magnetocardiographic setup.

It has much higher spatial resolution than the electrocardiogram. The patient can be clothed, and excellent evaluations of the heart can be made under conditions where it is difficult to attach electrodes to the chest, as with patients with skin problems, chest injuries, or burns, for example. Modern magnetocardiograms are being used by doctors to assess cardiac functioning, risk of sudden cardiac death, enlargement of the heart, risk of rejection of a heart transplant, and the effectiveness of various heart medications. Magnetocardiography can be substituted for stress tests when they are contraindicated. Figure 8.5 shows a modern magnetocardiogram setup.

Recent research indicates that the combined use of the electrocardiogram and the magnetocardiogram, called electromagnetocardiogram, can produce significant improvements in cardiac diagnosis (Malmivuo, 2004).

Brain Electricity and Magnetism

A few years after Einthoven received his Nobel Prize for the discovery of heart electricity, Hans Berger (1929) announced that much smaller electric fields could also be recorded from the brain, using electrodes attached to the scalp. His apparatus is shown in Figure 8.6A and some of the

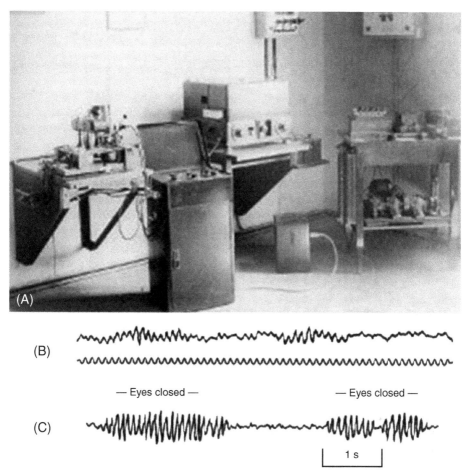

Figure 8.6 Electroencephalograms. (A) Apparatus used by Hans Berger to record electrical brain waves. (B) The first published electroencephalogram of a human being. The recording was made in 1926, but was not published until 1929. The lower line is a time pulse at 10 cycles per second (Berger, 1929). (C) The alpha rhythm of the human electroencephalogram. The alpha waves are much easier to observe when the eyes are closed (after Adrian and Matthews, 1934). Cohen (1972) found that the magnetoencephalograms recorded with a SQUID magnetometer are similar to electrical recordings such as these. *(A, Photo Deutsches Museum.)*

original recordings, dating from July 6, 1924, are shown in Figure 8.6B. A few years later, Lord Adrian and Sir Brian Matthews were able to show that the alpha rhythm of the human electroencephalogram is easy to record when the eyes are closed (Figure 8.6C). For his work on the functions of neurons, Adrian was awarded, jointly with Sir Charles Sherrington, the Nobel Prize in Physiology or Medicine in 1932. With some refinements, the recordings, which came to be known as electroencephalograms (EEGs), became a standard diagnostic method in neurology. Today the EEG is used in the clinical diagnosis of serious head injuries, brain tumors, cerebral infections, epilepsy, and various degenerative diseases of the nervous system. Berger became known as the 'Father of Electroencephalography'.

In 1972, Cohen was able to extend his SQUID measurements to the fields produced by the brain. The setup is shown in Figure 8.7. The MIT shielded room had the shape of a rhombicuboctrahedron. Five layers of shielding were necessary. Three were high-μ and two

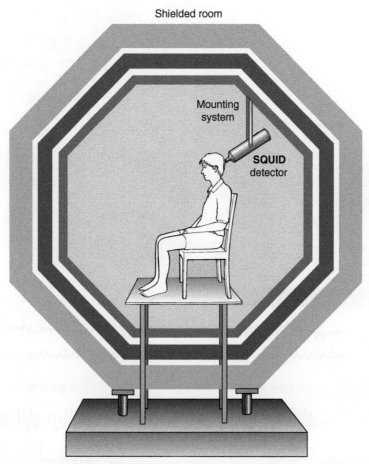

Figure 8.7 Shielded room used for studying the magnetic field of the brain. The SQUID detector is positioned close to but not touching the subject's head. Clothing must be free of magnetic material, such as zippers or nails in shoes. Shielded rooms such as this were manufactured by Takenaka Corporation. *(Illustration redrawn from Takenaka website: http://www.takenaka.co.jp/takenaka_e/techno/19_sldrm/19..sldrm.htm and used by kind permission of Nodoru Uenishi, Takenaka Corporation, New York.)*

were aluminum. (μ, the Greek letter mu, refers Mu-metal, which is a nickel–iron alloy (75% nickel, 15% iron, plus copper and molybdenum) that has very high magnetic permeability, making it very effective at screening static or low-frequency magnetic fields, which cannot be attenuated by other methods).

The brain fields are hundreds of times weaker than the heart's field, and a lot of tinkering and adjusting and engineering went into redesigning the SQUID so that it could detect these minute fields. The result was the first-ever recording of the biomagnetic field of the brain. These developments led to whole new fields in biomedicine, magnetoencephalography, and neuromagnetic imaging.

Because the first measurements were technically difficult to accomplish, the focus was on the alpha rhythm, which is a strong component of the brain waves. It is much easier to demonstrate strong alpha rhythms when the eyes are closed (Figure 8.6C). In later chapters we will return to the possible role of the alpha rhythm in healing.

Weak Versus Strong Fields

When Einthoven discovered the electric field of the heart, it was an extremely weak field and very difficult to measure. Because of progress in instrumentation, we now recognize that the heart produces the strongest field in the body. In comparison to the heart fields, the fields of the brain are weak. However, neural activities are involved in movements, thoughts and attitudes about ourselves and intentions, and therefore enable us to do everything we do. Hence 'strong versus weak' is more a statement about measuring instruments than about the biological importance of the different fields.

Measurement of the biomagnetic fields of the heart and brain led to a veritable explosion of research into biomagnetics. SQUID instruments became available commercially from more than a dozen manufacturers. These instruments are being used in medical research laboratories all over the world to explore aspects of the biological fields that scientists were certain did not exist a few decades ago (for reviews, see Hamaläinen et al., 1993; Koch, 2004). Some of the exciting work involves using arrays of SQUID detectors that can produce three-dimensional maps of the fields around the body. An early version of this instrumentation is shown in Figure 8.8 and more recent version in Figure 8.9.

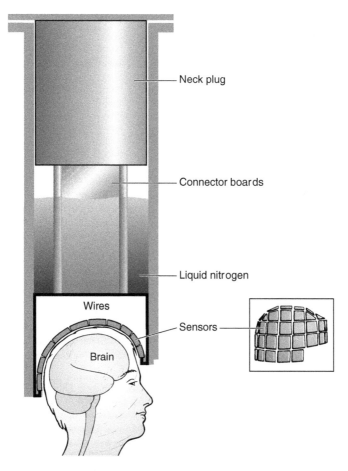

Figure 8.8 The 122-channel SQUID, "Neuromag-122" built in Helsinki, Finland. The sensors are wrapped around the head as shown. *After Hämäläinen et al., 1993, Fig. 41, p. 467, with permission from Reviews of Modern Physics and Dr. Risto Ilmoniemi.*

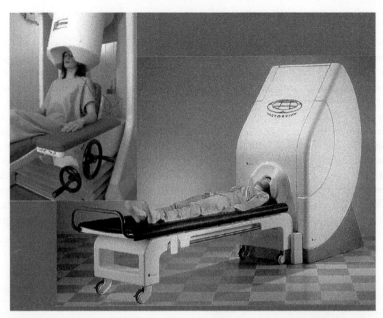

Figure 8.9   Modern magnetoencephalogram or neuromagnetic imager from Vectorview. *(Courtesy The Mind Research Network, Albuquerque, New Mexico).*

It turns out that biomagnetic fields are often better indicators of events taking place within the body than are electrical measurements at the skin surface. For example, biomagnetic fields produced by the brain pass undistorted through the cerebrospinal fluid, across the connective tissue covering of the brain (the dura), and through the skull bones and scalp. These tissues are virtually transparent to magnetic fields. In contrast, the electrical signals recorded with the electroencephalogram become distorted, smeared, and decreased in strength by a factor of about 10,000 as they pass through the surrounding tissues. EEGs therefore do not give as precise a representation of brain activity as MEGs. Electrical measurements are also compromised by intricate interactions between the skin and the electrode pickups, which can act as batteries and generate currents on their own. All in all, the MEG appears to provide more detail and better spatial localization than the EEG. The same advantages pertain to the magnetocardiogram.

Scientists realized that all of the classical electrical diagnostic tools have biomagnetic equivalents. For example, the eye acts as a battery and produces a substantial electrical field whose intensity depends on the amount of light falling on the retina. Records of this field are called electroretinograms. The magnetoretinogram is the corresponding record of the retina's biomagnetic field, detected in the space around the head.

Contractions of other muscles besides the heart produce electrical fields that are recorded by electromyography. The corresponding magnetic recordings are called magnetomyograms. Every muscle in the body produces magnetic pulses when it contracts. The larger muscles produce larger fields and the smaller muscles, such as those that move and focus the eyes, produce very tiny fields. This fact may be of interest to movement therapists, because we now know that any movement of any part of the body is 'broadcast' into the space around the body as a precise 'biomagnetic signature' of that movement. The relative strengths of the various biomagnetic fields produced by the human body are shown in Figure 8.10.

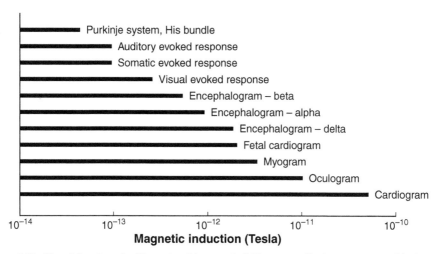

Figure 8.10   The relative strength of the various biomagnetic fields measured in the spaces around the human body. (Based on data presented in Figure 1 of Williamson & Kaufman 1981).

Effects of Practice on Brain Waves

An example of an interesting study using the multi-channel SQUID shown in Figure 8.8 is an investigation of the magnetic brain waves of musicians such as violinists and other string players (Elbert et al., 1995). It is known that the ways the body is used lead to corresponding alterations in the organization of the nervous system. Increased use of a part of the body results in enlargements in the representation of those parts in the motor and sensory portions of the cortex (Jenkins et al., 1990; Recanzone et al., 1992). This is referred to as cortical reorganization, or the recruitment of neurons into areas related to particular sensory and/or motor tasks. Practicing and performing with string and possibly other kinds of instruments involves considerable manual dexterity and sensory processing, particularly in fingering with the left hand. In comparison, the thumb of the left hand grasps the neck of the instrument. While the position and pressure of the thumb are frequently shifted, far less dexterity is required. And the tasks of the right hand, which manipulates the bow, also involve fewer precise finger movements. The hypothesis tested by Elbert and colleagues was that repeated and intense use of the fingers of the left hand, over years of practice, would increase the number of neurons and the size of the brain areas involved in movements and sensation of those fingers. Six violinists, two cellists, and a guitarist were studied. Six non-musicians served as controls.

Using an array of SQUID detectors such as the one shown in Figure 8.8, the investigators were able to map the surface or cortex of the brain and show that the biomagnetic fields produced by specific cortical regions were more intense in string musicians compared to non-performers. There was also a correlation between the number of years of practice and the intensity of the brain waves from the areas controlling skilled fingers. The number of nerve cells involved in controlling and sensing movement seems to increase with practice, as indicated by the biomagnetic output of the corresponding regions of the brain (Figure 8.11).

This is one of many studies completed or in progress that are enabling scientists to map the biomagnetic fields of the human body on a moment-to-moment basis and to determine how biofields correlate with physiological processes, behaviour, and human performance. To get an indication of what a rich and fascinating field this has become, look at the proceedings of the international Biomag conferences that have been held every 2 years since 1976.

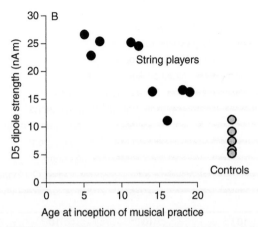

Figure 8.11   Elbert et al. (1995) measured the brain magnetic fields of string musicians with varying degrees of practice. Practice in fingering the instruments is correlated with a strong brain field, particularly for those cortical regions associated with moving and sensing with the fingers of the left hand.

HYPOTHESIS

It would obviously be fascinating to know if repeatedly practicing 'hands-on' methods – massage, Rolfing® or Structural Integration, Trager, reflexology, acupuncture, shiatsu, QiGong, cranial sacral, etc. – enhances the biomagnetic output from related areas of the brain, corresponding to increases the skill and sensitivity of touch, as practicing with a musical instrument does. Another hypothesis worthy of testing is that repeated practice of 'hands-off' methods, such as those that are often used in Reiki, Therapeutic Touch, Healing Touch, Polarity Therapy, and Aura Balancing, will also increase the biomagnetic output and sensitivity of the hands of the practitioners. Research of this kind could help us understand how the experienced energy therapist is both able to sense subtle aspects of a patient's biofield and is also able to project appropriate energies into injured or painful tissues to initiate a beneficial change.

The brain field, like the heart field, is not confined to the organ that produces it. We refer to 'brain waves' as though they are located in the brain, but they are not. The fields of all of the organs spread throughout the body and into the space around it. This was mentioned in Chapter 5 in relation to the sensing of the rhythms of the ovary (page 73). One of the primary channels for the flow of electrical waves through the body is the circulatory system. So, one could hypothesize that repeatedly practicing 'hands-on' work can also affect the biomagnetic output from a therapist's fingers and hands and the sophistication of their sensory perception via touch. In other words, *all* forms of therapeutic contact may involve far more than simple pressure on the skin.

Biomagnetic Fields and Senses

From the research done over the last few decades, we can definitely conclude that:

- Living organisms have biomagnetic fields around them.
- These fields change from moment to moment in relation to events taking place inside the body.
- The information contained in the biomagnetic fields give a more detailed representation of what is going on in the body than classical electrical diagnostic tools such as the electrocardiogram and the electroencephalogram.
- It can reasonably be hypothesized that the biofield is used as a fast communication system, assisting in integrating the body's diverse functions, although there is no objective evidence for this.

This should not be taken to suggest that the 'fields of life' are entirely magnetic. Other kinds of fields are also present (see Chapter 1).

It is one thing to say that the biofields accurately represent events taking place inside the body, and another for a person to claim he or she can see or feel those fields. However, it has now been predicted and shown that Josephson effects, the basis for the SQUID magnetic detector, also exist in living tissues (Del Giudice et al., 1989). This discovery provides a scientific basis for reports from energy therapists that they can not only sense the energy field of a patient, they can also use their senses to detect the parts of the body that are injured or painful.

There is an old idea that our technology recapitulates our biology – that all of our technological devices were first invented and perfected during millions of years of evolutionary experimentation with the laws and energies of nature. Perhaps there is a magnetic sense in the human body, a sense that can be developed and used in healing. From the information summarized in this chapter, and from the repeated experiences of a variety of energy therapists, this is not a preposterous idea.

We shall explore the application of biomagnetism in Polarity Therapy and related methods in subsequent chapters. First, though, we need to examine the circuits through which energy moves in the body and the kinds of energy that are involved.

References

Adrian, E.D., Matthews, B.H.C., 1934. The detection of the Berger rhythm: potential changes from the occipital lobes in man. Brain 57 (4), 24–385.

Anderson, P.W., Rowell, J.M., 1963. Probable observation of the Josephson superconducting tunneling effect. Phys. Rev. Lett. 10, 230–232.

Baule, G.M., McFee, R., 1963. Detection of the magnetic field of the heart. Am. Heart J. 66, 95–96.

Berger, H., 1929. Uber das Elektrenkephalogramm des Menschen. Archiv fur Psykchiatrica 87, 527–570.

Brockmeier, K., Burghoff, M., Koch, H., Schmitz, L., Zimmerman, R., 1995. ST segment changes in a healthy subject during pharmacological stress test using magnetocardiographic and electrocardiographic multi-channel recordings. In: Baumgartner, C., Deecke, L., Stroink, G., Williamson, S.J. (Eds.), Biomagnetism: Fundamental Research and Clinical Applications. Proceedings of the 9th International Conference on Biomagnetism. In: Studies in Applied Electromagnetics and Mechanics, Vol. 7. Elsevier Science, IOS Press, Amsterdam, pp. 633–636.

Brown, F.A. Jr, 1980. Free-running rhythms and biological clocks. A 1980 perspective. Unpublished manuscript.

Cohen, D., 1967. Magnetic fields around the torso: production by electrical activity of the human heart. Science 156, 652–654.

Cohen, D., 1972. Magnetoencephalography: detection of the brain's electrical activity with a superconducting magnetometer. Science 175, 664–666.

Cohen, D., Edelsack, E.A., Zimmerman, J.E., 1970. Magnetocardiograms taken inside a shielded room with a superconducting point-contact magnetometer. Appl. Phys. Lett. 16, 278–280.

Day, W., 1989. Bridge from Nowhere: A Story of Space, Motion, and the Structure of Matter. House of Tabs, East Lansing, MI.

Day, W., 1996. Bridge from Nowhere II. Rhombics Press, Cambridge, MA.

Del Giudice, E., Doglia, S., Milani, M., Smith, C.W., Vitiello, G., 1989. Magnetic flux quantization and Josephson behaviour in living systems. Phys. Scr. 40, 786–791.

Einthoven, W., 1906. Le telecardiogramme. Arch. Int. Physiol. 4, 132–164.

Elbert, T., Pantev, C., Weinbruch, C., Rockstroh, B., Taub, E., 1995. Increased cortical representation of the fingers of the left hand in string players. Science 270, 305–307.

Hamaläinen, M., Han, R., Ilmoniemi, R.J., Knuutila, J., Lounasmaa, O.V., 1993. Magnetoencephalography: theory, instrumentation, and applications to noninvasive studies of the working human brain. Rev. Mod. Phys. 65, 413–497.

Jenkins, W.M., Merzenich, M.M., Ochs, M.T., Allard, T., Guíc-Robles E., 1990. Functional reorganization of primary somatosensory cortex in adult owl monkeys after behaviorally controlled tactile stimulation. J Neurophysiol. 63 (1), 82–104.

Josephson, B.D., 1962. Possible new effects in superconductive tunneling. Phys. Lett. 1, 251–253.

Josephson, B.D., 1965. Supercurrents through barriers. Adv. Physiol. Educ. 14, 419–451.

Kaufman, L., Okada, Y., Tripp, J., Weinberg, H., 1984. Evoked neuromagnetic fields. Ann. N. Y. Acad. Sci. 425, 728.

Koch, H., 2004. Recent advances in magnetocardiography. J. Electrocardiol. 37, 117–122.

Langenberg, D.N., Scalapino, D.J., Taylor, B.N., 1966. The Josephson effects. Sci. Am. 214, 30–39.

Malmivuo, J.A., 2004. Bioelectromagnetism – relative merits of electric and magnetic measurements in cardiac studies. Conf. Proc. IEEE Eng. Med. Biol. Soc. 7, 5217.

Panvini, R.S., Weiler, T.J. (Eds.), 1998. Fundamental Particles and Interactions: Frontiers in Contemporary Physics: An International Lecture and Workshop Series at Vanderbilt University Nashville. American Institute of Physics Conference Proceedings, AIP Press, distributed by Springer, Secaucus, NJ.

Recanzone, G.H., Merzenich, M.M., Jenkins, W.M., Grajski, A., Dinse, H.R., 1992. Topographic reorganization of the hand representation in cortical area 3b owl monkeys trained in a frequency-discrimination task. J. Neurophysiol. 67 (5), 1031–1056.

Shapiro, S., 1963. Josephson currents in superconducting tunneling: the effect of microwaves and other observations. Phys. Rev. Lett. 11, 80–82.

Williamson, S.J., Kaufman, L., 1981. Biomagnetism. J. Magn. Magn. Mater. 22 (129–201), 132.

Wolff, M., 1993. Fundamental laws, microphysics, and cosmology. Phys. Essays 6, 181–203.

Wolff, M., 1997. Exploring the universe and the origin of its laws. Front. Perspect. 6 (2), 44–56.

Zimmerman, J.E., 1972. Josephson effect devices and low frequency field sensing. Cryogenics 12, 19–31.

Zimmerman, J.E., Thiene, P., Harding, J.T., 1970. Design and operation of stable rf-biased superconducting point-contact quantum devices, and a note on the properties of perfectly clean metal contacts. J. Appl. Phys. 41, 1572–1580.

CHAPTER 9

Regulatory Energetics

The transmission of excitation energies between molecules through electromagnetic coupling is not a mere matter of speculation.
Szent-Györgyi (1957)

Chapter Summary

In his lectures and conversations, Szent-Györgyi often stated that living processes are too rapid and subtle to be explained by slow moving nerve impulses and the random bumping about of molecules. If this is true, what kinds of communication and regulatory systems exist within the body that can operate faster than nerve impulses and chemical reactions? The question is significant because it relates to a wide variety of therapeutic approaches that seem to the well-educated observer to lie outside of conventional biomedicine. Is the problem with the therapies, or is the problem that normal science is missing something significant? This chapter will highlight a number of profoundly important phenomena that biomedical science does not delve into for historical reasons, with the result that a variety of potentially important communication mechanisms are not investigated. Moreover, various bodywork, energetic, and movement therapies have remained virtually incomprehensible to classically trained researchers and practitioners. However, this situation is changing.

A conclusion from extensive inquiry into complementary and alternative therapies and from basic biology is that each successful therapeutic approach works by interacting with one or more regulatory systems, and some of these have not been well characterized by conventional biomedicine. The result: Those steeped in the conventional paradigms are mystified by procedures that they cannot relate to on the basis of what they have learned. And what they have learned is not a complete picture. Energy medicine points toward a more complete picture.

In this chapter the vital issue of regulatory biology will be turned on its head: We will see that there are vast unknowns in the area of regulatory biology and regulatory biomedicine and that those who wish to explore the extremely important cutting edges of biological control processes will benefit immeasurably by studying methods that, at first sight, just don't seem to make sense on the basis of what we think we know.

Topics such as communication, control, regulation, coordination, integration, feedback, and energy flow are crucial to understanding living systems and the healing process. While much has been learned from the biochemical and molecular approaches, and there are many texts on these subjects, the conventional academic picture is very far from complete. A reason is that we are taught enough about different facets of regulation to get the impression that all of the problems have been solved. The problems have not been solved.

An Energetic Fabric

An intricate array of physiological processes is set in motion in response to any injury or disease. The body is designed to adjust extremely rapidly to changes in the environment and to cope with any damage or illness. These adjustments probably begin within an extremely short time period after a disturbance. This statement is founded on basic biology: Through an evolutionary process, living systems have taken advantage of, and made optimal use of, the various laws of physics and the various methods of regulation and control that are available to them. It is the body that is unable to adapt or the wound that does not heal on its own that presents the most common and significant challenge to any medical system. Failures in regulation simply mean that some of the vital communication processes are not functioning properly. The cells and systems 'know' what to do but are not doing what they were designed to do for some reason. One of the most important reasons is a breakdown in the communications and/or energy flows that are needed to maintain and restore wholeness. This book will explain precisely what we mean by wholeness, communications, and energy flows. In the past, these important terms have been used loosely and imprecisely, providing an opportunity for skeptics to dismiss them as insignificant. The study of energetics enables us to add scientific precision to the discussion. Hence, when we refer to energy flows, we need to define what kind of energy we are talking about and where and how it is flowing. By the time you have finished this book, you will have a detailed understanding of how at least some forms of energy move about within the body.

A universal teaching is that the nervous system is the master control and communication system in the body. Another class of widely studied regulatory mechanisms involves molecular messages: hormones, neurohormones, neurotransmitters, antigens, growth factors, cytokines, and intracellular messengers such as cyclic AMP and calcium. We shall see that Albert Szent-Györgyi was correct: There have to be additional communication and control systems that are just as important and vital as the nervous, hormonal, and second messenger systems. For example, a close look reveals that the nervous system actually plays only a small role in regulating the repair of an injury or in the body's response to a disease.

> *Much of the confusion that prevents physicians and other allopathic therapists from understanding complementary and alternative medicine arises because energy therapists have learned to work with vital communication and control systems that are not yet recognized by the prevailing medical paradigm, with its primary focus on nerves, biochemistry, and chemical messengers. As the energy story unfolds, we are acquiring valuable new information and concepts that cannot help but advance everyone's understanding of physiology and medicine and enhance the effectiveness and appreciation of all clinical approaches.*

Regulation Beyond Nerves and Chemical Messages

Albert Szent-Györgyi spent many years searching for the other systems in the living body that have to be present to account for life's speed and subtlety. To anticipate the material that will be presented in Chapter 11, Szent-Györgyi concluded that very small and highly mobile units such as electrons and protons have to be part of the picture of regulatory biology. He also recognized the importance of resonance and electromagnetic coupling between molecules (see his 1957 quote at the beginning of this chapter). A look at what we have been taught about regulations shows that something vital is missing from our conventional picture. For example, we are taught that living systems are regulated by a variety of types of messenger molecules such as hormones and growth factors. A fabric of diffusing regulatory molecules called cytokines regulates the response to injury. When these regulatory molecules reach a cell, they activate receptors on the cell surface that trigger other cascades of messages within the cell interior. These are called 'second messengers'. The scheme is illustrated in Figure 9.1.

> *Primary messengers such as hormones are viewed as being transported throughout the body via the circulatory system, and then through extracellular fluids by diffusion. Likewise, the second messengers are viewed as diffusing through the cell interior, which is viewed as a dilute solution. Both of these images are incomplete and inaccurate pictures of regulatory biology, and lead to much confusion.*

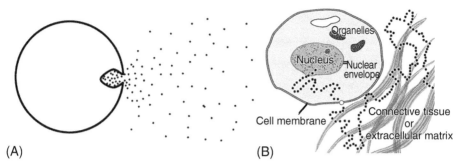

Figure 9.1 (A) The release of a signal molecule from a cell. Diffusion is generally in the direction of the concentration gradient. (B) The diffusion of a signal molecule to a receptor on the surface of a cell, followed by the diffusion of a second messenger within the cell to the site of action in the cell nucleus. These processes are far too slow to explain many aspects of life.

Diffusion of regulatory molecules is a relatively slow and random process because there is little motivation for molecular signals to move in any particular direction, i.e., toward or away from their respective receptors. The only directionality for diffusional processes is created by the gradient in concentration. Generally, the greater the difference in concentration, the faster diffusion takes place. And small molecules diffuse more rapidly than larger ones.

While molecules do tend to diffuse from regions of high concentration to regions of low concentration, statistically some molecules will move in the opposite direction. This means that when molecules are released from a source such as a secretory cell, as shown in Figure 9.1A, they tend to diffuse away in all directions. Their motions have little order to them; they bump and stagger about (Figure 9.2). Eventually signal molecules may encounter receptors on the surfaces of distant cells, activate the second messenger systems within the cells, and trigger changes in cell behaviour. Cellular processes are thought to be regulated up and down, depending on the concentration gradients of the messenger molecules. But there are profound problems with this picture.

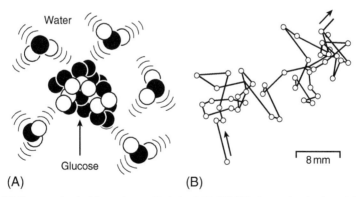

Figure 9.2 (A) Sugar molecule (glucose) magnified about 30,000,000 times, showing how it is jostled by the vibrating water molecules around it, drawn at about the same scale. The molecules are represented as 'space-filling' models, in which the atom is drawn as a sphere centred on the nucleus. Each sphere encloses a cloud of electrons. Space-filling models are useful because they show the effective size of the molecule, i.e., the approximate boundary through which other atoms cannot penetrate. (B) At body temperature, a sugar molecule travels more than 3 m/s, but it does not get far inside a cell because it keeps bumping into water and the other molecules around it. The jagged line represents the path taken by a single glucose molecule in a fraction of second.

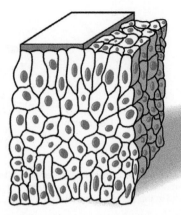

Figure 9.3 Cells in the body are generally packed closely together in layers called epithelia.

The basic fallacy of this scheme was summarized by Albrecht-Buehler (1990) in a valuable perspective entitled *In Defense of 'Nonmolecular' Cell Biology*. A key factor is that the cells in the body do not float about in a large volume of fluid. Instead, cells are packed close together within the various tissues. Many cells are organized into layers called epithelia. While some epithelia are only one cell thick, others consist of many cells packed closely together (Figure 9.3). If one considers the average fluid volume around an individual cell, the space available is such that a hormone with a concentration of $1\,pM$ (6×10^{11} molecules/l) will have a concentration of approximately eight molecules in the space surrounding an individual cell. In the region around the receptor, the hormone concentration, for all practical purposes, is approximately zero (Figure 9.4). Albrecht-Buehler (1990) concluded that our usual concept of concentration is essentially meaningless. The idea that hormones or other regulatory molecules can diffuse from some source, through the tissue fluids, to a receptor on the surface of a cell, and then activate a cellular process when the concentration of the regulatory molecule reaches a certain level, is highly improbable.

Moreover, the cell is often inaccurately viewed as a bag filled with a dilute solution of dissolved molecules. These molecules are also envisioned to diffuse about randomly until they have chance collisions with other molecules so that chemical reactions or regulatory interactions can take place. The problem with this model of the cell is that it is completely incorrect. Cells are not bags filled with dilute solutions of dissolved molecules. Cells are packed with filaments, fibres, tubules, and other organelles and other components that essentially fill the cytoplasm with barriers to molecular diffusion (see Chapter 11). Moreover, there is very little water available within cells that can act as solvent for the supposed dissolved molecules. A more realistic picture of the cell interior that is rarely, if ever, mentioned in basic texts of biology and medicine has been summarized in a review by Luby-Phelps (2000). Her conclusions:

- The cell interior is crowded, not dilute.
- Diffusion is restricted by binding and compartmentation.
- Enzymes are not dissolved but are organized into units.
- Most of the proteins are in solid form rather than dissolved.

This means that we must revise our perspectives on how intracellular 'second messenger' molecules move about within cells and how the various reactants involved in metabolism move about and interact with each other. When these revisions to our thinking are made, we will be better able to understand energy therapies, we will have new insights into regulatory biology, and we will expand our perspective of how quickly healing can take place.

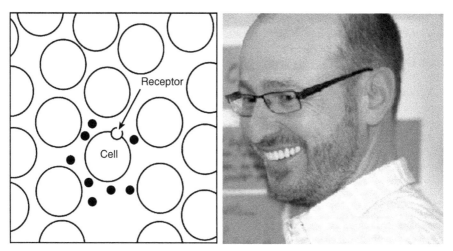

Figure 9.4 Albrecht-Buehler (1990) in a valuable perspective entitled *In Defense of 'Nonmolecular' Cell Biology* has raised a major argument against the view that regulations take place by diffusion of signal molecules to receptor sites on cells, where they activate cellular processes. While some epithelia are only one cell thick, others consist of many cells packed closely together (Figure 9.3). If one considers the average fluid volume around an individual cell, the actual space available is such that hormone molecules (black dots) with a concentration of 1 pM (6×10^{11} molecules/l) will have a concentration of approximately eight molecules in the space surrounding an individual cell. In the region around the receptor, the hormone concentration, for all practical purposes, is approximately zero. Albrecht-Buehler concluded that our usual concept of concentration is essentially meaningless.

To demonstrate the slowness of our conventional picture of regulation by diffusing signal molecules, consider what a pharmacologist would regard as a rapid reaction. Jump et al. (1984) demonstrated that the injection of a hormone produced by the thyroid gland, triiodothyronine (T3), at a dose sufficient to saturate all of the receptors throughout the body was followed within 20 min by a sharp increase in gene transcription, with levels rising about 10- to 15-fold above resting levels within 4 h. Other reactions can be even faster, with a lag time of less than 10 min (Narayan et al., 1984). While these reactions may seem rapid to a pharmacologist, in the scheme of regulatory processes that must adjust the body's physiology according to moment-to-moment changes in the environment, these are extremely slow reactions. They are suitable only for adjusting regulatory processes such as basal metabolic rate that vary relatively slowly. These are not the velocities of communication that would enable a quarterback to throw the pass that wins the Super Bowl. These are not the kinds of communications that enable a skater to perform a perfect triple axel that leads to a gold medal in the Olympics. And these are not the kinds of communications that enable us to respond quickly to an injury of any kind.

Other Models of Communication

The nervous system is capable of transmitting information at a variety of velocities, ranging from 0.5 to 120 m/s. Large nerve fibres are the fastest and can conduct an impulse the equivalent of the length of a football field in a second. While this may seem to be quite fast, conduction from one nerve to another involves synapses, and each of these introduces a delay of about 0.5 ms or 5 thousandths of a second.

Pressures for survival in predator-prey situations has driven the evolution of sensory-motor systems with extraordinary sensitivity and rapid responsiveness. These systems enable swift, precisely timed, incredibly coordinated and complex movements, such as those involved in peak dance or athletic performances or in the martial arts. Examples of performers operating in the state known as "the zone" are given in Murphy (1992), Oschman (2003) and Murphy and White (2012). Intricate neural processing is relatively slow, requiring signaling along many neurons and across many synapses. Other faster mechanisms must be involved. The visual system, for example, can require a quarter to half a second to deliver an image to the visual cortex (Jones, 2008; Nørretranders, 1991) though this is not how we perceive it. Nørretranders refers to an "illusion" created by adjusting the flows of sensory information so that we have a smoothly synchronized experience of the present moment of consciousness, even though the various sensory systems are transmitting information at different velocities. A related phenomenon is event-related desynchronization (ERD) discovered by Canadian neurophysiologists who reported that the normal sensori-motor brain rhythms recorded with electrodes touching the brain surface become desynchronized or blocked as much as 4 seconds before a movement (Jasper and Penfield, 1949). These temporal phenomena make it difficult to determine exactly how long it takes to process and react to a sensory input. Our experience is that we recognize familiar objects virtually instantaneously, but measuring the actual processing and response time is challenging. Reaction time is not a good measure as it includes both visual processing and neuromuscular responses.

Chapter 12 summarizes non-neural communication systems in the context of the unconscious mind and intuition. Some of these mechanisms operate much faster than nerves. A number of investigators have proposed electromagnetic or photonic communications, as Szent-Gyorgyi proposed in 1957 (see quote at the beginning of this chapter). A number of studies have demonstrated that cells can communicate with other cells that are physically separated by physical barriers that block chemical or electrical communications, as summarized by Prasad et al (2014) and Farhadi (2014). One study questioned the physical feasibility of electromagnetic communication between cells that lack bioluminescence (Kučera and Cifra, 2013). The conclusion was that the weak intensity of the emissions together with an unfavorable signal-to-noise ratio may rule-out photonic communication between cells. The authors of that report seem, however, to be unaware of recent research on biophotonics involving coherent biophoton emissions that are very much weaker than bioluminescence. Living cells amplify extremely weak electromagnetic fields and separate signals from large amounts of ambient noise. As mentioned in Chapter 3, scientists have been suspicious of reports that very tiny energy fields can have biological effects. It was generally accepted that extremely low energy photons, too weak to change the temperature within a cell, and therefore unable to affect cell chemistry, could not possibly have biological effects. Recent research has explained how this is possible. Pall (2013) summarized 23 studies demonstrating that voltage-gated calcium channels, which regulate a vast number of cellular processes, are activated virtually instantaneously by very weak photons. Pall's study marks a turning-point in "frequency medicine" involving the application of low-energy oscillating fields from medical devices, essential oils, botanical and homeopathic remedies, pharmaceuticals, the voice, and the human hand.

Lock and Key Model

The interaction of messengers with receptors, enzymes with substrates, and antibodies with antigens has been analogized with a simple lock and key model. The messenger is the key and the receptor is the lock (Figure 9.5A). Within the cell, the metabolic substrate (a term biochemists use to describe a molecule upon which an enzyme acts, such as glucose that is broken down in a metabolic pathway) is the key and the enzyme is the lock. Since everyone has used keys and locks, the image is easy to grasp. But images that are easy to grasp can be deceptive and can create the impression that a question has been completely answered, when there may be much more to the story.

Lock and key model

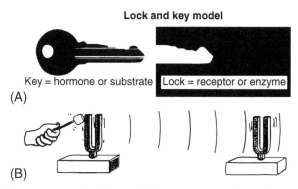

(A)

(B)

Figure 9.5 (A) The lock and key model used to describe hormone–receptor interactions or substrate–enzyme interactions. Since everyone has used keys and locks, the image is easy to grasp. But is it a complete and accurate image? Another method of molecular interaction that is seldom discussed involves electromagnetic resonance. (B) A musical analogy is provided by the 'tuning fork effect' in which the vibrations of one tuning fork causes another nearby tuning fork tuned to the same note to vibrate.

With the molecular lock and key model, we are dealing with things we cannot see because they are too small, so we have to infer the picture from various kinds of evidence obtained with molecular and biochemical techniques. We can isolate hormones and receptors, and we can isolate enzymes and substrates, for example, and we can determine that their molecular structures match in ways that allow them to fit together or bind to each other. But we must always remember that when we isolate the components of a living system we are no longer dealing with an intact system. And when we study the behaviour of the components in a certain way, other modes of behaviour become invisible. We always need to ask if the intact living system really behaves the way we think it does from study of the parts in isolation; we must always ask if our method of observation limits our perspectives on the process. The mature scientist knows the answers to these questions.

Random diffusion is far too slow and far too imprecise to regulate living processes in an orderly and timely manner. Diffusion of regulatory molecules and diffusion of metabolites within cells are processes that are too slow to allow the organism to adapt to rapid changes in its environment. If random diffusion is the mechanism involved in cellular metabolism, it would take about 10,000 years for you to digest your breakfast!

Spectroscopy: The Webwork of Molecular Electromagnetic Fields

There is a way for regulatory molecules to communicate without touching. Every object has a certain natural or resonant frequency. Strike it, bump it, pluck it, or heat it and it will tend to vibrate at a specific frequency. This applies to a bone, a piece of wood, a molecule, an atom, an electron, or a string on a musical instrument. When two objects have similar natural frequencies, they can interact without touching; their vibrations can become coupled or entrained. For electromagnetic interactions between molecules, the word 'resonance' is used more often than entrainment. In the older literature you will find the term 'sympathetic vibrations'.

At any temperature above absolute zero, molecules are vibrating intensely. Because molecules contain electrically charged atoms, their vibrations give rise to electromagnetic fields that can travel throughout the body. Recall Ampère's law from Chapter 2 and Maxwell's electromagnetism from Chapter 3. When charges move, magnetic fields are created in the surrounding region, and when charges oscillate, electromagnetic fields are produced that can travel considerable distances (e.g., Figure 3.4). There is no mystery here, because the emission of electromagnetic fields by vibrating molecules is the basis for spectroscopy, a well-established and highly refined technology that enables us to determine the detailed structure of atoms and molecules. Spectroscopy is so sophisticated that we know the wavelengths of the emission spectra of the various elements in nature to a hundredth of an Ångström, a unit of measure that represents one ten-millionth of a millimeter, or 1×10^{-10} m. These spectra can be found in some of the most widely accessed tables in the world, found in *The Handbook of Chemistry and Physics* (Haynes, 2014).

Not only does each vibrating molecule emit a characteristic set of electromagnetic frequencies, similar molecules a distance away will also absorb the same frequency from their environment. Such absorptions can be measured to provide an absorption spectrum. What is important for regulatory communications within an organism is that similarly shaped molecules will resonate with each other. The mechanical or musical analogy to this is called the tuning fork effect (Figure 9.5B).

The conventional model of regulations, with molecular signals diffusing from a source to a receptor, lacks an important feature: feedback. The cybernetic concept of regulatory systems (Wiener, 1948) suggests that ideal regulation involves a closed loop between the signal source and the receptor and back to the source, to inform the source that the message has been received. Resonant molecular information transfer has feedback built into it in the form of co-resonance. Albert Szent-Györgyi (1957) described it this way: "If two systems, capable of similar oscillation, are coupled, then they make 'coupled oscillators' and the oscillations will tend to pass back and forth between the two."

If you ask a chemist to identify an unknown material, the first step will be to obtain an absorption or emission spectrum of the substance and determine the molecular/atomic structure from the frequencies absorbed or emitted. Figure 9.6, for example, shows the emission spectrum of a fluorescent lamp. The many peaks identified on the spectrum are produced by the electromagnetic emissions from mercury. Spectroscopy is a fundamental tool in analytical chemistry and is also used by astronomers to determine the chemical composition of distant stars. Most large telescopes have spectrometers attached to them.

Spectroscopy provides much of the information we have on atomic and molecular behaviour. For a listing of books and review articles on this important subject, see Sauer (1995). Spectroscopy is possible because of the resonant interactions taking place in atoms and molecules.

Next we look at the kinds of motions taking place within and between molecules that make spectroscopy such a powerful tool. A molecule contains various charged components: protons, electrons, and side groups such as the amino acids shown in Figure 9.7. Each of these charges has an electric field around it. When a charge moves or rotates, the electric field moves or rotates, and this sets up electromagnetic fields that are radiated into the environment. The opposite is also true: Specific frequencies in the environment can be absorbed by a molecule, including movements of the component parts. Figure 9.7 shows the basic unit of the protein backbone, called a peptide group. These units are repeated again and again to create proteins of various sizes, shapes, and functions.

The carbon–nitrogen bond of the peptide group is rigid, while the adjacent bonds are essentially free to rotate (Pauling, 1960). This is important because it explains the flexibility of the protein backbone, which enables proteins to assume different shapes as they carry out their functions.

Computer simulation can be used to determine how proteins fold and twist as they perform their functions. The bonds between the atoms are treated as though they are springs. High-speed computers determine the forces acting on the parts. Beginning with the average 'ball-and-stick' structure, the computer calculates the bends and twists taking place from instant to instant as a result of the jiggling of surrounding molecules (inset, Figure 9.7).

Gilson and colleagues (1994) used computer molecular dynamics simulations to study important neurochemical reactions. They showed how acetylcholine gets to the active site deep within the acetylcholinesterase enzyme. The enzyme has a 'back door' with an electric field that attracts acetylcholine into the active site and then allows the products of the reaction, choline and acetate, to escape. The process is illustrated on the cover of the 4 March 1994 issue of *Science*.

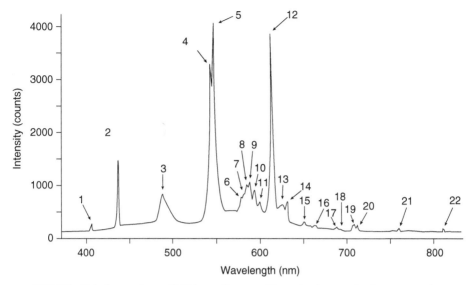

Figure 9.6 Emission spectrum of light from a fluorescent lamp showing prominent mercury peaks.

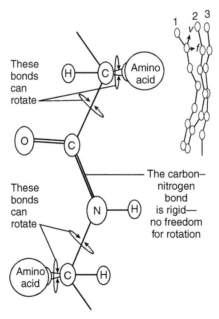

Figure 9.7 The basic unit of the protein backbone, the peptide group. These units are repeated again and again to create proteins of various sizes, shapes, and functions. The C–N bond of the peptide group is rigid, while the adjacent bonds can rotate (Pauling, 1960). Bending and rotation of these bonds allow the protein backbone to assume different shapes. The inset shows three successive shapes of a protein segment, as determined by molecular dynamics simulation, at 10^{-15}-s intervals. The computer determines shape changes on the basis of forces (f) and velocities (v) created by interactions with surrounding molecules. *(Inset after Karplus and McCammon (1986). The dynamics of proteins. Scientific American 254, 45, with permission from Scientific American.)*

Ball-and-stick images of molecules (such as those shown in Figure 9.7) create the false impression that the atoms within a molecule are fixed in position. Actually, such drawings show the average structure. In real life, molecules change their shapes extremely rapidly, with time intervals measured in trillionths of a second. This is shown in the inset of Figure 9.7.

A substance such as water, appearing colorless to the eye, absorbs strongly at a variety of frequencies that we cannot see. We shall see in chapter 15 how such absorptions may be involved in homeopathic and related vibrational medicines. Different kinds of motions taking place within molecules result in the emission or absorption of different types of energy fields as shown in Figure 9.8.

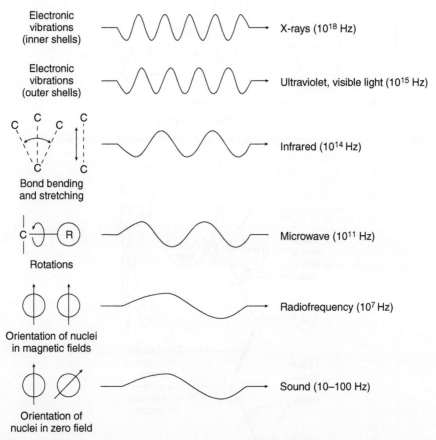

Figure 9.8 Movements within molecules and the kinds of electromagnetic fields they emit or absorb. The highest frequency and highest energy motions are those of the innermost electrons, which resonate in the X-ray region of the electromagnetic spectrum. The outermost electrons, which are responsible for most of the physical and chemical properties of an atom, resonate at the ultraviolet and visible portions of the spectrum. Bond bending and stretching involves infrared light. Bond rotations resonate at microwave frequencies. The spins and orientations of atomic nuclei correspond to vibrations in the radiofrequency and sound portions of the spectrum. Usually the frequencies absorbed by a molecule are identical with the frequencies emitted when the molecule is excited. This reciprocity of absorption and emission is known as Kirchhoff's principle. Energy is absorbed by the reverse of the process by which emissions are produced, i.e., the absorbed energy causes particular motions to be set up within the molecule. The boundaries between the different frequency regions are not sharply defined. The illustration is a simplification in that it does not show the couplings that take place between different activities, such as between vibrations and rotations. For more details, see a chart of the electromagnetic spectrum. *(Modified from Whiffen DH: Spectroscopy, John Wiley & Sons, 1966.)*

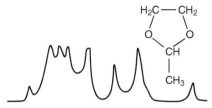

Figure 9.9   The infrared absorption spectrum of 2-methyl dioxolane and its molecular structure. *(From Whiffen DH: Spectroscopy, John Wiley & Sons, 1966.)*

Spectrometers of various kinds are used to measure the emissions and absorptions of molecules. Technically the radiation or absorption pattern is called a spectrum (a graph of energy intensity versus frequency or wavelength). Figure 9.9 shows a typical infrared absorption spectrum of a compound. Each peak represents a frequency that is absorbed by bending or stretching or rotation of a particular bond within the molecule.

Every molecule in the body, and the molecules in every homeopathic, herbal, or aromatherapy preparation, vibrate in specific ways and emit characteristic energy spectra. Complex molecules contain thousands or even millions of atoms, and their spectra can be quite intricate. The spectrum is an electromagnetic 'signature' or 'fingerprint' of a molecule that is an extremely precise representation of the motions of the particles within it. So characteristic are these fingerprints that a chemist can use them to identify an unknown substance.

In terms of vibrations, the human body can be compared to a symphony orchestra. Each molecule corresponds to a particular instrument. Each bend, rotation, or stretch of a chemical bond has a certain resonant frequency and will give off certain frequencies or 'notes' if it is energized. Since molecules, water, and dissolved ions are constantly bumping into each other at body temperature (Figure 9.2), all parts are constantly jiggling and absorbing and emitting characteristic frequencies.

While a chemical process, such as the breaking of a bond, may look superficially like a mechanical event, at a deeper level the event is better described as a series of vibratory energetic interactions. This is one level at which the various energy therapies may have their effects.

A soprano shatters a crystal goblet by singing a high note coinciding with the natural frequency of the goblet. The atoms in the glass vibrate so strongly that they cannot hold together, and the goblet breaks. The same thing can happen to a molecule. Figure 9.10 shows a molecule of hydrogen peroxide, H_2O_2, being fractured by vibrations. Sometimes this is called 'molecular surgery'.

The oxygen–oxygen (O–O) bond of hydrogen peroxide is broken selectively with an electromagnetic field of a specific frequency. The wavy arrow in the drawing represents a photon of laser light that energizes the O–H bond (i.e., it makes the bond vibrate violently) just as a tuning fork vibrates when you strike it. The vibrations are rapidly conducted or redistributed throughout the molecule, and the O–O bond, which is weaker than the O–H bond, breaks.

'Molecular surgery' of this kind is important to bodywork because it provides a biophysical basis for controversial vibrational therapies in which toxins, such as agent orange or DDT, which have been stored in the body, can be broken apart by energy fields emitted by the hands, the voice, oscillating microcurrents, musical instruments, or by crystals. When such a complex molecule is 'shattered' by vibrations, its fragments can be detoxified and excreted from the body.

Vibratory Interactions Between Molecules

Molecules and their vibrations orchestrate all living processes. Every event taking place within the body involves molecules performing tasks on other molecules. Regardless of technique or philosophy, all healing affects molecules.

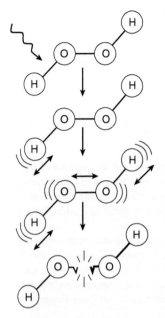

Figure 9.10 Molecular surgery, in which the O–O bond of hydrogen peroxide, H_2O_2, is broken apart by a specific frequency of laser light. The wavy arrow represents a photon of light that energizes the O–H bond (i.e., it makes it vibrate violently). The vibrations are rapidly redistributed throughout the molecule, and the O–O bond, which is weaker than the O–H bond, breaks. The experiment was done by Fleming and Crim of the University of Wisconsin (see Crim, 1990). *(Ball, K., 1994. Designing the molecular world: chemistry at the frontier. Princeton University Press, Princeton, NJ.)*

No one has ever seen a molecule: They are simply too small. Even the most powerful microscopes give us only a fuzzy outline of molecular shape. In spite of this, we have a detailed knowledge of how molecules are constructed and carry out their functions. How can this be?

Molecules are composed of atoms, which are made up of electrons. Virtually all of our knowledge about molecules, and about matter in general, has come from studying the ways light interacts with electrons.

Figure 9.11 shows a resonant interaction between two nearby proteins. The rotation of a charged amino acid sets up an electromagnetic field that entrains rotations of the corresponding amino acid on a second protein. The second protein also emits an electromagnetic field that affects other proteins. As a result, molecular motions and energy fields join together to form a continuous or collective energy system. We shall see below that the crystal-like organization of molecules in living systems enhances this phenomenon.

The ability of molecules to transmit and receive electromagnetic signals has been discussed above. Spectroscopy provides a detailed explanation of the importance of both the emission and the absorption of electromagnetic fields by molecules. The processes are analogous to the radio transmitter and receiver shown in Figure 3.4 with the additional feature that the molecules are the antennas.

In Chapter 10 we will see the evidence that there are much faster ways for biochemical reactions to take place within cells. Metabolites do not have to rely on slow random diffusion to interact. Many of the enzymes within cells are not dissolved, but are assembled into units so that the products of a reaction can be handed from enzyme to enzyme in the sequence, much like the steps in an automobile assembly plant (Figure 10.7B). This enables biochemical processes to operate at extremely high velocities. While many chemists suspected that such velocities might be very high, few thought it would ever be possible to measure them. Remarkably, Ahmed Zewail was able to do this, using a technology he developed that came to be known as femtochemistry or femtosecond spectroscopy. Zewail received the Nobel Prize in 1999 for his accomplishments. His measurements showed that the velocity of atoms in chemical reactions is actually comparable to that of a rifle bullet, 1000 m/s (Nordén, 1999). Recall from above that the fastest nerves conduct at 120 m/s.

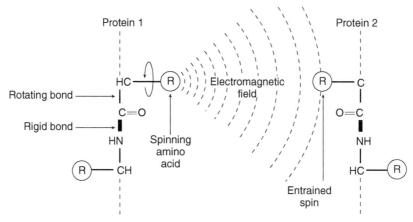

Figure 9.11 The rotations of a charged portion of the protein molecule on the left set up an electromagnetic field that brings about complementary motions in the protein to the right, even though the two molecules are not touching. It is the oscillating electric component of the electromagnetic field that makes the amino acid of protein 2 oscillate in synchrony with the corresponding amino acid of protein 1.

The Field of the Body

Just as molecules produce energy fields due to the movements of their charges, fields are produced by larger objects such as cells, tissues, and organs. This has been one of the most controversial and confusing aspects of the story of energy medicine. For a long time, sensitive individuals and experienced therapists have reported that they can sense a person's 'energy field' a distance from the body. Moreover, therapists report that they can use this sense to locate painful or injured areas and can project energy into a part of a person's body to relieve pain or trigger a healing response. Some people seem to be born with a heightened sensitivity to such fields; others can acquire the ability with practice. Many therapeutic schools teach these techniques.

Western medicine and biology have regarded such claims with great skepticism. Energy fields in and around the body have been regarded as either nonexistent or too weak to be important. Practitioners who utilize energy field interactions every day in their practices have had to endure disrespectful designations of their work as new-age psycho-babble, quackery, and the like. However, over the last few decades, scientists have developed more than adequate measurable and logical connections between biological energy fields and generally accepted scientific knowledge.

That such fields exist within the body has been known for more than a century, since the work of Einthoven and his contemporaries that led to the modern electrocardiogram. Einthoven's early electrocardiograph weighed 600 pounds and required five people to operate (Figure 9.12). Einthoven is credited with the discovery that different forms of heart disease reveal themselves in the characteristic traces of the electrocardiographic recording. He did not believe, however, that the fluctuations in the electric field of the heart have any biological importance. This point was disputed in Chapter 8

A modern electrocardiogram, using electronic microcircuitry, is the Holter Monitor, named after its inventor, a biophysicist, Dr. Norman J. Holter. The device weighs less than one pound and can record the electric field generated by a patient's heart for 24 h or more (Figure 9.13).

It is a law of physics that the flow of electricity, such as that generated by the heart or other organs and tissues in the body, must produce magnetic fields in the surrounding space (Chapter 2). Successful measurements of these fields were described in Chapter 8. Not only are we documenting the existence of such fields, but researchers now understand how the fields are generated and how

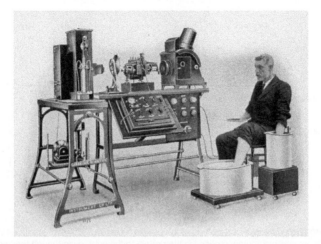

Figure 9.12 Photograph of an early electrocardiograph made by the Cambridge Scientific Instrument Company. The 'electrodes' connecting the device to the patient are buckets of saltwater, one for each hand and one for the left foot.

Holter Monitor

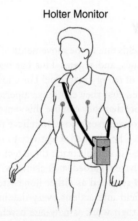

Figure 9.13 A modern electrocardiographic recorder called a Holter Monitor can record the electric field generated by the heart for 24 h or more. *(Courtesy of Midmark Corporation.)*

they are altered by disease and disorder. We are also beginning to understand the biophysical mechanisms that enable the discerning therapist to sense and manipulate energy fields for the benefit of the patient.

While there will always be skeptics, they cannot base their doubts on a lack of relevant science. The fields generated by the various organs are termed *biomagnetic fields* because they are of biological origin. The study of such fields is now an established set of disciplines, as evidenced by 520,000 web pages on bio-magnetism, 376,000 on magneto-biology, 320,000,000 on magneto-cardiology, and 400,000 on magnetoencephalography.* Our ideas about energy fields have gone from skepticism to the point where physicians are using information from biomagnetic fields to make therapeutic decisions. During the past century, the electric field of the heart has progressed from a phenomenon that

---

*These figures correct as at November 2014.

was very weak, and therefore very difficult to measure, to an appreciation that the heart produces the largest field of the body. Our concepts of weak versus strong energetic influences have more to do with the sensitivity of measuring technologies than with the biological significance.

Finally, we can view the fabric of the biofield as a communication system. Every event taking place in the body involves the production of electric or bioelectric current flows, and these flows must give rise to characteristic biomagnetic fields in the space around the body. Each organ generates electrical activity that is conducted through the surrounding extracellular spaces and also through the circulatory system because the blood is a good conductor. These electric fields travel at velocities that are far faster than nerve impulses. The velocities are comparable to the speed of light, some 300,000,000 m/s. Since the circulation reaches every part of the organism, it contains a complex of electrical activity that represents a composite of all of the activities taking place in the various organs and tissues. In a sense, every organ has a way of 'knowing' what every other organ is doing through the patterns of bioelectric fields 'circulating' in the blood.

A Physical Matrix

In addition to the webwork of electromagnetic and energy field interactions between parts of the body, there is a physical fabric composed of the molecules that form the cells and tissues and organs. The system is called the *living matrix*. The crucial piece of evidence that gave rise to this concept was the discovery that the molecular fabric within every cell is connected across the cell surface to the surrounding extracellular connective tissue system. The scientist who made this important discovery is seldom mentioned. His name is Mark Bretscher, and he did the research at the Medical Research Council in Cambridge, England, in 1973. He made his discovery by asking a question that had not been asked before. He was studying a protein associated with the membranes of red blood cells and wanted to know whether these proteins were on the inside of the membrane or on the outside. What he discovered was that the protein he studied extended across the cell surface, forming a link between the cell interior and the exterior.

Since nobody had ever thought about proteins extending across the cell surface, Bretscher's discovery was greeted with the customary skepticism. However, it was not long before the finding was confirmed. This marked a turning point in the study of cell biology because it established an important physical link between the cell interior, including the nucleus, and the cell exterior. It was soon discovered that transmembrane proteins are widespread and that they play key roles in integrating cellular activities with processes taking place outside the cell. Hence these proteins came to be called *integrins*. By 1997, Horwitz stated in a review article, 'Discovered only recently, these adhesive cell surface molecules have quickly revealed themselves to be critical to proper functioning of the body and to life itself'. Detailed research has shown that integrins are not individual molecules but complex assemblies that are responsible for adhesion of cells to each other as well as receptors for various kinds of signal molecules.

The integrin concept was also a turning point in helping us comprehend the significance of the term *holistic*. From a structural and functional perspective, the integrins link the connective tissue system with the cellular domains throughout the body. From a biological perspective, the integrins provide a physical and energetic connection between the domains of physiology and cell biology. From the perspective of complementary and alternative medicine, the integrins complete the picture of the body as a whole system. Moreover, this complete system is thoroughly definable from a molecular perspective, since most of the major components of the matrix have been extracted and characterized individually. Here is a gigantic connection between reductionism, the study of isolated parts, and holism, the study of how those parts go together to make an organism. Holistic therapists quickly relate to the living matrix concept because it helps explain some of the remarkable therapeutic accomplishments that come from regarding the body as an interconnected system.

The Dual Nervous System

An important part of the living matrix is the connective tissue surrounding the nerves and organizing the space within the brain. The perineural system is the connective tissue covering the nerves as they course through the various tissues. We shall see in Chapter 11 that the perineural system is an energetic and informational system with key roles in regulating the repair of injured or damaged tissue. The term *dual nervous system* comes from the work of Dr. Robert O. Becker. In contrast to the high-speed digital signals transmitted through neurons, the perineural system generates slow waves of direct current that actually regulate the nervous system and that also play a key role in regeneration and repair (see Figure 11.13).

The Fabric of Space

At a much finer scale we find an even larger component of the living body, even more pervasive than the living matrix. This is the domain of space, which was formerly referred to as 'empty' space or the quantum vacuum. Below the level of molecules and atoms and subatomic particles is a micro world discernable through the methods of quantum physics. When viewed at the Planck length, 10^{-33} cm, we encounter the basic aspects of energy and matter in the universe. We are unable to see this world with our limited senses. We can only imagine what is going on and must temper our imaginations with indirect evidence from particle and mathematical physics and cosmology, because this domain extends throughout our bodies and is completely continuous with all space everywhere. The activities taking place in space reflect what is going on everywhere within us and everywhere in the cosmos. We now know that the 'quantum vacuum' is far from empty. It has been described as a turbulent froth, the subquantum foam, an absolute fullness, an infinitely coherent field of luminosity and the embedding space for electromagnetism (Comings, 2007).

Some Conclusions

We have explored some of the energetic fabrics or matrices within and around us. Each contributes to the web of interconnected regulatory pathways that enable us to function on a moment-to-moment basis to enable us to adjust to changes in our surroundings, and that also enable us to repair and regenerate after injury or disease. The velocities of these regulatory processes range from very slow to extremely rapid to virtually instantaneous. The following chapters will discuss each of these systems in more detail. The purpose here was to introduce the essential concepts that are emerging in energy medicine.

References

Albrecht-Buehler, G., 1990. In defense of 'nonmolecular' cell biology. Int. Rev. Cytol. 120, 191–241.
Allen, H.C., Cross, P.C., 1963. Molecular Vib-rotors. John Wiley, New York.
Ball, K., 1994. Designing the molecular world: chemistry at the frontier. Princeton University Press, Princeton, NJ.
Comings, M., 2007. The quantum plenum: the hidden key to life, energetics and sentience. Bridges: The quarterly magazine of the International Society for the Study of Subtle Energies and Energy Medicine 17 (1), 4–13, 20.
Crim, F.F., 1990. State- and bond-selected unimolecular reactions. Science 249, 1387.
Farhadi, A., 2014. Non-chemical distant cellular interactions as a potential cofounder of cell biology experiments. Frontiers in Physiology 5, article 405.
Gilson, M.K., Straatsma, T.P., McCammon, J.A., et al., 1994. Open 'back door' in a molecular dynamics simulation of acetylcholinesterase. Science 263, 1276–1278.
Haynes, W.M. (Ed.), 2014. CRC Handbook of Chemistry and Physics, 95th Edition, CRC Press, Boca Raton, FL.

Horwitz, A.F., 1997. Integrins and health. Discovered only recently, these adhesive cell surface molecules have quickly revealed themselves to be critical to proper functioning of the body and to life itself. Sci. Am. 276, 68–75.

Jasper, H.H., Penfield, W., 1949. Electrocortiograms in man: effect of the vountary movement upon the electrical activity of the precentral gyrus. Archiv für Psychiatrie und Nervenkrankheiten, vereingt mit Zeitschrifte für die gesamte Neurologie und Psychiatrie 183, 163–174.

Jones, J.P., 2008. An investigation of the acupuncture process using medical imaging. Presentation at Tai Sophia, now Maryland University of Integrative Health, Laurel, MD.

Jump, D.B., Narayan, P., Towle, H., Oppenheimer, J.H., 1984. Rapid effects of triiodothyronine on hepatic gene expression. Hybridization analysis of tissue-specific triiodothyronine regulation of mRNAS14. J. Biol. Chem. 259, 2789–2797.

Karplus, M., McGammon, J.A., 1986. The dynamics of proteins: the incessant motions that underlay a protein's function are explored in computer simulations. Scientific American 254, 42–51.

Kučera, O., Cifra, M., 2013. Cell-to-cell signaling through light: just a ghost of chance? Cell Communication and Signaling 11, 87.

Luby-Phelps, K., 2000. Cytoarchitecture and physical properties of cytoplasm: volume, viscosity, diffusion, intracellular surface area. Int. Rev. Cytol. 192, 189–221.

Murphy, M., 1992. The Future of the Body. Explorations into the further evolution of human nature. Jeremy P. Tarcher/Perigee, Los Angeles, CA.

Murphy, M., White, R.A., 2012. In the Zone: Transcendent Experience in Sports. Open Road Media, New York, NY.

Narayan, P., Liaw, C.W., Towle, H.C., 1984. Rapid induction of a specific nuclear mRNA precursor by thyroid hormone. Proc. Natl. Acad. Sci. U.S.A. 81, 4687–4691.

Nordén, B., 1999. The Nobel Prize in chemistry 1999. Presentation speech, December 10, 1999. In: Grenthe, I. (Ed.), Nobel Lectures, Chemistry 1996–2000. World Scientific Publishing Co, Singapore, 2003.

Nørretranders, T., 1991. The User Illusion. Viking/Penguin, New York.

Oschman, J.L., 2003. Energy medicine in therapeutics and human performance. Butterworth Heineman, Oxford.

Pall, M.L., 2013. Electromagnetic fields act via activation of voltage-gated calcium channels to produce beneficial or adverse effects. J. Cell. Mol. Med 17 (8), 958–965.

Pauling, L., 1960. The nature of the chemical bond and the structure of molecules and crystals. 3rd eds., Cornell University Press, Ithaca, N.

Prasad, A., Rossi, C., Lamponi, S., Pospíšil, P., Foletti, A., 2014. New perspective in cell communication: potential role of ultra-weak photon emission. J. Photochem. Photobiol. B. http://dx.doi.org/10.1016/j.jphotobiol.2014.03.004 [Epub ahead f print].

Sauer, K. (Ed.), 1995. Biochemical spectroscopy. Methods in Enzymology 246. Academic Press, New York.

Slater-Hammel, A.T., Stumpner, R.L., 1950. Batting reaction-time. Res. Q. 21, 353–356.

Szent-Györgyi, A., 1957. Bioenergetics. Academic Press, New York.

CHAPTER 10

Energy 'Circuits' in the Body

Nature has neither kernel nor shell – she is everything at once.
Goethe

When we look at any one thing in the world, we find it is hitched to everything else.
John Muir

The moment one gives close attention to anything, even a blade of grass, it becomes a mysterious, awesome, indescribably magnificent world in itself.
Henry Miller

Chapter Summary

The chapter begins with a scientific perspective on the term *holism*. The reductionist perspective says that the organism is too complex to be studied whole and must be separated into smaller and smaller parts for study. The holistic perspective is that the information from study of the parts becomes even more valuable when the parts are viewed in context – in their relationships with other parts. The living matrix concept provides a basis for a unifying picture of the relations between the thousands of parts of the living organism that have been so thoroughly studied over the past century of sustained reductionist research. Holism and reductionism are actually complementary viewpoints, in the same sense that Niels Bohr used complementarity to resolve the wave-particle duality. To understand any one system requires understanding the living body as a whole and to understand the body as a whole requires understanding each system (Figure 10.1).

The living matrix is a physical fabric, with essential roles in movement and support, but it is also an electronic circuit with the capability of transferring both energy and information very rapidly from place to place. As an electronic system, the matrix also has the capacity to process information, as in an electronic computer or other printed circuit device.

A key aspect of the matrix is that its components are highly arrayed, i.e., they are primarily in a liquid crystalline form. Giant arrays of collagen molecules form the structural fabric of the body – the connective tissues, bones, and fascia. Connective tissue called tendons connect to the contractile fibres inside of muscle – another highly crystalline material. The bones are also composed crystalline collagen interspersed with mineral crystals called apatite. Finally, the surfaces of cells are composed of liquid crystalline arrays of phospholipids, and the interiors of cells are packed with various fibres that often have a crystalline configuration. Importantly from an energetic perspective, these molecular arrays also organize vast numbers of water molecules. These arrangements have profound significance from a quantum physics and quantum biology perspective.

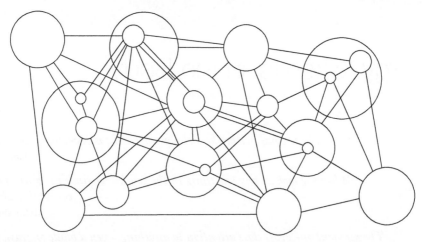

Figure 10.1   Strictly speaking, every system is itself a system composed of systems, every system is a member of a system, and the forces between systems are themselves systems. To understand any one system requires understanding the living body as a whole and to understand the body as a whole requires understanding each system; no one part of the system is more fundamental than any other (Maitland, 1980).

Introducing Holism

> *If nature puts two things together, she produces something new with new qualities, which cannot be expressed in terms of qualities of the components. When going from electrons and protons to atoms, from here to molecules, molecular aggregates, etc., up to the cell or the whole animal, at every level we find something new, a new breathtaking vista. Whenever we separate two things, we lose something, something which may have been the most essential feature.*

Szent-Györgyi (1963)

This chapter and the one that follows will bring the reader to a clear understanding of the important term *holistic*. For some it is a term that is identified with flaky new-age alternative medicine *twilight zone* gobbledygook. However, such negativity is no longer warranted, for what is emerging is a unifying picture of the relationships between the 10,000 or so different named parts that make up a human being. The point of the science of holism is that one could spend a lifetime studying the properties of these parts without getting a glimpse of what life and health really are.

In contrast, the science of reductionism states that the whole is too complex to study, so we must begin by studying the separate parts. A holistic/reductionist dichotomy exists in our present medical culture. Here we will learn that both of these perspectives are essential and that enormous opportunity comes from integrating both holistic and reductionist pictures. We might think that this would require us to gather and interpret an overwhelming amount of detailed information and could leave us more confused than ever. However, we can be spared such an endless journey by finding logical ways to organize the key pieces of discovery and information that have been obtained from a century or so of reductionist science and an equal period of investigation from the holistic perspective. The intellectual challenge is to understand the living body as a whole while being aware of each system. There are many pieces to this puzzle, but the problem becomes easier if one uses the matrix or continuum concept and energetics as frameworks for the exploration. We shall see that many facts and discoveries and concepts can be organized coherently in this way.

Attempts at the interpretation and synthesis of a diversity of information and insights are invariably speculative. It is easy for skeptics to raise many objections. It is inevitable that new ideas will emerge, and some of them may turn out to be inaccurate or incomplete. Skepticism is important, is not to be avoided, and is actually an essential part of the scientific and synthetic processes.

The word *holistic* is from the Greek, Őλος, holos, meaning all, entire, or total. It is a scientific concept stating that the properties of a system, whether it is biological, chemical, social, economic, mental, or linguistic, cannot be explained by the properties of its component parts. Instead, systems can acquire new properties that are not expected or predicted from the study of the behaviours of the parts. Some of these new properties arise when similar or dissimilar materials combine to form composites. These unexpected behaviours can be extraordinary. Life in all its intricate beauty is an example. These are called emergent or whole systems or collective or synergistic properties – each of these terms is the name of a distinct and scholarly field of inquiry.

The holistic principle was concisely summarized by Aristotle in his *Metaphysics*: 'The whole is more than the sum of its parts' (McKeon, 2001). It is the principle that gave rise to the modern sciences of chaos, complexity, and complex adaptive systems. The holistic approach is very old and is a fundamental part of science that continues to be at the forefront of new discovery.

Reductionism in science and medicine says that a complex system can be understood through study of its parts. Those who negate holism as an unsound fuzzy new-age concept, as a contributor to quackery and holistic mysticism, can point to the great successes of reductionist science and the resulting advances in medicine. Some whose clinical perspective is holistic are equally suspicious of reductionism. While these superficially polarized perspectives have been argued endlessly, the simple fact is that holism and reductionism are complementary viewpoints, much like the wave and particle concepts in quantum physics. Complementarity was developed by Niels Bohr (Nobel Prize in Physics in 1922). Complementarity is the idea that things can have a dual nature (as the electron is both particle and wave), but we can only experience one aspect at a time. Both perspectives are essential to get a complete picture of a system. But it might seem to be intellectually challenging to hold a holistic perspective and a reductionist perspective in focus at the same time. Arguments that one is better than the other are not productive. A philosopher/bodyworker, Jeffrey Maitland, has nicely summarized the situation (Figure 10.1).

Recently the public has come to understand and appreciate the practical value of holistic and whole-person approaches, and more and more scientists are shifting some of their research perspectives in this direction. Scientists who have written eloquently about this field are Fritjof Capra (1984, 2000, 2004), Ervin László (1996), Alicia Juarrero (2002), and Rustum Roy (2002).

The matrix perspective has resonated throughout the world of holistic therapies, with over 27,000 web pages specifically mentioning the living matrix as it is described below.[1] Scientists and physicians are now looking at the living matrix as a convenient and scientifically accurate paradigm to help them understand what lies ahead in the field of medicine through the integration of reductionist biomedicine with its holistic complements. The living matrix concept of the cell and its environment that is presented next would be a good place for students of medicine and medical research to begin.

Defining Matrix

INTRODUCING THE LIVING MATRIX

We shall see that the diverse molecules in the body are woven together into a single continuous fabric called the *living matrix*. This is a truly remarkable material, with properties and possibilities that have been explored by those who wish to go beyond what everyone agrees are the limits to our potential as living beings.

---

[1]From inserting 'living matrix' and 'James Oschman' in Google.

While the living matrix is a physical fabric, with essential roles in movement and support, it is far more. It is an electronic circuit with capabilities that make the inventions of the electronic age look like children's toys. Many of the remarkable experiences we are glimpsing with holistic and energetic therapies can be accounted for by the electronic, photonic, and other 'solid state' properties of the living matrix and the ways these properties can be sensed and influenced by therapists. Solid-state physics is the study of solid matter, using methods such as quantum mechanics, crystallography and electromagnetism. It studies how the properties of solids arise from atomic and quantum properties, and provides the theoretical basis for transistors and other semiconductor devices. This represents one line of exploration that is leading us to explanations of and cures for conditions that are currently considered incurable. It expands the possibilities of modern medicine and the medicine of the future.

From Biomagnetism to Semiconduction

The energy fields described in Chapter 8 provide a logical connection between the various therapies employing energetic concepts and one of the most exciting areas of biomedical research – biomagnetism. Mention was made of the laws of physics that state that when charges flow, magnetic fields are created in the surrounding spaces (Chapter 2). Now we need to explore precisely what these charges are and where they are flowing.

Willem Einthoven made a temporary simplifying assumption when he was attempting to understand how the electrical activity of the heart is conducted to the skin surface (Einthoven et al., 1913). The simplifying assumption was that the human body is essentially a bag filled with a conductive salt solution. This assumption was very important because it made it possible to calculate the electrical aspects of the cardiac cycle on the basis of measurements taken at the skin surface. The problem with this simplifying assumption is that eventually it was forgotten that it was a tentative assumption, and it came to be accepted as a truth. Einthoven's assumption has evolved into a statement that can be found in many places in the academic literature: The human body is a volume conductor. This means that all electrical phenomena associated with life can be explained on the basis of ionic charges moving about in a salt solution.

Oversimplified assumptions plague science and, in this case, provide one of the reasons some of the discoveries in this chapter and the next one are unfamiliar to most readers.

Assume a Spherical Cow

The spherical cow (Figure 10.2) arises from a story that is often told in physics classes. It explains how a simplifying assumption can evolve from an approximation to an accepted truth. The story draws attention to a method widely used by scientists: They make simplifying assumptions to make it easier to tackle problems that would otherwise be too complex. Such assumptions have played key roles in helping us understand a wide variety of biological and medical problems. For example, the early work on the electrocardiogram required a simplifying assumption so that theoretical work could proceed.

A difficulty arises, however, when we forget that an assumption is an assumption and is meant to be tentative. Over a period of time, an assumption can go through several stages:

1. To simplify our calculations, we assume a spherical cow.
2. It can be assumed that cows are spherical.
3. Cows are spherical.

This type of problem occurs again and again in science. It is always instructive to examine tentative assumptions about living systems that were temporarily useful but that have gradually come to be taken as facts. The tendency to retain the definitions of terms that were acceptable in early stages of a study or science is called *meaning invariance*. It creates very serious logical problems over time because a re-examination of a certain meaning could require revision of widely accepted concepts. Philosopher of science Paul Feyerabend wrote:

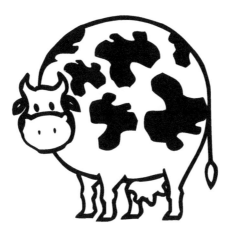

Figure 10.2 The spherical cow comes from a story that is often told in physics classes. A farmer is having trouble getting enough milk from his cows and consults a physicist. After pondering the problem for a while, the physicist begins his analysis with the statement, 'Assume a spherical cow'. This illustrates a situation that arises frequently in science: A tentative assumption is made to simplify calculations. It begins with, 'assume a spherical cow'; progresses to 'it can be assumed that cows are spherical'; and finally leads to 'cows are spherical'. Here we are exploring the progression from 'tentatively assume the body is a volume conductor' to 'the body is a volume conductor'.

... any form of meaning invariance is bound to lead to difficulties when the task arises either of giving a proper account of the growth of knowledge, and of discoveries contributing to this growth, or of establishing correlations between entities which are described with the help of what we will later call incommensurable [unmeasurable] concepts ... it will usually turn out that a solution of these problems is deemed satisfactory only if it leaves unchanged the meanings of certain key terms and it is exactly this condition, the condition of meaning invariance, which makes them insoluble.

FEYERABEND (1981)

In other words, we are discouraged from discussing electronic conduction in living tissues because it would be inconsistent or incompatible with the volume conductor assumption and all of its consequences and implications, which extend throughout the fields of physiology and medicine. On the same subject, Northrop commented:

One of the basic problems in the unification of scientific knowledge is that of clarifying the relation between those concepts which a given science uses in the early natural history stage of its development and those which enter into its final and more theoretical formulations as a verified deductive theory.

NORTHROP (1959)

The volume conductor assumption totally confuses our conceptualization of ourselves, our health, disease, and the healing process. The volume conductor assumption is one confusion that perpetuates an illusionary barrier to the integration of conventional biomedicine with complementary and alternative therapies and vice versa. The mobile electron has many potential roles in vital processes such as bioenergetics, regulation, consciousness, and communication, but any recognition of its importance would require a rather extensive revision of many textbooks. Some think that such a revision is long overdue.

Assumptions and Deductive Logic

The dictionary tells us that an *assumption* is a tentative proposition that is taken for granted. In other words, assumptions are treated for the sake of a given discussion as if they are true. In logic, in the context of deductive reasoning, an assumption is made in the expectation that it will be discharged in due course, once the goals that necessitated the assumption have been achieved or when more details are known so that more realistic assumptions can be made. Logical processes that begin with simplifying approximations must, of necessity, give rise to simplified or approximate answers. Some philosophers who explore the methods of science recognize that virtually all scientific discoveries are based on assumptions or approximations of one kind or another and that scientific truth is therefore always relative or approximate (e.g., Ratcliffe, 1983; Singer, 1986). To understand anything about electronic biology, we must appropriately discharge the idea that the volume conductor applies in all conditions when energy and information move from place to place and replace it with assumptions that are closer to reality and that can therefore lead us to conclusions that are closer to reality.

Once we get past the assumption that the volume conductor approximation applies in all circumstances, we can see that there are energetic circuits in the living organism that are much faster than those involving bulky and relatively slow-moving ions, nerve impulses, and molecules. Energy and information can stream through electronic, protonic, and photonic circuits to every nook and cranny of the body. These flows probably play key roles in conscious and unconscious processing that will be discussed in Chapter 12. These flows can be influenced by energy fields in the environment, including the energy fields produced by the hands of therapists and by medical devices of various kinds. Moreover, disease and disorder alter these flows in predictable and correctable ways.

Electricity Versus Electronics

Next we clarify the distinction between biological electricity and biological electronics.

Biological electricity is usually conceptualized as a large-scale phenomenon arising from the movements of charged ions such as sodium, potassium, calcium, magnesium, and chloride. It is understood from the perspective of the volume conductor assumption just described. In virtually all cases, this kind of physiological electricity is thought to arise because of the large electrical polarity across cell membranes and across layers of cells called epithelia, and the ability of these membranes to temporarily depolarize and then repolarize. This is the process that is thought to enable nerves to conduct signals from place to place within the body. A wave of depolarization also goes along the surface of a muscle cell and triggers it to contract. The large electrical fields and measurable magnetic fields detected by the electrocardiogram, as well as the electroretinogram, electromyogram, and electroencephalogram, arise primarily because of the electrical currents that flow as these organs carry out their activities (see Chapter 8). Less known but just as important are slow waves of electrical depolarization that are set up across the skin in response to injury. These are called injury potentials, and they are important in triggering and guiding tissue repair as was described in Chapter 6.

Biological electricity is widely studied by many different scientists, including electrobiologists, physiologists, and neurophysiologists. Much is known about the subject because electrical currents are relatively easy to measure.

In contrast, biological electronics refers to a relatively new topic of research. It deals with the flows of much smaller entities than ions. These are mainly electrons, protons, and the space where an electron is missing, called a *hole*.

For a familiar example, consider the electrical appliances in your home and the wiring that brings electrical power to them. Contrast this with the far more subtle electronic processes taking place within your computer or cellular telephone. These devices contain miniature electronic circuits that utilize far smaller amounts of power to carry out sophisticated tasks at very high speed. This is possible because of advances in solid state physics and electronics and the use of semiconductor devices. We are now going to look at the corresponding subtle semiconducting circuitry that has been discovered in living systems. We begin by taking a close look at cells.

Cell and Tissue Structure: The 'Living Matrix'

One of the most important developments in recent science is a better understanding of the structure and energetics of the material substrate of the body – the living substance that is touched and interacted with in all therapeutic approaches. For surgeons as well as for the hands-on therapist, the energetic properties of this living substance have both conceptual and practical consequences. To understand the new developments, we begin with breakthroughs in our understandings of the cell.

A few decades ago, the living cell was visualized as a membrane-bound bag containing a solution of molecules. Figure 10.3 shows a cell as it is often illustrated in texts. Note that adjacent to the cell is a fibrous material called the connective tissue or extracellular matrix. This matrix contains large amounts of a fascinating protein called collagen. In the drawings in most texts, both the space between the connective tissue and the cell and the cell interior appear almost 'empty' except for a few organelles such as the nucleus and mitochondria floating about in the 'cytosol'. We shall see that this term, *cytosol*, is misleading. Illustrations such as Figure 10.3 are widely used in introductory and advanced texts, including those used in medical schools, even though they omit one of the most important attributes of cell and tissue structure: the cytoskeleton.

One reason the image shown in Figure 10.3 has persisted and can still be found in modern texts has to do with the ways cells are studied. The breakthrough that has made it possible for modern biochemists and cell biologists to research the components of cells is a sophisticated fractionation procedure. The method (Figure 10.4) was developed by Albert Claude, Christian de Duve, and George Palade at the Rockefeller University in New York, who received the Nobel Prize in Physiology or Medicine in 1974 for their remarkable discoveries.

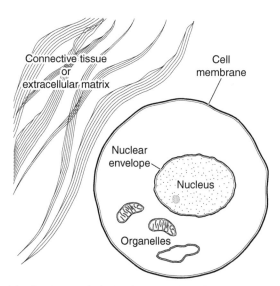

Figure 10.3 A cell as it is often incorrectly depicted in texts. The cell is drawn as a membrane-bound bag assumed to contain a solution of molecules. Adjacent to the cell but separate from it is a fibrous material, called the connective tissue or extracellular matrix. In the drawings in most texts, both the space between the connective tissue and the cell, and the cell interior appear almost 'empty' except for a few organelles such as the nucleus and mitochondria floating about in the "cytosol." The image omits the most important attributes of cell and tissue structure: the continuity of the nuclear matrix, cytoskeleton, and the connective tissue matrix.

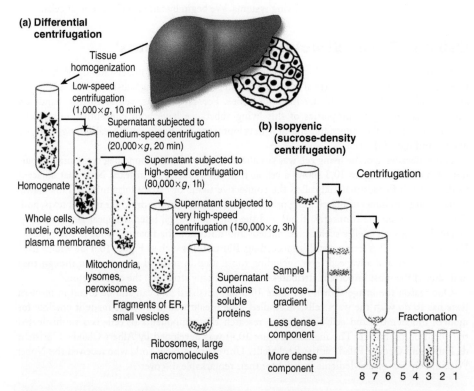

Figure 10.4 (A) Cellular components can be separated and isolated by homogenizing the tissue and passing the homogenate through a series of centrifugations at different speeds. (B) Individual organelles such as mitochondria can be separated and purified by the methods shown in A, and other techniques such as sucrose-density centrifugation (B) can fracture the organelles and separate out their molecular constituents, such as the mitochondrial enzymes involved in electron transport.

Microscopy had already revealed that cells contain a number of different components, but it was very difficult to determine what they were and what their functions were. The 1974 Nobel Prize was significant because it was the first prize in the field of cell biology. To quote the Nobel Presentation Speech:

> There are no earlier Prize Winners in this field, simply because it is one that has been newly created, largely by the Prize Winners themselves ... The components of the cell are so small that it was not possible to study their inner structure, their mutual relations or their different roles. To take a metaphor from an earlier Prize Winner, the cell was like a mother's work basket, in that it contained objects strewn about in no discernible order and evidently ... with no recognizable functions. But, if the cell is a work basket, it is one on a very tiny scale indeed, having a volume corresponding to a millionth of that of a pin's head. The various components responsible for the functions of the cell correspond in their turn to a millionth of this millionth, and are far below the resolving powers of the light microscope. Nor would it have helped if researchers had used larger experimental animals: the cells of the elephant are not larger than those of the mouse.

EDSTRÖM (1992)

With the fractionation methods developed by Claude, de Duve, and Palade, it became possible to separate the various cell components so that the behaviour of each could be studied separately. Gradually the various organelles were isolated and their separate functions determined. These included the nucleus, mitochondria, ribosomes, lysosomes, endoplasmic reticulum, Golgi apparatus, and various kinds of filaments and fibres that constitute the cytoskeleton and nuclear matrix. Further fractionation separated the individual organelles into their molecular constituents. These techniques made it possible to show that lysosomes, for example, contain degradative enzymes, mitochondria contain the enzymes involved in oxidative metabolism, chloroplasts contain the photosynthetic pigments, and so on.

The focus of modern biochemistry and molecular biology has been the study of the soluble proteins, the enzymes, and other reactants, called substrates, found in the final supernatant (Figure 10.4). Our concepts of cell metabolism are based on the chemical reactions that can be carried out by cell-free extracts of these soluble enzymes. For example, glucose can be added to such an extract, and it will be metabolized into various other compounds through a 10-step enzymatic sequence called glycolysis:

1. Hexokinase
2. Glucose-6-phosphate isomerase
3. 6-Phosphofructokinase
4. Fructose biphosphate aldolase
5. Triosephosphate isomerase
6. Glyceraldehyde-3-phosphate dehydrogenase
7. Phosphoglycerate kinase
8. Phosphoglycerate mutase
9. Phosphopyruvate hydratase
10. Pyruvate kinase

The result of this series of reactions is the production of adenosine triphosphate (ATP), which powers the activities of life, such as:

- Muscle contraction
- Nerve transmission
- Cellular metabolism
- Cell division
- Active transport
- Osmotic work

The individual enzymes involved in sugar metabolism can be isolated and studied, as was described above. With some exceptions, biochemists discard the solid material, the insoluble fabric of cells and tissues, that collects in the bottoms of the centrifuge tubes. As a consequence, the biochemical view of cells is as follows:

- The cell interior is a dilute solution containing dissolved enzymes.
- Molecules diffuse randomly from place to place within cells.
- Biochemical processes take place when there are chance encounters between enzymes and substrates.

In fact, we shall see that these widely held views are inaccurate (reviewed by Luby-Phelps, 2000):

- The cell interior is actually crowded, filled with matrix, not dilute.
- Diffusion within the cell is restricted by binding of the molecules to structures and compartmentation.
- Many of the enzymes are organized into functional units, like the steps in an automobile assembly plant, so that reactions can proceed much faster than by random diffusion. These functional units are called metabolons.
- Nearly half of the protein is solid rather than dissolved.

Take a close look at glycolysis, the sequential breakdown of sugar molecules by the 10 'soluble' enzymes listed above (Figure 10.5A). Glycolysis and other biochemical pathways can take place

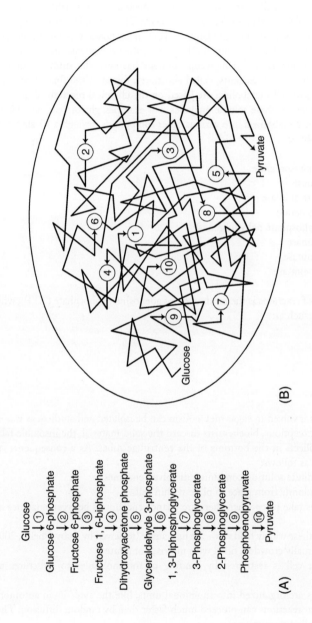

(A)

Glucose
↓①
Glucose 6-phosphate
↓②
Fructose 6-phosphate
↓③
Fructose 1, 6-biphosphate
↓④
Dihydroxyacetone phosphate
↓⑤
Glyceraldehyde 3-phosphate
↓⑥
1, 3-Diphosphoglycerate
↓⑦
3-Phosphoglycerate
↓⑧
2-Phosphoglycerate
↓⑨
Phosphoenolpyruvate
↓⑩
Pyruvate

(B)

Figure 10.5 Glycolysis, the process by which sugar (glucose) is metabolized to pyruvate. (A) shows the series of 10 steps performed by a sequence of 9 enzymes. (B) depicts the conventional model of glycolysis in which the various enzymes and their metabolic products are envisioned to float about in the cytosol. Presumably the glucose molecule diffuses through the cytosol until it more or less accidentally bumps into the first enzyme, which then converts it to glucose 6-phosphate. The products of the subsequent enzymatic steps are likewise presumed to diffuse randomly until they encounter the next enzyme in the sequence. It is stated in the text that if this is the basis for cellular metabolism, it would take you 10,000 years to derive nourishment from your breakfast.

in a cell-free extract prepared as shown in Figure 10.4, but this is probably not what is happening in intact cells. The way this is thought to take place in the intact cell is shown in Figure 10.5B. To correspond to the reactions taking place in the test tube, the cell interior is referred to as the 'cytosol'; this is where glycolysis is thought to take place. The glucose enters the cell and diffuses randomly until it has a chance encounter with enzyme 1, hexokinase. This enzyme attaches a phosphate to position 6 of the glucose molecule, producing glucose 6-phosphate. This molecule is then rearranged into fructose 6-phosphate by glucose phosphate isomerase, and so on. This is the first process in most of carbohydrate catabolism, it is the foundation of both aerobic and anaerobic respiration, and it is known to take place in many types of cells in nearly all organisms. Glycolysis, through anaerobic respiration, is the main energy source in many organisms.

The biochemical image of life is summarized as follows: There are 'particles', the enzymes, proteins, amino acids, sugars, etc., that randomly diffuse about within the membrane-bounded volume of the cell. When appropriate molecules chance to bump into each other, they interact, and chemical bonds are formed or broken. In this way, chemical energy is liberated from molecules such as glucose, and the resulting energy is used to assemble or break down living structures, toxins are broken down, and life's activities are carried out. Figure 10.5B shows this 'random walk' image of the steps in glycolysis.

Edelmann (2002) has developed a way of preparing tissues for electron microscopy that avoids dehydration. The images show that there is virtually no empty space within cells (Figure 10.6).

The torrent of information and clinical applications developed from the 'molecular soup' view of the cell led to an attitude that 'there are only a few problems remaining, and we will soon be able to answer all of them, using this same, incredibly successful, approach'. Physiologists seized the 'bag of solution' model of cell structure and also adopted the 'volume conductor' model of the extracellular and intracellular fluids. The appeal of these simplifications was that it made it possible to carry out calculations needed to test various theoretical models of cell and tissue function. Decades of research have been carried out with the underlying assumption that substances crossing a layer of cells, such as the intestinal wall, simply diffuse through the fluid compartments inside the cells and then enter an extracellular medium that is likewise a solution. The result is a substantial case of 'meaning invariance' (see page 11) that makes it difficult to look at alternative perspectives because of the amount of revision it would take to sort out the existing confusion in all areas of physiology and medicine.

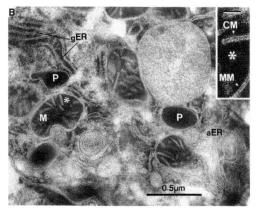

Figure 10.6 Early electron microscopy confirmed that cells contain substantial amounts of 'empty' space. It was assumed that this was the cytosol, the places where the particles are dissolved or suspended, and where metabolism takes place. However, a more realistic look at the structure within cells has come from the research of Edelmann (2002) who has found a way of preparing tissues for electron microscopy that avoids dehydration. The images show that there is virtually no empty space within cells.

The Cell Is Not a Bag

This section may be the most valuable part of the book because it explains the connections between the effects of hands-on bodywork and biochemistry. Our understanding is changing slowly but dramatically because of the discovery that the cell is *not* a bag of solution as was shown in Figures 10.3 and 10.5B. The more closely biologists and microscopists look at cells, the more structures they find. With better preparation techniques, electron microscopists began to see within cells the material that the biochemists had been discarding when they purified the 'soluble' enzymes. Figure 10.7A summarizes the view of the cell that emerges when information on actual cell structure is taken into consideration. This image includes the nuclear matrix, the cytoskeleton, and the connections between the cytoskeleton and the extracellular matrix, called integrins. The entire living matrix can be summarized as a matrix within a matrix within a matrix.

We now know that the cell is so filled with filaments, microfilaments, and microtubules – collectively called the cytoplasmic matrix or cytoskeleton – that there is little space left for a solution of randomly diffusing 'billiard ball' molecules (Figure 10.5B). Moreover, there is very little solvent water inside cells that can dissolve the so-called soluble enzymes. Virtually all the cell water is bound and structured. Water is associated in particular and important ways to the cellular framework (see, e.g., Cope, 1967; Corongiu and Clementi, 1981; Damadian, 1971; Ling, 1992) and most of the protein is insoluble.

Many of the enzymes that were previously thought to be floating about within the cytoplasmic 'soup' or 'cytosol' are actually attached to the matrix (Figure 10.7B). This has been suspected since the work of Arnold and Pette (1968) who suggested that under the physiological conditions thought to prevail in a muscle cell, 100% of the aldolase (the fourth enzyme in the glycolytic pathway) is bound to actomyosin. The studies identified other enzymes in the pathway that are bound. These include the third, sixth, and the tenth glycolytic enzyme. Figure 10.7 shows the binding of aldolase and another enzyme, troponin, to the actin thin filament in muscle (Masters, 1981). Reed and Cox (1966) suggested the association of enzymes with structures has the advantage of increased efficiency and control. Atkinson (1969) suggested that the solvent capacity of the cell may be so limited that it is not possible to adequately dissolve or solvate or suspend all of the 'soluble' enzymes and metabolites. Sols and Marco (1970) suggested that metabolic intermediates may also be protein bound. Hence, when looking at the new view of cell structure shown in Figure 10.7A, it should be recognized that there is little space for random diffusion and convection of enzymes and metabolites. Many studies have shown that the rates of diffusion of small molecules are much lower within the cell interior compared to aqueous solutions (Dick, 1964; Fenichel and Horowitz, 1963; Harris, 1957; Harris and Prankerd, 1957; Ling and Cope, 1969). Duncan and Storey (1992) proposed that the association of glycolytic enzymes with structural elements of the cell may physically position the glycolytic pathway to facilitate the transfer of ATP to the places that use ATP as an energy source.

Living matter seems to be a system of water and organic matter, which forms one single inseparable unit, a system, as the cogwheels do in a watch.

SZENT-GYÖRGYI (1957)

The relationships of enzyme sequences and their associations with elements of the matrix have been formalized by giving them a name, the *metabolon*. A metabolon is defined as a functional complex of several sequential enzymes for a particular metabolic pathway that are held in position by noncovalent bonds. The term was first proposed by Paul Srere (1985). The efficiency of the arrangement arises because the product of one enzyme is channelled directly into the active site of a second enzyme, where it acts as a substrate (Figure 10.7B).

Research on metabolons continues. For example, evidence has been obtained for a metabolon involving at least the first two, and possibly the first three, enzymes of arginine biosynthesis

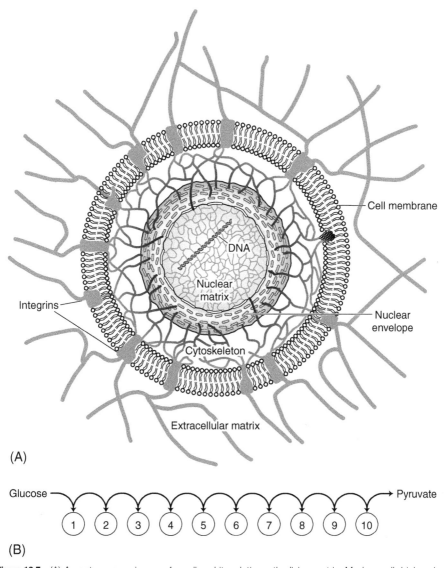

Figure 10.7 (A) A contemporary image of a cell and its relations: the living matrix. Modern cell biology has recognized that the cell interior is virtually filled with fibers and tubes and filaments, collectively called the cytoskeleton or cytoplasmic matrix. Likewise, the nucleus contains a matrix that supports the genetic material. Linkers called integrins extend across the cell surface, connecting the cytoskeleton with the extracellular matrix. The entire system is termed the living matrix. (B) shows a more realistic model of a biochemical pathway, glycolysis, in which the enzymes are organized in sequence along the cytoskeletal structures. The reaction sequence can proceed very rapidly because reactants are passed from one enzyme to the next to the next, as in an assembly line. These assemblies have been called "metabolons" by Srere (1985).

(Abadjieva et al., 2001). It is possible that all of the enzymes of glycolysis are bound in sequence, as shown in Figure 10.7B. These tiny metabolic factories are often attached to structures within the cell and nucleus (also see Ingber, 1993). These attachments are delicate. Biochemical homogenization techniques detach enzymes and other proteins from the cellular and nuclear scaffolds that support them in actual living cells. 'Solution biochemistry', while quite instructive, is actually the study of an artefact:

The empirical fact that a given molecule appears primarily in the 'soluble' fraction may divert attention from the cataclysmic violence of the most gentle homogenization procedure.

McCONKEY (1982)

Most textbooks still oversimplify biochemistry by showing metabolic pathways as linear sequences of steps (Figure 10.5A), without mentioning the essential *structural* or *solid state* context in which the chemistry of life takes place.

Continuum

Soon after the cytoskeleton became a popular subject for research, it was realized that the cellular matrix is connected, across the cell surface, with the connective tissue system or extracellular matrix (also shown in Figure 10.7A). A whole class of 'trans-membrane' linking molecules, or 'integrins', has been discovered. Virtually unmentioned in most descriptions of the integrins (e.g., Horwitz, 1997) is the name of the scientist who first observed them. His name is Mark Bretscher. He was studying the proteins in the membrane of the red blood cell and found that one of them extended from the inside of the cell to the outside (Bretscher, 1975). This was a new and rather startling concept at the time.

Likewise, it is now recognized that the cytoplasmic matrix also links to the nuclear envelope, nuclear matrix, and genes (e.g., Maniotis et al., 1997).

These are important discoveries for our understanding of structure and function and for biomedicine. The boundaries between the cell environment, the cell interior, and the genetic material are not as distinct or as impermeable as we once thought. As a hands-on therapist, what you touch is not merely the skin – you contact a continuous interconnected webwork that extends throughout the body. Indeed, the skin is one of the first tissues in which this structural continuity was documented (Figure 10.8, Ellison and Garrod, 1984).

The entire interconnected system has been called the connective tissue–cytoskeleton (Oschman, 1994), the tissue-tensegrity matrix (see Chapter 11, Figure 11.16) (Pienta and Coffey, 1991), or simply, the *living matrix*. A popular acupuncture text refers to 'the web that has no weaver' (Kaptchuk, 1983).

The living matrix is a continuous and dynamic 'supramolecular' webwork, extending into every nook and cranny of the body: a nuclear matrix within a cellular matrix within a connective tissue matrix. The term *supramolecular* refers to the area of chemistry that focuses on the noncovalent bonding interactions of similar or different molecules to form larger structures. While traditional chemistry focuses on strong or covalent bonds, supramolecular chemistry examines the weaker and reversible noncovalent interactions between molecules that enable complexes composed of many molecules to form.

In essence, when you touch a human body, you are touching a continuously interconnected system, composed of virtually all of the molecules in the body linked together in an intricate webwork. The living matrix has no fundamental unit or central aspect, no part that is primary or most basic. The properties of the whole network depend upon the integrated activities of all of the components. Beneficial or harmful effects on one part of the system can and do spread to others.

This is an important image of the structure of the living body. Our images shape our therapeutic successes because they can give rise to specific intentions and techniques. For example, techniques that stretch the fascia, such as massage, Active Isolated Stretching, Unwinding, Structural Integration, or Rolfing and many others, change the tensions in the living matrix network and thereby alter cellular biochemistry. In the next chapter, we will look at the direct evidence for the relationship between matrix tension and biochemistry, which is part of the work pioneered by Donald Ingber and colleagues. We will also see in Chapter 14 that acupuncture fits into this scheme because of the way matrix fibres wind around the acupuncture needle when it is twisted.

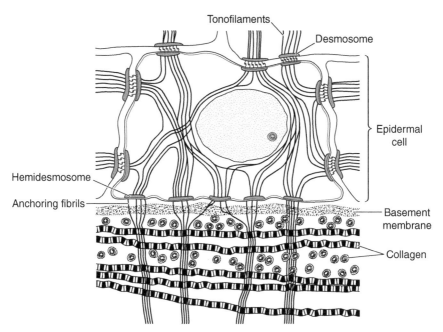

Figure 10.8 The epidermal-dermal continuum. Ellison and Garrod (1984) and others cited by them have described the epidermal-dermal junction in detail. Adjacent epidermal cells are attached to each other by desmosomes, and are anchored to the dermal connective tissue by hemidesmosomes. All of the anchors are traversed by tonofilaments, which form a continuous fibrous matrix joining together all epidermal cells throughout the skin. Anchoring fibrils link the cellular matrix with the connective tissue. The dermal connective tisssue is part of a continuous integrated system extending throughout the body. The cytoskeletons of all other cells in the body are similarly linked to the connective tissue system. (*From Ellison, J., Garrod, D.R., 1984. Anchoring filaments of the amphibian epidermal junction traverse the basal lamina entirely from the plasma membrane of hemidesmosomes to the dermis. J. Cell Sci. 72, 163–172*).

Intentions are not trivial, because they give rise to specific patterns of electrical and magnetic activity in the nervous system of the therapist that can spread through their body and into the body of a patient they are touching (see pages 226–229 in Oschman 2000).

While it is obviously useful to study the various individual parts and systems in the body, each component can be regarded as a local domain or subdivision of a continuous web. The shape, form, mechanical, energetic, and functional characteristics of every cell, tissue, or organ arise because of local variations in the properties of the matrix. The genome, within the nuclear matrix, is a subdivision of this network.

Information Flows

A legacy of the mechanism/vitalism argument and the reductionist approach was a tendency to disregard the overall coordination or integration of the body, such as the systemic regulations proposed in acupuncture theory and the other regulations discussed in Chapter 9. By its very nature, the reductionist approach assumes that it is virtually impossible to study phenomena at the level of the whole organism, simply because it is too complex. To make sense out of it, life must be taken apart and studied one piece at a time. The reassembly of the parts into a whole is a process that must be put off until some vague and distant future date, when we have come to understand all of the parts. A 'general systems theory' was developed (von Bertalanffy, 1971), but few physiologists took active interest in it. The time has now come to put together the pieces that so many scientists have laboured to understand and to synthesize the bigger picture.

Simply stated, in order to survive, complex living systems require an intricate web of informational processes. Each component must be able to quickly and appropriately adjust its activities in relation to what the other parts are doing. One distinguished physiologist, Edward F. Adolph, took a deep look at the mechanisms of physiological integration:

The biology of wholeness is the study of the body as an integrated, coordinated, successful system. No parts or properties are uncorrelated, all are demonstrably interlinked. And the links are not single chains, but a great number of crisscrossed pathways.

ADOLPH (1982)

When scientists think of regulations, they usually begin with the nervous system. The discovery of neurohormones led to an understanding of how neural and hormonal systems interact. Chemical regulations are usually viewed in the same manner as cell metabolism – i.e., controlling substances (hormones) diffuse through the extracellular matrix until they happen to bump into 'target' cells, upon which they exert their influences. Recall Chapter 9 and Figure 9.1.

A simplistic view is that some hormones react with cell surfaces, while others cross the cell membrane and exert their effects on the cell interior. We now know that many hormones or other signal molecules deliver messages to cell surfaces and that this then causes the production of 'second messengers' within the cells that activate cellular activities (see, e.g., Rasmussen, 1981). Hence, communication in living systems involves two main languages: chemical and energetic. Chemical regulations are carried out by hormones, various 'factors' (e.g., growth factor, epithelial growth factor) and the various 'second messengers' within cells. In contrast, energetic interactions are of two kinds, electrical and electronic. The electrical activities of nerves and muscles are well known, but there are many other kinds of energetic signaling systems. Some remain to be discovered.

We shall see that an even more profound realization is emerging. The entire living matrix is simultaneously a mechanical, vibrational or oscillatory, energetic, electronic, photonic and informational network (Oschman, 1994; Pienta and Coffey, 1991). Hence the entire composite of physiological and regulatory processes we refer to as the 'living state' takes place within the context of a continuous communicating living matrix.

A sensible design for a living system is one in which every cell receives information on the activities taking place in every other part of the body:

The integrated human body is the sum of thousands of physiological processes and traits working together. Each breath and each heartbeat involves the working together of countless events. Huge numbers of functions are carried on simultaneously. The parts and processes within an organism are woven together with great intricacy. Coordination occurs at a thousand points. If there were no integration of activities, life would be a random jumble of physical and chemical events that reaches no known accomplishment. In actuality, each process is of consequence to the whole.

ADOLPH (1982)

Physiological integration is possible because every cell and every molecule fine-tunes its activities appropriately. While the diffusion of chemicals from place to place is one important means of communication, it is far too slow a process to account for the rapid and subtle aspects of the living process. We are now discerning that the living matrix itself is a high-speed communication network linking every part with every other.

Matrix Dynamics: Signaling and Cell Crawling

Recently there has been tremendous excitement in the research community about the properties of the living matrix. The excitement arises because the matrix has key roles in defence and repair. Moreover, it is through this matrix that nutrients, hormones, and other signal molecules, toxins, and waste products diffuse to and from all cells. Obviously, the properties of this system, its 'open-ness' to the flows of various materials and signals, are essential to life.

One of the conclusions from studying the various complementary therapies in relation to con-ventional medicine is that the latter has become focused on the various organs and systems and has given relatively scant attention to the ways in which they communicate with each other via the living matrix. In contrast, complementary therapists often solve health problems by first attending to the 'quality' of the matrix, meaning the way the flesh looks and feels to the touch and the ways it moves. Areas that have been injured can be left with scars or densities that hinder the flows of blood, nutrients, energy, information flows, and cell migrations. These are often palpable to the holistic therapist or the experienced physician. Structural bodywork procedures systematically resolve these remnants of old injuries, enabling the lymphatic, circulatory, nervous, and other communicating systems to work better.

The molecules that link the cell interior with the extracellular matrix have come to be called *integrins*.

> *Integrins are a class of adhesion molecules that 'glue' cells in place. Surprisingly, at a fundamental level, they also regulate most functions of the body. The author reveals the hidden role of integrins in arthritis, heart disease, stroke, osteoporosis, and the spread of cancer.*
>
> HORWITZ (1997)

The living matrix is a dynamic rather than a fixed system. The connections between adjacent cells, and between the cells and the substrate, are labile rather than permanent. Connections form, break, and reform as cells change shape and/or crawl about. Specific connectors, called tono-filaments, desmosomes, hemidesmosomes, integrins, connexins, and anchoring filaments, are all labile structures that can disconnect, retract, dissolve, and reform (Gabbiani et al., 1978; Krawczyk and Wilgram, 1973). These reversible adhesions enable epidermal cells, fibroblasts, osteoblasts, myoblasts, and other 'generative' cells to move about when necessary to repair (re-epithialize) dam-aged skin and restore other tissues. Amoeboid motions enable the various leukocytes to migrate to sites of infection or into tumors for resorption of 'non-self' material. All of these activities are enhanced by bodywork, energetic and movement therapies.

Solid State Biochemistry

As discussed above, modern biochemistry and cell biology were founded on the study of reactions taking place in solution. The discovery of the pervasive cytoskeleton, with its dynamic intercon-nections with the nuclear and connective tissue matrices, has advanced our understanding of *solid state biochemistry*.

The development of this field obviously does not reject the beautiful and profoundly important work done by biochemists and molecular biologists on the 'soluble' enzymes and their activities. Instead, solid state biochemistry opens up the study of additional processes taking place on and in the solid fibres and filaments that constitute living cells and tissues. This approach also opens up a deeper understanding of the effects of hands-on, structural, energetic, and biomechanical therapies on processes taking place throughout the body.

Solution biochemistry required that the molecules within the cell diffuse about more or less randomly until they bump into appropriate enzymes (Figure 10.5B). Solid state biochemistry rec-ognizes that chemical reactions proceed in a much more orderly and rapid manner if the enzymes are organized on a structural framework (Figure 10.7B). The actual velocity of such reactions has been measured by a remarkable technique called *femtosecond spectroscopy*. The developers of the approach, Ahmed H. Zewail and his colleagues at the California Institute of Technology, received the Nobel Prize in Chemistry in 1999. To understand their discovery, consider what an athletic event on TV would be like without 'slow motion' revealing precisely how a goal was scored? The same is true of chemical reactions. Zewail and his colleagues developed a method for studying atoms and molecules in 'slow motion' during a reaction to see the details of the breaking of chemical bonds and the formation of new ones. The method uses what has to be the world's fastest camera. Using femtosecond spectroscopy, Zewail discovered that atoms move at a speed of the order of 1000 m/s – about as fast as a rifle bullet. Few scientists believed that it would ever be possible to see such fast events. This is one of the achievements of solid state biochemistry – understanding the velocities chemical reactions can achieve if they do not have to rely on random diffusion to bring the reactants together.

The living matrix concept opens up the possibilities for global control: Signals travelling *in* the matrix can regulate or fine-tune matrix-associated enzymes, metabolons, throughout the organism. Here we distinguish between messages that travel *through* the matrix, as by diffusion through the interstitial fluid lying between its fibres, and messages travelling *in* the matrix itself, as by electronic conduction along protein backbones, or by hopping of protons in the layers of water associated with the protein surface (Ho and Knight, 1998). The mechanisms involved in matrix communication are dealt with in the next sections.

To understand the therapeutic significance of solid state biochemistry and matrix regulation, we begin with an examination of the high degree of order, or regularity, or crystallinity present in cells and tissues.

Crystalline Arrays in Cells and Tissues: Piezoelectricity

We do not intuitively consider biological materials to be crystalline, because when we think of crystals we usually think of hard materials, such as diamond or agate. Living crystals are composed of long, thin, pliable molecules and are soft and flexible. To be more precise, they are liquid crystals (e.g., Bouligand, 1978). Crystalline arrangements are the rule and not the exception in living systems. Figure 16.2 gives some important examples.

Physicists know a great deal about the properties of crystals. The information they have obtained is of considerable medical importance. For example, certain kinds of crystals are piezoelectric, that is, they generate electric fields when they are compressed or stretched. Many piezoelectric materials are also thermoelectric – they generate electric fields when their temperature changes. One consequence of these two solid state properties, piezoelectricity and thermoelectricity, is that touching the body can cause the tissue to produce electric fields, and these fields, in turn, can interact with physiological processes.

Physiologists have recognized the importance of the piezoelectric effect and have studied the generation of electricity by bone. Each step you take compresses bones in the legs and throughout the skeleton and generates characteristic electrical fields. The piezoelectric effect is not, however, confined to bone. Virtually all of the tissues in the body generate electric fields when they are compressed or stretched (Oschman, 1981). The piezoelectric effect is partly responsible for these electric fields. Another source of such fields is a phenomenon known as the streaming potential. The relative contribution of these two ways of generating electric fields in tissues has been studied (e.g., MacGinitie, 1995). Figure 10.9 compares the two phenomena.

The important point is that when a bone or cartilage is compressed, when a tendon or ligament stretches, or when the skin is stretched or bent, as at a joint, minute electric pulsations are set up. These oscillations and their harmonics (harmonics are multiples of the fundamental frequency) are precisely representative of the forces acting on the tissues involved. In other words, they contain information on the precise nature of the movements taking place. This information is electrically and electronically conducted through the surrounding living matrix. One of the roles of this information is in the control of form.

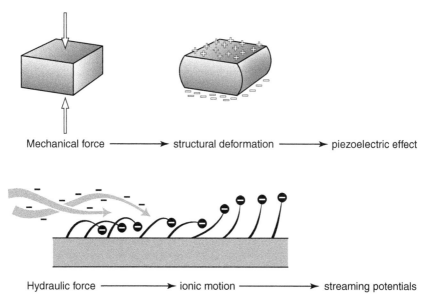

Mechanical force ⟶ structural deformation ⟶ piezoelectric effect

Hydraulic force ⟶ ionic motion ⟶ streaming potentials

Figure 10.9 Two methods by which movements generate electricity in tissues. The upper drawing shows the generation of piezoelectric or pressure electricity by the deformation of a crystalline structure. The lower drawing shows the way streaming potentials are developed by the flow of fluid containing charged ions over electrically charged surfaces. The charge is built up by the electrostatic interactions between the fixed tissue charge and the mobile charge. Potentials of this type are generated by both blood flow and propulsion of extracellular fluids through the extracellular matrix, as a result of tissue deformation. The streaming potentials can interact additively or subtractively with piezoelectric potential. *From Buchwald H, Varco RL: Metabolic Surgery. New York: Grune & Stratton; 1978.)*

The Control of Body Structure: Metabolic Regeneration

The therapeutic and physiological importance of the piezoelectric and other solid state electronic properties of tissues is that they provide a framework for understanding how the body adapts to the ways it is used (Oschman, 1989).

There was a time when biologists had assumed that the structure of the adult body is relatively fixed and permanent, although a few scientists had suggested that a small portion of the dietary intake might be used to repair and replace structures that undergo wear and tear. This picture changed dramatically with the publication of a little book in 1942 with the title *The Dynamic State of Body Constituents*. The book contained three Dunham Lectures that had been presented at Harvard University by Rudolph Schoenheimer, MD, of Columbia University. In these lectures Schoenheimer described his pioneering studies in which radioactive isotopes were used to label organic compounds that could be incorporated into the diets of animals. The labels could be traced to see if the compounds appeared in the tissues of the animal or were excreted. To everyone's great surprise, Schoenheimer and his colleagues discovered that a large fraction of the isotopically labelled compounds were incorporated into the tissues.

Ratner (1979), a colleague of Schoenheimer, reviewed the way this inquiry evolved since Schoenheimer's 1942 publication. Schoenheimer had developed the concept of 'metabolic regeneration', which stood the test of time. The large molecules in the body, such as fats and proteins, are constantly being assembled and disassembled. The various bonds or linkages that hold them together are constantly being opened, enabling their building blocks (fatty acids and amino acids, respectively) to be liberated. The fragments then enter what has been called the metabolic 'pool', which is also fed by absorption of the same materials from the digestive tract. This pool is located within the sponge-like interstices of the meshwork of the connective tissue and cytoplasmic ground substance shown in Figures 11.3 and 11.4. Some of the molecules in this pool are degraded and excreted, while others are inserted back into large molecules such as the collagen in connective tissue.

All of the reactions involved are balanced so precisely that the body components remain nearly constant in quantity, position, and structure. The lytic or degradative enzymes that take structures apart are balanced by synthetic or generative reactions. And these enzymes are themselves proteins that are constantly being assembled and taken apart. The process is controlled by the cell nucleus, which fine-tunes the rates of production and degradation of the enzymes.

The situation is analogous to a brick wall held together by a water-soluble cement so that bricks can easily be removed and replaced without changing the size and shape of the wall. Should the wall for some reason be called upon to carry an extra load, additional bricks and cement can be added to strengthen the structure. This is accomplished by bringing in more bricklayers (enzymes for synthesis) so that the rate of assembly exceeds the rate of removal.

A question that has arisen is why nature, which is usually so economical in the use of materials and energy, chose to engage in the costly process of continual turnover of the molecules of which the body is composed. The rate of turnover seems beyond that needed for repair of worn-out parts. Some molecules have a half-life of only 19 min (Schimke and Doyle, 1970). The biochemists who have studied this problem have not ventured an explanation, except for some speculations that protein turnover might enable an animal to adapt to changes in diet, hormone levels, or starvation. But from the perspective of energetics there is an obvious explanation: Nature has allowed for rapid adaptive change in the structure of an organism in response to changes in the way the organism interacts energetically with its environment. Changes in diet are only one of many such interactions. The healing of wounds, physical or emotional, is another. For example, Pickup (1978) suggested that behaviourally mediated patterns of stress can bring about increases in collagen density in connective tissues. And the degree to which the body is moving and interacting with the gravity field is another important influence on structure.

Athletes, musicians, dancers, and other performers experience the progressive adaptations of structure, function, motion, and availability of energy that occur when an activity is practiced again and again. An extreme example is the body-builder, who through the stimulus of constant exertion brings about a dramatic alteration in body form. Not only do the muscles increase in size and strength, but the other components of the myofascial system increase as well. The delicate skill of the concert violinist is an example of the same phenomenon – the gradual perfection of form and motion as the body adjusts to the way it is used.

By what mechanism are these remarkably orderly and concerted changes in structure coordinated? At present it is thought that the electric fields produced during movements provide information that directs the activities of 'generative' cells (e.g., Bassett, 1971; Bassett et al., 1964). These are the osteoblasts, myoblasts, perivascular cells, fibroblasts, and other cells that deposit or reabsorb collagen and other components of the connective tissue and thereby reform tissues so they can adapt to the ways the body is used. This regulatory concept dates back to Wolff in 1892 (see Bassett, 1968):

The form of the bone (or other connective tissue) being given, the bone elements (collagen) place or displace themselves in the direction of the functional pressure and increase or decrease their mass to reflect the amount of functional pressure.

WOLFF'S LAW, FROM BASSETT (1968)

Robert O. Becker, MD, summarized the consequences of Wolff's law:

When a bone is bent, one side is compressed and the other side is stretched. When it's bent consistently in one direction, extra bone grows to shore up the compressed side, and some is absorbed from the stretched side. It's as though a bridge could sense that most of its traffic was in one lane and could put up extra beams and cables on that side while dismantling them from the other. As a result, a tennis player or baseball pitcher has heavier and differently contoured bones in the racket arm or pitching arm than in the other one.

BECKER AND SELDEN (1985)

Again, these concepts are highly relevant to the hands-on, energetic, or movement therapist and to the practitioner of energy psychology. There is a scientific basis for progressive changes in body structure that take place because of the ways in which individuals use their bodies in relation to gravity because of habits, emotional states, or injuries. There is also a scientific basis for restorative measures that correct gravity-related disorders, whether they are caused by habitual patterns of movement, injury or emotional trauma (Oschman, 1997; Rolf, 1962) (see Chapters 11 and 12 in Oschman, 2000).

The flexibility and adaptability of human structure was well understood by Dr. Ida P. Rolf:

Human bodies can change toward orderliness, or they can change away from it ... bodies are amazingly plastic media.

ROLF (1977)

By what mechanism are orderly and concerted changes in structure coordinated? At present it is thought that communication between the various tissues and cells is, at least in part, mediated by the electric fields produced by the piezoelectric effect and streaming potentials, as described on page 166 of this chapter. This signaling system provides the link between the ways we use our bodies and carry loads and our body structure. A stimulus for research on this topic has been the discovery by Robert O. Becker and others that weak electrical currents can facilitate the healing of bone fractures and regeneration of limbs, to be discussed in detail in Chapter 15 (see Figures 15.1 and 15.2). It is thought that cells such as fibroblasts and osteoblasts utilize information contained in the minute bioelectric signals generated by the piezoelectric effect to determine the rates of production of enzymes that are responsible for the synthetic and degradative processes that were given the name metabolic regeneration by Schoenheimer. We will see in Chapter 15 that the application of minute artificial electrical fields can facilitate bone healing and regeneration by augmenting the natural piezoelectric fields that are poorly conducted through injured or disordered tissues. At the same time, therapeutic fields can help reorganize disordered tissues, improving their conductivity. This is a classic example of a positive feedback loop in which improvements in a process increase the rate of improvement.

Properties of the Living Matrix

On the basis of the information presented so far, we can begin to form a picture of the energetic systems in the living body. The living matrix continuum includes all of the connective tissues and all of the cytoskeletons and cell nuclei throughout the body. We can summarize its properties as follows:

- All of the great systems of the body – the circulation, the nervous system, the musculoskeletal system, the digestive tract, the various organs and glands – are everywhere covered with material that is but a part of a continuous connective tissue fabric.
- The connective tissues form a mechanical continuum, extending throughout the animal body, even into the innermost parts of each cell. Tensions or compressions in one part affect the whole.
- The connective tissues determine the overall shape of the organism as well as the detailed architecture of all of its parts.
- All movement of the body as a whole or of its smallest parts is created by tensions conducted through the connective tissue fabric. Individual cells move about by generating tensions in their cytoskeletons, tensions that are transmitted to the connective tissue substrate.

- Each tension, each compression, each movement causes the crystalline lattice of the connective tissues to generate piezoelectric, bioelectric, bioelectronic, biomagnetic and probably biophotonic signals that are precisely characteristic of those tensions, compressions, and movements.
- The connective tissue fabric is a semiconducting communication network that conducts bioelectronic signals between every part of the body and every other part. Optimal health can be visualized as arising from optimizing all of these communications.
- The connective tissue and its extensions into every cell and nucleus, the living matrix, is the largest and most pervasive organ system in the body because it is the material that all of the other organ systems are made of. It is the background, the common denominator, life's mater and matrix, mother and medium, that enables all therapies to have their effects.

Circuits and Meridians

That the human body is composed of electronic circuits is not widely appreciated, and this is part of the reason some of the phenomena found in alternative medicine have been difficult to grasp. Electronic circuits can be designed to do many things – this is the wonder of our present age of technology. Life has tested all possible combinations of electronic and quantum electronic tricks and has mastered all of them for its purposes, through the honing process of evolution. The next chapter will detail the discovery of the electronic and other solid state properties of living matter.

Information about biological electronics has been with us for a long time, but it has not been widely appreciated. Figure 11.10 shows the image of a circuit diagram laid over a salamander that was used as the logo for a scientific conference on mechanisms of growth control, clinical applications, held at the State University of New York Upstate Medical Center in 1979. Regeneration of limbs has long been a goal of a number of clinical researchers and alternative therapists. The attainment of this goal will require a more detailed understanding of the regulatory processes taking place in the matrix than we presently have.

The best introduction to the electronic circuitry of the human body is to be found in the study of acupuncture. We take a close look at this in Chapter 14, describing how energy and information circulate within the 'living matrix'.

Conclusions

Interconnectivity is a concept that is used in numerous fields such as cybernetics, biology, ecology, network theory, complex adaptive systems and nonlinear dynamics. The concept can be summarized: All parts of a system interact with and rely on one another simply by the fact that they are parts of the same system. The fundamental discoveries providing the basis for the various energetic therapies have taken place in a wide variety of disciplines. With a few exceptions, the remarkable generalizations – the 'big picture' – emerging from the individual discoveries has been virtually invisible to the participants in the search for knowledge. What has been discovered is the scientific basis for the interconnectedness and continuity and integrated functioning of the parts of the living organism. This interconnectedness is based upon careful study of the structure and function of cells and tissues. It provides a basis for the streaming of energy and information throughout the living body.

References

Abadjieva, A., Pauwels, K., Hilven, P., Crabeel, M., 2001. Discovery of a new yeast metabolon involving the two first enzymes of arginine biosynthesis: acetylglutamate synthase activity and regulation requires complex formation with acetylglutamate kinase. Paper Presented at the Meeting of the Benelux Yeast Research Groups Leuven, Belgium, 4 May 2001 Yesterday 2001, 1:or008.

Adolph, E.F., 1982. Physiological integrations in action. Physiologist 25 (2), 1–67, (April) supplement.

Arnold, H., Pette, D., 1968. Binding of glycolytic enzymes to structure proteins of the muscle. Eur. J. Biochem. 6, 163–171.

Atkinson, D.E., 1969. Limitation of metabolite concentrations and the conservation of solvent capacity in the living cell. Curr. Top. Cell. Regul. 1, 29.

Bassett, C.A.L., 1968. Biologic significance of piezoelectricity. Calcif. Tissue Res. 1, 252–272.

Bassett, C.A.L., 1971. Effect of forces on skeletal tissues. In: Downey, J.A., Darling, R.C. (Eds.), Physiological Basis of Rehabilitation Medicine. W.B. Saunders, Philadelphia, pp. 283–316.

Bassett, C.A.L., Pawluk, R.J., Becker, R.O., 1964. Effects of electric currents on bone formation in vivo. Nature (London) 204, 652–654.

Bouligand, Y., 1978. Liquid crystals and their analogs in biological systems. In: Liebert, L. (Ed.), Liquid Crystals. In: Solid State Physics, Academic Press, New York, NY. 14. pp. 259–294 (supplement).

Bretscher, M., 1975. C-Terminal region of the major erythrocyte sialoglycoprotein is on the cytoplasmic side of the membrane. J. Mol. Biol. 98, 831–833.

Capra, F., 1984. The Turning Point: Science, Society, and the Rising Culture. Bantam, New York, NY.

Capra, F., 2000. The Tao of Physics: An Exploration of the Parallels between Modern Physics and Eastern Mysticism (25th Anniversary Edition). Shambhala Publications, Inc., Boston, MA.

Capra, F., 2004. The Hidden Connections: A Science for Sustainable Living. Anchor, New York, NY.

Cope, F.W., 1967. A theory of cell hydration governed by adsorption of water on cell proteins rather than by osmotic pressure. Bull. Math. Biophys. 29, 583–596.

Corongiu, G., Clementi, E., 1981. Simulations of the solvent structure for macromolecules. I. Solvation of B-DNA double helix at T=300 K. Biopolymers 20, 551–571.

Damadian, R., 1971. Tumor detection by nuclear magnetic resonance. Science 171 (19), 1151–1153.

Dick, D.A.T., 1964. The permeability coefficient of water in the cell membrane and the diffusion coefficient in the cell interior. J. Theor. Biol. 7, 504–531.

Duncan, J.A., Storey, K.B., 1992. Subcellular enzyme binding and the regulation of glycolysis in anoxic turtle brain. Am. J. Physiol. 262 (3 Pt. 2), R517–R523.

Edelmann, L., 2002. Freeze-dried and resin-embedded biological material is well suited for ultrastructure research. J. Microsc. 207 (1), 5–26.

Edström J-E 1992 Presentation Speech for The Nobel Prize in Physiology or Medicine, 1974 From Nobel Lectures, Physiology or Medicine 1971-1980, translated from the Swedish text. Lindsten J ed, World Scientific Publishing Co., Singapore.

Einthoven, W., Fahr, G., de Waart, A., 1913. Über die Richtung und die manifeste Grösse der Potentialschwankungen im menschlichen Herzen und über den Einfluss der Herzlage auf die Form des Elektrokardiogramms. Pflugers Arch Gesamte Physiol Menschen Tiere 150, 275–315.

Ellison, J., Garrod, D.R., 1984. Anchoring filaments of the amphibian epidermal junction traverse the basal lamina entirely from the plasma membrane of hemidesmosomes to the dermis. J. Cell Sci. 72, 163–172.

Fenichel, I.R., Horowitz, S.B., 1963. The transport of nonelectrolytes in muscle as a diffusional process in cytoplasm. Acta Physiol. Scand. 60 (suppl. 221), 1–63.

Feyerabend, P., 1981. Realism, Rationalism and Scientific Method: Philosophical Papers, vol. 1. Cambridge University Press, Cambridge, UK, p. 185.

Gabbiani, G., Chaponnier, C., Huttner, I., 1978. Cytoplasmic filaments and gap junctions in epithelial cells and myofibroblasts during wound healing. J. Cell Biol. 76 (3), 561–568.

Harris, E.J., 1957. Permeation and diffusion of K ions in frog muscle. J. Gen. Physiol. 41, 169–195.

Harris, E.J., Prankerd, T.A.J., 1957. Diffusion and permeation of cations in human and dog erythrocytes. J. Gen. Physiol. 41, 197–218.

Ho, M.-W., Knight, D.P., 1998. The acupuncture system and the liquid crystalline collagen fibers of the connective tissues. Am. J. Chin. Med. 26 (3–4), 1–13.

Horwitz, A.F., 1997. Integrins and health. Discovered only recently, these adhesive cell surface molecules have quickly revealed themselves to be critical to proper functioning of the body and to life itself. Sci. Am. 276, 68–75.

Ingber, D.E., 1993. The riddle of morphogenesis: a question of solution chemistry or molecular cell engineering? Cell 75, 1249–1252.

Juarrero, A., 2002. Dynamics in Action: Intentional Behavior as a Complex System. A Bradford Book, MIT Press, Cambridge, MA.

Kaptchuk, T.J., 1983. The Web That Has No Weaver: Understanding Chinese Medicine. Congdon & Weed, New York, NY.

Krawczyk, W.S., Wilgram, G.F., 1973. Hemidesmosome and desmosome morphogenesis during epidermal wound healing. J. Ultrastruct. Res. 45, 93.

László, E., 1996. The Systems View of the World: A Holistic Vision for Our Time. Hampton Press, New York, NY.

Ling, G.N., 1992. A Revolution in the Physiology of the Living Cell. Krieger Publishing Company, Malabar, FL.

Ling, G.N., Cope, F.W., 1969. Potassium ion: is the bulk of intracellular K adsorbed? Science 163, 1335–1336.

Luby-Phelps, K., 2000. Cytoarchitecture and physical properties of cytoplasm: volume, viscosity diffusion, intracellular surface area. Int. Rev. Cytol. 192, 189–221.

MacGinitie, L.A., 1995. Streaming and piezoelectric potentials in connective tissues. In: Blank, M. (Ed.), Electromagnetic Fields: Biological Interactions and Mechanisms. Advances in Chemistry Series, 250. American Chemical Society, Washington, DC, pp. 125–142 ch 8.

Maitland, J., 1980. A phenomenology of fascia. Somatics Vol. III, #1(Autumn)15–21.

Maniotis, A.J., Chen, C.S., Ingber, D.E., 1997. Demonstration of mechanical connections between integrins, cytoskeletal filaments, and nucleoplasm that stabilize nuclear structure. Proc. Natl. Acad. Sci. U.S.A. 94, 849–854.

Masters, C.J., 1981. Interactions between soluble enzymes and subcellular structure. CRC Crit. Rev. Biochem. 11 (2), 105–143.

McConkey, E.H., 1982. Molecular evolution, intracellular organization, and the quinary structure of proteins. Proc. Natl. Acad. Sci. U.S.A. 79 (10), 3236–3240 (Part 1: Biological Sciences).

McKeon, R. (Ed.), 2001. The Basic Works of Aristotle. Modern Library, Random House, New York, NY.

Northrop, F.S.C., 1959. The two kinds of deductively formulated theory. In: The Logic of the Sciences and the Humanities. Asher A., ed. Meridian Books, New Haven, CT, p. 102, ch 6.

Oschman JL 1981 The connective tissue and myofascial systems. In: readings on the scientific basis of bodywork, energetic, and movement therapies. NORA Press, P.O. Box 5101, Dover, NH 03821, USA. E-mail: joschman@aol.com.; web page: www.bodywork-res.com.

Oschman, J.L., 1989. How the body maintains its shape. Rolf Lines (news magazine for Rolf Institute members) 17 (3), 27.

Oschman, J.L., 1994. A biophysical basis for acupuncture. In: Proceedings of the First Symposium of the Society for Acupuncture Research, Winston Salem, NC, Jan 23-24, 1993. The Society for Acupuncture Research/Paradigm Publications, Brookline, MA.

Oschman, J.L., 1997. What is healing energy? Part 5: gravity, structure, and emotions. J. Bodyw. Mov. Ther. 1 (5), 297–309.

Oschman, J.L., 2000. Energy Medicine: the scientific basis. Churchill Livingstone, Edinburgh, page 47.

Pickup, A.J., 1978. Collagen and behaviour: a model for progressive debilitation. IRCS. J. Med. Sci. 6, 499–502.

Pienta, K.J., Coffey, D., 1991. Cellular harmonic information transfer through a tissue tensegrity-matrix system. Med. Hypotheses 34, 88–95.

Rasmussen, H., 1981. Calcium and cAMP As Synarchic Messengers. John Wiley & Sons, New York, NY.

Ratcliffe, J.W., 1983. Notions of validity in qualitative research methodology. Sci. Commun. 5 (2), 147–167.

Ratner, S., 1979. The dynamic state of body proteins. Ann. N. Y. Acad. Sci. 325, 189–209.

Reed, L.J., Cox, D.J., 1966. Macromolecular organization of enzyme systems. Annu. Rev. Biochem. 35, 57–84.

Rolf, I.P., 1962. Structural integration gravity: an unexplored factor in a more human use of human beings. J. Inst. Compar. Study History Philos. Sci. 1, 3–20 (Available from the Rolf Institute, Boulder, Colorado. Tel: (1)800-530-8875).

Roy, R., 2002. Science and whole person medicine: enormous potential in a new relationship. Bull. Sci. Technol. Soc. 22 (5), 374–390.

Schimke, R.T., Doyle, D., 1970. Control of enzyme levels in animal tissues. Annu. Rev. Biochem. 39, 929–976.

Schoenheimer, R., 1942. The Dynamic State of Body Constituents. Harvard University Press, Cambridge, MA.

Singer, E.A., 1986. Mind as a Behavior. AMS Press, Brooklyn, NY.

Sols, A., Marco, R., 1970. Concentrations of metabolites and binding sites. Implications in metabolic regulation. Curr. Top. Cell. Regul. 2, 227.

Srere, P.A., 1985. The metabolon. Trends Biochem. Sci. 10, 109–110.

Szent-Györgyi, A., 1957. Bioenergetics. Academic Press, New York, NY, pp. 38–39.

Szent-Györgyi, A., 1963. Lost in the twentieth century. Annu. Rev. Biochem. 32, 1–14.

von Bertalanffy, L., 1971. General System Theory. Foundations, Development, Applications (revised and enlarged edition). Penguin, London.

CHAPTER 11

The Living Matrix: Ten Perspectives

Chapter Summary

Now we look at the living matrix from a variety of different, but related, views. As with an elaborate sculpture, every perspective gives a different image. Every branch of science and human inquiry has to be taken into account for a thorough study of the living matrix, which is the fundamental material that gives rise to the living state – that fundamentally enables us to do what we do. Alfred Pischinger and Hartmut Heine (Figure 11.1) referred to this as the largest system penetrating the organism completely because it touches all of the other systems. It is actually impossible to take in all perspectives at once, especially since there are undoubtedly other perspectives we do not yet know about. Therefore, achieving a full and complete synthesis will always be an approximation. Attempting to do this is nonetheless a very worthwhile endeavour because it leads to increased clarity on the real nature of life. Moreover, each perspective has important clinical implications, and each perspective is worthy of further research.

The discoveries summarized in this chapter help explain how energy and information circulate within the body to power and regulate dynamic living processes. The present view is that the entire living matrix forms an electronic, protonic, and photonic network reaching into every part of the body. A number of prominent scientists and clinicians have contributed valuable insights. Our goal is to synthesize these diverse perspectives. We shall summarize the work of Andrew Taylor Still, Alfred Pischinger, Hartmut Heine, Albert Szent-Györgyi, Robert O. Becker, Herbert Fröhlich, Donald Ingber, K.J. Pienta, Donald S. Coffey, Thomas Hanna, Mae-Wan Ho, David P. Knight, Mark F. Barnes, Gerald Pollack, and last, the author.

Andrew Taylor Still and the Connective Tissue

In Chapter 4, it was pointed out that Andrew Taylor Still (1828–1917) originated many of the concepts that are now used in a wide variety of complementary and alternative therapies. His gift to the world, osteopathy, continues to evolve and to set high standards for quality and effective healthcare. It is always fascinating to explore the discoveries of insightful people who have done their basic research using their sensitive hands, long before scientific instruments were available. For example, A.T. Still determined that the brain is an electric 'dynamo' because he could feel its electrical activity through his sensitive fingers. He reported this in 1908, more than a dozen years before Hans Berger (1873–1941) published the first electroencephalogram, which was recorded in 1924 (see Figure 8.6 for his apparatus and recordings).

We will look at some of Andrew Taylor Still's comments about the connective tissue. His focus is on the fascia. First we define this material:

Fascia is the soft tissue component of the connective tissue system that permeates the human body. Fascia interpenetrates and surrounds muscles, bones, organs, nerves, blood vessels and other structures. Fascia is an uninterrupted, three-dimensional web of tissue that extends from head to toe, from front to back, from interior to exterior. It is responsible for maintaining structural integrity; for providing support and protection; and acts as a shock absorber. Fascia has an

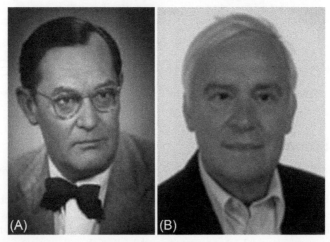

Figure 11.1   Alfred Pischinger (A) and Hartmut Heine (B), authors of *Matrix and Matrix Regulation: Basis for a Holistic Theory in Medicine.*

essential role in hemodynamics (blood flow) and biochemical processes, and provides the matrix that allows for intercellular communication. Fascia functions as the body's first line of defense against pathogenic agents and infections. After injury, it is the fascia that creates an environment for tissue repair.

PAOLETTI (2006)

Still's writing style will now be viewed as somewhat antiquated, but his passion and sensitive clinical observations are profound. In the next section, describing the work of Alfred Pischinger and colleagues, we will see that many of Still's insights have been confirmed and elaborated upon by modern research and clinical experience:

- *The fascia is the place to look for the cause of disease and the place to consult and begin the action of remedies in all diseases.*
- *As soon as we pass through the skin we enter the fascia. In it we find cells, glands, blood and other vessels, with nerves running to and from every part. Here we could spend an eternity with our present mental capacity, before we could comprehend even a superficial knowledge of the powers and uses of the fascia in the laboratory of animal life.*
- *I have thought for many years that the lymphatics and cellular system of the fascia ... do get filled up with impure and unhealthy fluids, long before any disease makes its appearance, and that the procedure of changes known as fermentation, with its electromagnetic disturbances, were the cause of at least ninety per cent of the diseases that we labor to relieve.*
- *There is no real difference between structure and function; they are the two sides of the same coin. If structure does not tell us anything about function, it means we have not looked at it correctly.*
- *This life is surely too short to solve the uses of the fascia in animal forms. It penetrates even its own finest fibers to supply and assist their gliding elasticity. Turn the visions of our mind to follow those infinitely fine fibers. You see the fascia, and in your wonder and surprise you exclaim: 'Omnipresent in man and in all other living beings of the land and sea. We see all the beauties of life on exhibition in the wonders found in the fascia ... the framework of life, the dwelling place in which life sojourns ... the places in which diseases germinate and develop the seeds of sickness and death ... going with and covering all muscles, tendons and fibers and separating them even to the last fiber.*
- *Each muscle plays its part in active life. Each fiber of all muscles owes its pliability to that yielding septum-washer that allows all muscles to glide over and around all adjacent muscles and*

ligaments without friction or jar. It not only lubricates the fibers, but gives nourishment to all parts of the body. Its nerves are so abundant that no atom of flesh fails to get the nerve and blood supply therefrom.

The most recent elaborations of the concepts Still put forward, and those advanced by a long line of other pioneers (Figure 4.6) as well as by modern fascia researchers from around the world, are recorded in *Fascia Research, Basic Science and Implications for Conventional and Complementary Health Care*, the proceedings of three International Fascia Research Congresses (Findley and Schleip, 2007; Huijing et al., 2009; Chaitow et al., 2012).

Alfred Pischinger and Hartmut Heine: The Extracellular Matrix and Ground Regulation

In 1975, Alfred Pischinger and Hartmut Heine published an important book about the whole-body regulatory system consisting of the capillaries, connective tissue, ground substance (matrix), extracellular fluid, and terminal autonomic axons. This seminal work was the culmination of years of Pischinger's research as Professor of Histology and Embryology in Vienna. Eight editions of his book have been published in German, and a newer translation is now available in both English (Pischinger, 2007) and as an updated version in German (Pischinger, 2004). Pischinger's theories have profound clinical implications and his applications and are worthy of careful study by any-one interested in clinical medicine and physiology. Professor Hartmut Heine contributed to the evolution of Pischinger's research, and he and his colleagues continue the work at the University of Frankfurt in Germany (e.g., Heine and Förster, 2004).

Pischinger and Heine recognized that the 'ground regulation system' (Figure 11.2) is respon-sible for all vital functions, including nutrition of cells, removal of wastes, inflammation, and de-fence and repair processes. The smallest common denominator of life in the vertebrate organism is therefore a triad: capillary-matrix-cell, as shown in Figure 11.2.

> *The concept of a cell is, strictly speaking, only a morphological abstraction. Seen from a biological viewpoint, a cell cannot be considered by itself without taking its environment into account.*
>
> PISCHINGER (2007)

This statement reveals the weakness of the popular concept of cellular pathology that has dominated Western medicine since it was first put forward by Virchow (1871). This is the idea that all illness arises in cells and is therefore only treatable by biochemical/pharmaco-logical approaches that affect cellular metabolism as viewed through the biochemical 'cytosol'

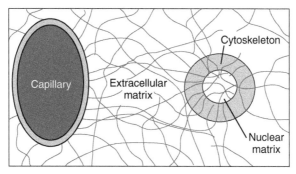

Figure 11.2 The ground regulation system of Pischinger and Heine is a triad consisting of the capillary, matrix, and cells.

model. What characterizes the complementary and alternative therapies is the importance placed on the quality of the matrix. This is one of many concepts that are fundamental to complementary and alternative medicine but that are virtually unknown in conventional Western biomedicine. This lack of awareness is unjustified and hampers advancement of medical science. It is not due to any fundamental flaw in Pischinger's logic or to a conspiracy of some kind. It is simply due to the omission of these concepts in medical school education.

Pischinger and Heine's triad has unique capacities for whole-person healing. The network of polymers between cells, the so-called ground substance, is continuously regenerated by the fibroblasts (Figure 11.3). This is also referred to as the extracellular matrix (ECM), which provides architectural support and anchorage for all cells. The ECM consists of a complex meshwork of highly cross-linked proteins and extends into organs and as specialized forms, such as basement membranes underlying epithelia, vascular endothelium, and surrounding certain other tissues and cell types.

The ECM is a remarkable assembly of molecules known as proteoglycans and hyaluronans (Figures 11.3 and 11.4). The basic unit in the ground substance is called the matrisome (Figure 11.3C). The subscript 'n' after the brackets [matrisome]$_n$ is an enormous number, because the matrisome is replicated throughout the body. There is no part of the body that lacks this substance. It has key roles in sensing, storing, distributing, and interpreting information and using this information to adjust energy flows. We shall see in Chapter 17 that the matrisomes are also thought to be stores of electrons needed for preventing the spread of inflammation when there is an injury.

The matrix and its associated water molecules form the oldest and most pervasive information and defence system in nature. By 'oldest' we are referring to the fact that the living matrix, including the matrisomes, has had a very much longer evolutionary history than the nervous system. It began with the extracellular sugar polymer coatings of individual bacteria, viruses, and protozoa, which extended the 'reach' of the individual cell into its environment. In the human body, then, the matrix extends the reach of every cell to its neighbours and beyond, to all other cells in the organism. It will not be surprising, then, if the matrix proves to be far more sophisticated than the nervous system in its ability to capture, store, and process information. The matrix extends into every cell and nucleus in the form of the cytoskeleton and nuclear matrix (Figure 10.7A). Referring to the complex behaviours of protozoa such as paramecium, the distinguished British neurophysiologist, C.S. Sherrington (1951) said, 'of nerve there is no trace. But the cell framework, the cytoskeleton might serve.'

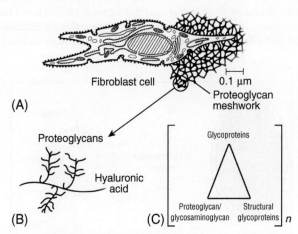

Figure 11.3 The network of proteoglycan polymers between cells, the so-called ground substance, is continuously regenerated by the fibroblasts. (A) The extracellular matrix is composed of the proteoglycans and hyaluronic acid. The basic unit in the ground substance is called the matrisome (C).

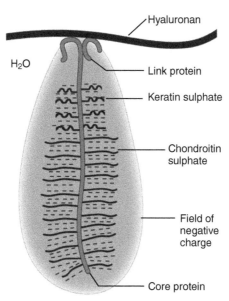

Figure 11.4 Negative charges on the ground substance bind water and ions. Excess hydrogen ions (acid pH) displace water and ions needed for normal physiology. *(Lee RP: Interface: Mechanisms of Spirit in Osteopathy, Stillness Press LLC, 2005.)*

The triad of Pischinger and Heine (Figure 11.2) can allow for organized or non-chaotic energy to spread suddenly throughout the organism. Such 'phase changes' are probably the most important events that can happen to a patient – the sudden whole-body sensation of lightness and lift that takes place as the whole system shifts into a new level of functioning. While rare, these are profound and emotional experiences of wholeness and whole-body integration and may account for the phenomenon of spontaneous healing, to be discussed in chapter 13.

Oxygen and nutrients from the blood wend their way through the interstices of the matrix to every cell in the body. Likewise, the waste products of metabolism diffuse from cells to the capillaries via the matrix. The matrix is the locus of the pathways that allow cells to communicate with each other. Any interference or blockage in these pathways can set the stage for disease. Toxins can accumulate in the matrix and can impact functioning. Here Pischinger is in complete agreement with A.T. Still: Most effective therapeutic approaches restore or enhance signaling and energy flows in the matrix and thereby prevent or treat disease.

Pischinger recognized the importance of the pH of the matrix fluids. Negative charges on the polyelectrolytes of the matrix (Figure 11.4) bind water and ions. Excess hydrogen ions (acid pH) displace the water and ions in this body-wide storage depot. This reservoir is essential to maintain a wide variety of functions. Acidity and the consequent dehydration of the matrix compromise cell-to-cell communications, flexibility, and range of motion at joints.

The relations between capillaries, connective tissue, ground substance, extracellular fluid, and terminal autonomic axons mentioned at the beginning of this section are summarized in Figure 11.5. For a more recent perspective on the matrisome, see Hynes and Naba (2011).

There is a basic electrostatic 'tone' to the whole connective tissue matrix system. This affects tissue elastic properties and impacts the delivery of hormones, neurotransmitters, neuropeptides, and pharmacological agents to all cells. The interstitial pH also influences the lubrication of joints, the ability of muscles to glide over each other and the freedom of cells to migrate from place to place. Inflammation compromises matrix functioning by causing swelling and reduction in range of motion. It also produces redness, pain, and heat.

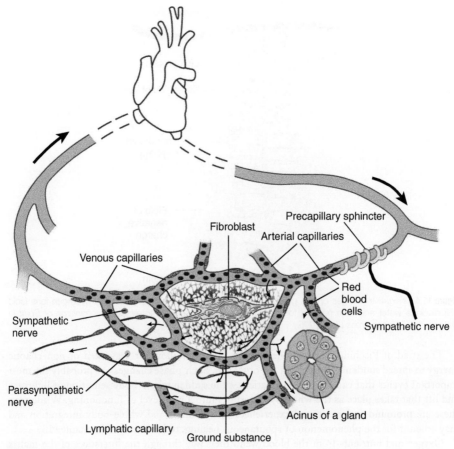

Figure 11.5   Relations between capillaries, connective tissue, ground substance, extracellular fluid, and terminal autonomic axons, based on Pischinger (2007).

Albert Szent-Györgyi: Electronic Conduction and Semiconduction

Albert Szent-Györgyi (Figure 11.6), who received the Nobel Prize in 1937 for the synthesis of vitamin C, was certain that the random bumping about of molecules (Figures 9.1 and 10.5B) was far too slow to explain the speed and subtlety of life. He looked for something that could move about rapidly within the living structure and focused on electrons, protons, and energy fields. Szent-Györgyi researched the insoluble scaffoldings that other biochemists routinely discarded (Figure 11.7). In 1941 he made a remarkable suggestion: The proteins in the body are semiconductors. He stated:

> *If a great number of atoms be arranged with regularity in close proximity, as for example in a crystal lattice, single electrons cease to belong to one or two atoms only, and belong instead to the whole system. A great number of molecules may join to form energy continua, along which energy, namely excited electrons, may travel a certain distance.*

SZENT-GYÖRGYI (1941)

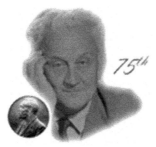

Figure 11.6 Portrait of Albert Szent-Györgyi published in 2012 to celebrate the 75th anniversary of his Nobel Prize award for the synthesis of Vitamin C.

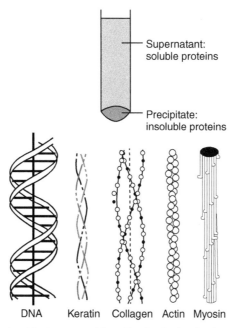

Figure 11.7 Traditional biochemistry focuses mainly on the dissolved molecules, while discarding the solids. The discarded material includes DNA, keratin, collagen, actin, and myosin.

To comprehend the implications of Szent-Györgyi's idea, it is important to understand the nature of conductors, insulators, and semiconductors (Figure 11.8). Insulators are materials in which the orbitals of the atoms are complete, i.e., there are no extra electrons that are free to move about, to participate in reactions or electrical conduction. Examples are teflon, rubber-like polymers, and most plastics (Figure 11.8A). Conductors are substances, such as metallic wires, that readily conduct electricity. Metals have a number of interesting properties that arise because they have free electrons that are not fixed in place but can move about (Figure 11.8B). Semiconductors lie between conductors and insulators in terms of their ability to conduct electricity. Collagen is an example of a biological semiconductor (Figure 11.8C). Other proteins can form semiconducting networks because of their periodic double bonds (Figure 11.8C). Each double bond contributes one electron that is mobile; it free to move about in the protein fabric. Since the living matrix is continuous throughout the organism, these electrons can go anywhere. What is extraordinary about semiconductors is that their conduction can be precisely controlled. This makes it possible to use semiconductors to make

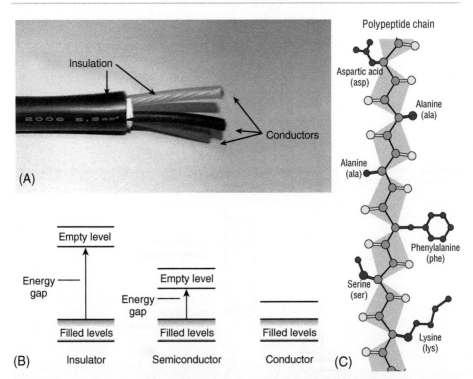

Figure 11.8 Conductors, insulators, and semiconductors. (A) is a standard electrical wire, showing the conductors and insulation that prevents the conductors from touching each other and causing a short circuit. (B) is a common scheme of the electrical properties of insulators, semiconductors, and conductors. In the insulator there is a large energy gap between the electrons in the atom and the 'empty level' where electrons can move about. In the conductor there is virtually no energy gap, so ordinary electrons can move into the empty or conduction zone. The semiconductor has a small energy gap, so that at normal temperatures some electrons can easily make the transition to the empty level where conduction can take place. (C) the double bonds, C = O, in a protein contain two electrons. Szent-Györgyi suggested that one of these pi electrons stabilizes the protein structure while the other one is somewhat delocalized and free to move about.

miniature electronic devices, such as switches, amplifiers, detectors, oscillators, rectifiers, and memory devices – the stuff our modern electronic computers and cell phones and other devices are made of.

The concept of semiconduction in living systems was vigorously opposed, but it was eventually shown to be entirely correct (Rosenberg and Postow, 1969). Virtually all of the molecules forming the living matrix are semiconductors. The modern global nanoelectronics enterprise has been built up substantially by using semiconducting proteins and has acknowledged Szent-Györgyi's seminal work in this field (see Hush, 2003).

In Chapter 1, we mentioned Szent-Györgyi's (1988) statement that, 'Molecules do not have to touch each other to interact. Energy can flow through ... the electromagnetic field.' He continued, 'The electromagnetic field, along with water, forms the matrix of life. Water ... can form structures that transmit energy.' The structures he was referring to are the layers of water intimately associated with the proteins in the living matrix. Thanks to contemporary research, we can now visualize the way water is organized in relationship to collagen, which is the major protein found in connective tissue (Figure 11.9). The importance of the water associated with proteins and other components of the matrix cannot be overestimated. Each fibre of the living matrix, both outside and inside cells and nuclei and the genetic material, is surrounded by organized layers of water that can serve as separate channels of communication and energy flow. While electrons flow through the fibres (electricity), protons flow through the water layer. This proton flow has been called 'proticity' (Mitchell, 1976).

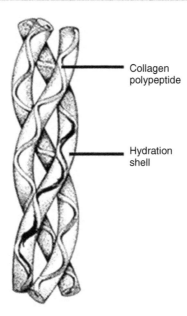

Figure 11.9   The collagen triple helix, showing the protein molecules and their hydration.

Robert O. Becker: Regeneration

The idea of the circuitry of the body deserves investigation for a variety of important reasons. One of these is the subject of regeneration of limbs, of obvious importance in a world in which warfare and accidents can lead to tragic loss of limbs.

Robert O. Becker was a pioneer in the study of limb regeneration. In 1979, he organized a conference on *Mechanisms of Growth Control, Clinical Applications*. The meeting was held on September 26–28 at the State University of New York Upstate Medical Centre. The logo for the conference (Figure 11.10) was an electronic circuit superimposed over the body of a salamander, a popular animal for regeneration research because of its ability to rapidly regenerate limbs and even the heart (Libbin et al., 1979; Mele and Sessions, 2014).

Rahul Sarpeshkar: Cell-Inspired Electronics

The transfer of information and insights between biology and technology has taken a quantum leap with the research of MIT scientist, Rahul Sarpeshkar (2010) (Figure 11.11).

A single cell in the human body is approximately 10,000 times more energy-efficient than any transistor, the fundamental building block of electronic chips and integrated circuits. In 1 second, a cell performs about 10 million energy-consuming chemical reactions, requiring about 1 picowatt (one-millionth-millionth of a watt) of power. Sarpeshkar is now applying principles learned from study of living cells to the design of low-power, highly parallel, hybrid analog-digital electronic circuits. Such circuits have enormous potential for many areas of medicine, biology, and technology. Specifically, they can be used to create miniature ultra-fast supercomputers and other devices, while at the same time helping resolve some difficult medical issues such as regeneration, spontaneous healing, inflammation, and the causes of serious conditions such as cancer and cardiovascular disease.

In his recent book, *Ultra Low Power Bioelectronics*, Sarpeshkar (2010) outlines the deep under-lying similarities between chemical reactions that occur in a cell and the flow of current through

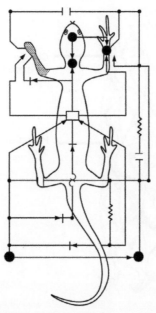

Figure 11.10 Logo for Robert O. Becker's 1979 conference: *Mechanisms of Growth Control, Clinical Applications*, held on September 26-28, 1979, at the State University of New York Upstate Medical Center. An electronic circuit is superimposed over the body of a salamander, a popular animal for research on regeneration.

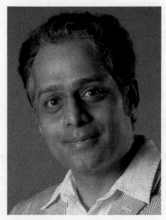

Figure 11.11 Rahul Sarpeshkar, MIT professor and author of *Ultra Low Power Bioelectronics: Fundamentals, Biomedical Applications, and Bio-Inspired Systems* (2010).

an analog electronic circuit. He discusses how biological cells perform reliable computations in the presence of noise (referring to random variations in both internal and environmental signals).

> *Circuits are a language for representing and trying to understand almost anything, whether it be networks in biology or cars ... there's a unified way of looking at the biological world through circuits that is very powerful.*

SARPESHKAR (2010)

Circuit designers already know hundreds of strategies to run analog circuits at low power, amplify signals, and reduce noise, which have helped them design low-power electronics such as mobile phones, mp3 players, and laptop computers. Electrical engineering has devoted 50 years to studying the design of complex systems, and we can now start to think of biology in the same way. Sarpeshkar has created a new field that he has called cytomorphic or cell-inspired or cell-transforming electronics, which has expanded neuromorphic to cytomorphic electronics, based on his analysis of the equations that govern the dynamics of chemical reactions and the flow of electrons through analog circuits. He has found that those equations, which predict the behaviour of both chemical reactions and electronic circuits, are astonishingly similar.

In a paper presented at a 2009 Institute of Electrical and Electronics Engineers (IEEE) symposium on Biological Circuits and Systems, Sarpeshkar described how a genetic network reaction can be simulated on a chip (Sarpeshkar, 2010).

Robert O. Becker: The Perineural Control System

In a series of important articles, Robert O. Becker described the properties of the connective tissue layer surrounding the nervous system, called the perineurium. Nearly every nerve fibre in the body, down to its finest terminations, is completely encased in perineural cells of one type or another. Becker recognized a 'dual nervous system' composed of the classical digital (all or none) nerve network, the focus of modern neurophysiology, and the evolutionarily more ancient perineural system, which operates on direct current (Figure 11.12). The perineural system is a distinct communication system. It sets up a low voltage current, the current of injury that controls injury repair. Pulsations of the direct current field in the brain, the so-called brain waves, direct the overall operation of the nervous system, and may regulate consciousness. This subject is also discussed in Chapters 14 and 15.

One of Becker's important discoveries is that the perineural system is sensitive to magnetic fields. The basis for this research is a magnetic phenomenon known as 'the transverse Hall effect', which indicates that semiconduction is taking place. This discovery simultaneously confirmed Szent-Györgyi's suggestion of semiconduction in the living matrix and gave a basis for the use of magnets and biomagnetic fields in healing (Becker, 1990, 1991; Oschman and Oschman, 1995). Becker concluded that the acupuncture points and meridians are input channels for the system that regulates tissue repair. With Maria Reichmanis, Becker showed that the meridians are low-resistance pathways through the body. He thought they had 'cable properties' much like transmission lines used for telephone and cable television, and required periodic 'booster amplifiers' to maintain signal integrity. Oschman (1994) agreed that the acupuncture points might be booster amplifiers and suggested that they may also be analogous to microprocessors located at nodes in a computer network. Nerve impulses are self-regenerating, whereas transmission through the meridians may lose strength over distance, as with any transmission line.

Herbert Fröhlich: Biological Coherence

Another area of research complements the work of Szent-Györgyi and Becker. Biophysicists have discovered in living matter a profoundly important vibratory phenomenon that further opens acupuncture and other energy therapies to academic inquiry. The individual most closely associated with this field is Herbert Fröhlich (Fröhlich, 1988). To make Fröhlich's discoveries more accessible to the non-scientist, Oschman and Oschman (1998) has published a review and commentary summarizing this work and relating the concepts to complementary therapies. There is also an extensive discussion of Fröhlich's work in Oschman (2003).

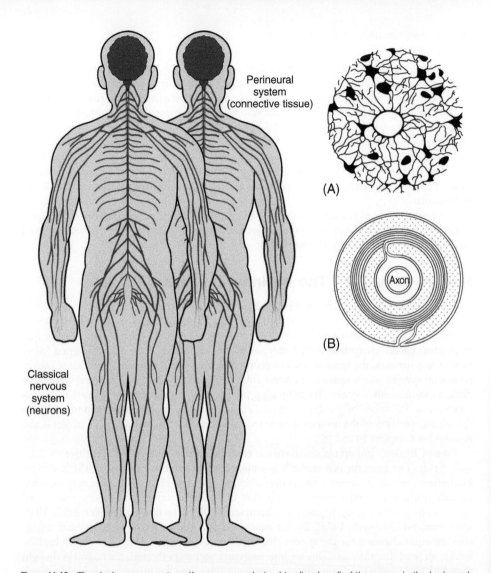

Perineural
system
(connective tissue)

(A)

Axon

(B)

Classical
nervous
system
(neurons)

Figure 11.12 The dual nervous system. If a way were devised to dissolve all of the nerves in the brain and throughout the body, it would appear to the naked eye that nothing was missing. The brain and the spinal cord and all of the peripheral nerves would be intact down to their smallest terminations. This is because the central nervous system is composed of two separate types of cells: the nerve cells, or 'neurons', and the 'perineural cells' (Becker 1990, 1991). The 'classical' nervous system is composed of neurons conducting information from place to place as electrical impulses. The signals are digital or 'all or none' in nature. Signals may be individual spikes, or trains of pulses. Digital systems provide high speed, high volume information transfer. In terms of evolution and phylogeny, this nervous system is a relatively recent innovation. This system is responsible for sensation and movement, and communications are 'point-to-point'. In contrast, the perineural nervous system is composed of perineural cells that conduct information from place to place as relatively slowly varying direct currents. These slow waves are analog rather than digital. Analog systems cannot transmit large amounts of data, but are ideally suited for precise control of individual functions. Some of these oscillations are maintained by pacemakers (e.g. brain waves). In terms of evolution and phylogeny, the perineural system is ancient. This system is responsible for overall regulation of the classical nervous system, and for regulating wound healing and injury repair. Instead of point-to-point signaling, information propagated by this system spreads throughout the body. The insets show examples of perineural cells. (A) Fibrous astrocytes with end feet around a small blood vessel. (B) A Schwann cell surrounding an axon in the peripheral nervous system. (Inset A from Glees 1955 Neurologia: Morphology and Function, with permission from Blackwell Science Ltd. Inset B is adapted from Fawcett 1994, Fig. 11.21, p. 335, with permission from Arnold.)

In the late 1960s, Fröhlich predicted, on the basis of quantum physics, that the living matrix must produce coherent or laser-like oscillations (Fröhlich, 1968). His prediction was confirmed in a number of laboratories. Of course, energy therapists of many schools have always recognized the importance of vibratory phenomena (including sound and light) in healing, but academic molecular science was focused on other matters.

From the work of Fröhlich and others, we now know that all parts of the living matrix set up vibrations that move about within the organism and that are radiated into the environment. These vibrations or oscillations occur at many different frequencies, including visible and near-visible light frequencies. Aspects of this vibratory communication will be considered in the next two sections of this chapter. These are not subtle phenomena; they can be large, or even gigantic, in scale. Moreover, their effects are not trivial, because living matter is highly organized and exceedingly sensitive to the information conveyed by coherent signals.

Coherent vibrations recognize no boundaries, at the surface of a molecule, cell, or organism – they are collective or cooperative properties of the entire being (Figure 11.13). As such, they are likely to serve as signals that integrate processes, such as growth, injury repair, defence, and the functioning of the organism as a whole. Each molecule, cell, tissue, and organ has an ideal

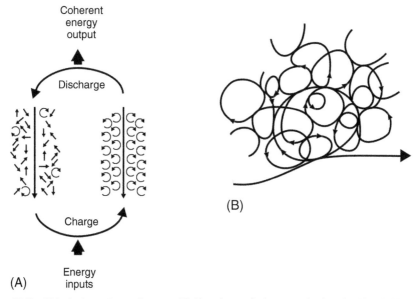

Figure 11.13 Biological quantum coherence. (A) The charge-discharge cycle described by Fröhlich, from Oschman (2003). Filamentous proteins such as collagen have electric charges along their length. Water molecules are also electrically charged because the oxygen atom is negative relative to the hydrogen atoms. Del Giudice and colleagues (1988) made a detailed mathematical application of quantum field theory (QFT) to these assemblies. Water molecules can vibrate or spin in various planes. As electrons are semi-conducted along the protein, the motions of nearby water molecules become temporarily correlated or coherent. As the charge moves away, the water molecules become less ordered. This rapid oscillation or cycle of order/disorder creates soliton waves (Hyman et al., 1981) that create electromagnetic fields. Since connective tissue consists of very large numbers of collagen molecules packed tightly together in a liquid crystalline arrangement, these fields can be substantial, and can couple to other parts of the organism. (B) Mae-Wan Ho (1997) has described how energy and information can move about efficiently within the organism through a cascade of cyclic quantum coherent waves. Energy and information input into any of the body's systems can be readily delocalized over all systems; conversely energy and information from all systems can become concentrated into any single system.

resonant frequency that coordinates its activities. By manipulating and balancing the vibratory circuits, complementary therapists are able to directly influence the body's systemic defence and repair mechanisms.

Donald Ingber, Stephen Levin, and Tom Flemons: Biotensegrity

These individuals have contributed importantly to our understandings of biomechanics and solid state biochemistry at different levels of scale. Their work has involved showing how tissue, cellular, and nuclear architecture can be described as tensegrity systems (Figure 11.14A). In collaboration between Ingber and his colleagues, the experiment described in Figure 11.14B showed that the cytoskeleton behaves like a tensegrity structure (Heidemann, 1993).

Tensegrity is a useful architectural and energetic concept developed by Kenneth Snelson and Buckminster Fuller (see Pugh, 1976). Tensegrity concepts underlie geodesic domes, tents, sailing vessels, and various stick-and-wire sculptures, toy models, bones, and cranes (Figure 11.14). Tensegrity also provides a valuable perspective for therapists who work with the body from a structural, movement, biomechanical, or solid-state perspective. We return to this subject later in this chapter.

A tensegrity system is characterized by a continuous tensional network (tendons) supported by a discontinuous set of compressive elements (struts). One might be inclined to place bones in the strut category, but this is only an approximation, because bones contain both compressive and tensile fibres and are therefore tensegrity systems themselves (Figure 11.14A). For practical purposes, bones are much stiffer than the soft tissues, and act more or less as struts suspended in the connective tissue networks. Attach tendons and muscles to the bones, and one has a three dimensional tensegrity network that supports and moves the body. A complete drawing of the tensegrity system in a rabbit is shown in Figure 11.14D. This simplified illustration was made by drawing each muscle-tendon combination as a single straight line.

Orthopedic surgeon Steven M. Levin, MD, coined the term *biotensegrity* and published a series of fascinating articles on the application of the principle to the human body and biomechanics (Levin, 1981, 1986, 1990, 1995, 1997).

Tom Flemons devised a number of anatomical/tensegrity models that are very revealing about the design of joints that are under tension rather than compression. Flemons (2006) has constructed a tensegrity model of the whole:

> *The complete tensegrity skeleton can walk, sit, stretch, and contort. It will stand self-supporting with all of the compression elements (bones) floating in the web of tension that is woven around it from top to bottom.*
>
> FLEMONS (2006)

Ingber and his colleagues have brought both tensegrity and solid state biochemistry concepts into biomedicine by describing how physical forces exerted on tensegrous molecular scaffolds regulate the biochemical pathways involved in determining biological patterns – the 'blueprint' Harold Saxton Burr was seeking (see Chapter 5 and Ingber, 1993a,b; Wang et al., 1993) as well as cell behaviour. This work is important to the therapist because it describes how various kinds of manipulative methods can influence biochemical processes in important ways.

Ingber's work with tensegrity provides a conceptual link between the structural systems and the energy-informational systems we have been discussing. The body as a whole and the various parts, including the interiors of all cells and nuclei, can be visualized as tensegrity systems (Ingber, 1998; Oschman, 1996; Oschman and Oschman, 1988).

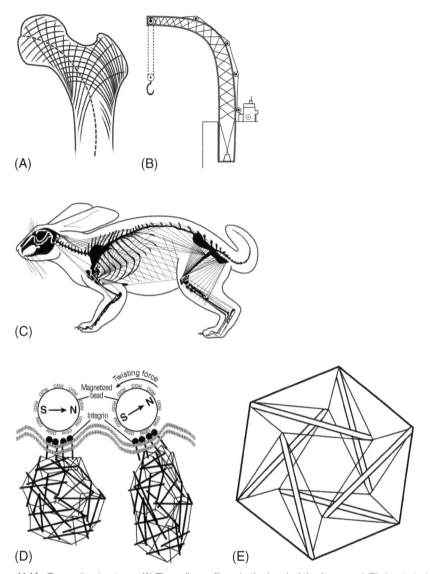

Figure 11.14 Tensegrity structures. (A) The collagen fibers in the head of the femur and (B) the struts in a crane employ a combination of tension resisting and compression elements. (C) The tensegrity system of a rabbit, created by replacing each muscle-tendon unit with a single straight line. (Reproduced from a figure drawn from life or redrawn from another figure by Miss ER Turlington and Miss JID de Vere in Young Z, 1957, The Life of Mammals, Oxford University Press, New York, with kind permission from Oxford University Press. (D) Experiment demonstrating that the cytoskeleton behaves as a tensegrity structure. Magnetic beads coated with integrin antibodies attached to integrins spanning the cell surface. The beads twist in a magnetic field, and the measurable relationship between the twisting force and the extent of bead twisting indicates that the cytoskeleton has a tensegity structure. From Heidemann, 1993, with kind permission from Science and the American Association for the Advancement of Science, and from the artist, Deborah Moulton. (E) The cell is held together by tensegrity. (*Adapted from Levine, J., 1985. The man who says yes. Johns Hopkins Mag. 36 (1 and 2), 34).*

Tensegrity accounts for the ability of the body to absorb impacts without being damaged. Mechanical energy is conducted away from a site of impact through the tensegrous living matrix. The more flexible and balanced the network (the better the tensional integrity), the more readily it absorbs shocks and converts them to information rather than damage. This concept is useful for practitioners who work with athletes and other performers: Flexible and well-organized fascia and myofascial relationships enhance performance and reduce the incidence or severity of injuries.

Tensegrity also accounts for the fact that inflexibility or shortening in one tissue influences structure and movement in other parts. While a therapist may focus on improving flexibility and/ or mobility of a particular part of the body, the effects can and do spread to other areas. This is, in part, due to the tensional integrity of the system, but it is also due to the fact that the tensional system is a vibratory continuum. This can be demonstrated with a tensegrity model by plucking one of the tendons. This will cause the entire network to vibrate.

Since the living tensegrity network is simultaneously a mechanical and a vibratory continuum, restrictions in one part have both structural and energetic consequences for the entire organism. Structural integrity, vibratory integrity, and energetic or informational integrity go hand in hand. One cannot influence the structural system without influencing the energetic/informational system and vice versa. Ingber's work shows how these systems interact with biochemical pathways.

K.J. Pienta and D.S. Coffey: The Vibratory Matrix

The ideas presented here are leading to a new image of the way the organism functions in health and disease. The abstract (below) of a 1991 paper by Pienta and Coffey, entitled 'Cellular harmonic information transfer through a tissue tensegrity-matrix system', combines the concepts of the living matrix, vibratory and resonant interactions, cellular and tissue continuity, piezoelectricity, solid state biochemistry, coherence, and tensegrity to paint a picture of the regulation of living systems. The structures involved in their concept are illustrated in Figure 11.15:

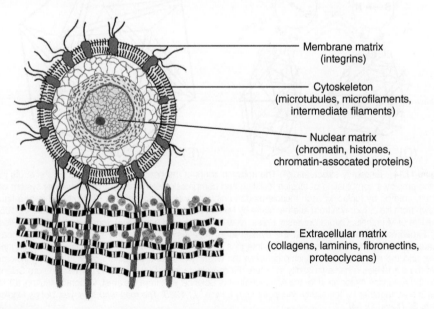

Membrane matrix
(integrins)

Cytoskeleton
(microtubules, microfilaments,
intermediate filaments)

Nuclear matrix
(chromatin, histones,
chromatin-assocated proteins)

Extracellular matrix
(collagens, laminins, fibronectins,
proteoclycans)

Figure 11.15 The tissue tensegrity as described by Pienta and Coffey (1991). Reproduced with permission from Medical Hypotheses. *(Adapted from Pienta KJ, Coffey DS: Cellular harmonic information transfer through a tissue tensegrity–matrix system, Med Hypotheses 1991 Jan;34(1):88–95)*

Cells and intracellular elements are capable of vibrating in a dynamic manner with complex harmonics, the frequency of which can now be measured and analyzed in a quantitative manner by Fourier analysis (and by other methods). Cellular events such as changes in shape, membrane ruffling, motility, and signal transduction occur within spatial and temporal harmonics that have potential regulatory importance. These vibrations can be altered by growth factors and the process of carcinogenesis. It is important to understand the mechanism by which this vibrational information is transferred directly throughout the cell [and throughout the organism].

From these observations we propose that vibrational information is transferred through a tissue tensegrity-matrix which acts as a coupled harmonic oscillator operating as a signal transducing system from the cell periphery to the nucleus and ultimately to the DNA. The vibrational interactions occur through a tissue matrix system consisting of the nuclear matrix, the cytoskeleton, and the extracellular matrix that is poised to couple the biological oscillations of the cell from the peripheral membrane to the DNA through a tensegrity-matrix structure. Tensegrity has been defined as a structural system composed of discontinuous compression elements connected by continuous tension cables, which interact in a dynamic fashion. A tensegrity tissue matrix system allows for specific transfer of information through the cell (and throughout the organism) by direct transmission of vibrational chemomechanical energy through harmonic wave motion. (Bracketed additions are author's.)

PIENTA AND COFFEY (1991)

Thomas Hanna, Mae-Wan Ho, David P. Knight, John F. Barnes, Gerald Pollack: Soma, Consciousness, and the Water-Collagen Matrix

In 1988, Thomas Hanna, PhD (1928–1990), introduced the Greek term *soma* into the world of bodywork and movement therapies. Hanna created a school of 'somatics' and a set of simple exercises that enhance flexibility and ease of movement. According to Hanna, soma represents the body of life, the body experienced from within, the original cybernetic system. Cybernetics, in turn, is another term defined by Norbert Wiener (1965) in his book of that title as the study of control and communication in animals and machines. The term *cybernetics* stems from the Greek Κυβερνήτης (*kybernetes*, steersman, governor, pilot, or rudder – the same root as government). The goal of cybernetics is to understand and define the functions and processes of systems that have goals and that have chains of communication linking action and sensation in ways that continually compare what is taking place with the desired goal.

Hanna's reference to the original cybernetic system is profoundly relevant to the study of the connective tissue and living matrix. Whether in an amoeba or in the human body, the matrix forms a self-guiding system that continually strives to achieve stability and balance by constantly adapting to its environment. An important aspect of adaptation was described in the last chapter: the way the body form adjusts to the ways it is used. The ancient somatic systems that accomplish this exist in protozoa and other microorganisms and thereby predate the evolution of the nervous system.

A modern conceptualization of somatic principles emerged from the work of Ho and Knight (1998). Taking into consideration semiconduction and proticity in the living matrix, they proposed that 'memory is dynamically distributed' throughout the body. The concepts of information processing proposed by Oschman (1994), semiconduction proposed by Szent-Györgyi, proticity proposed by Mitchell, as well as others, led to a remarkable conclusion. Ho and Knight (1998) proposed there is a body consciousness, possessing all of the hallmarks of consciousness – sentience, intercommunication, and memory, existing alongside 'brain consciousness'. They propose that 'brain consciousness', which we usually consider to be the only consciousness, is embedded within this 'matrix consciousness' and is coupled to it. In the context of such a system the acupuncture meridians are regarded as a specialized information network, based on liquid crystalline resonant pathways, that link and coordinate the various structures and functions within the organism, separate from or along with neural communications. Support for a role of the meridians in consciousness also comes from a variety of energy psychology techniques that will be discussed in Chapter 12.

John F. Barnes (1990) synthesized these concepts in an effort to understand the deeper significance of changes in connective tissue brought about by myofascial release and other approaches. A key point he derived from Pischinger is that all vital activity and information exchange takes place in the matrix, not in the nervous system. It is in this extracellular environment that all of the primary regulating processes take place. The matrix is a good candidate for the 'operating system' of the body. In a computer, the operating system coordinates the operations of the various components: the keyboard, the hard drive, the screen, printer, modem, and any other devices. The operating system works quietly in the background without making itself known until something goes wrong, at which point the computer or the program being used must be restarted. Similarly, the human body must have the equivalent of an operating system that manages the countless tasks that take place on an instant-to-instant basis, as was described so eloquently by E.F. Adolph, as quoted in Chapter 10. It is these matrix regulations and communications, and not just neural communications, that make life possible. Most importantly, if the matrix functions are interfered with, the defence and repair systems are compromised. What every bodyworker understands, however, is that the matrix compensates for trauma and injury in a way that can leave the individual unaware that anything is wrong. These compensations cause excess strain on parts of the system that were initially undamaged. This strain can accumulate and lead to breakdown. However, the felt problem may be a distance from the original injury site.

References

Barnes, J.F., 1990. Myofascial Release: The Search for Excellence – A Comprehensive Evaluatory and Treatment Approach. 10th ed. Rehabilitation Services, Inc., Malvern, PA.

Becker, R.O., 1990. The machine brain and properties of the mind. Subtle Energies 113, 79–97.

Becker, R.O., 1991. Evidence for a primitive DC electrical analog system controlling brain function. Subtle Energies 2 (1), 71–88.

Chaitow, L., Findley, T.W., Schleip, R. (Eds.), 2012. Fascia Research, Basic Science and Implications for Conventional and Complementary Health Care. Kiener, Munich.

Del Giudice, E., Doglia, S., Milani, M., Vitiello, G., 1988. Structures, Correlations and Electromagnetic Interactions in Living Matter: Theory and Applications. In: Frohlich, H. (Ed.), Biological Coherence and Response to External Stimuli. Published by Springer-Verlag, Berlin, pp. 49–64.

Findley, T.W., Schleip, R. (Eds.), 2007. Fascia Research, Basic Science and Implications for Conventional and Complementary Health Care. Elsevier GmbH, Munich.

Flemons, T.E., 2006. http://www.intensiondesigns.com/.

Fröhlich, H., 1968. Bose condensation of strongly excited longitudinal electric modes. Phys. Lett. 26A, 402–403.

Fröhlich, H. (Ed.), 1988. Biological Coherence and Response to External Stimuli. Springer Verlag, Berlin.

Hanna, T., 1988. Somatics: Reawakening the Mind's Control of Movement, Flexibility and Health. Addison-Wesley, New York.

Heidemann, S.R., 1993. A new twist on integrins and the cytoskeleton. Science 260, 1080–1081.

Heine, H., Förster, J., 2004. Histophysiology of mast cells in skin and other organs. Arch. Dermatol. Res. 253 (3), 225–228.

Ho, M.-W., 1997. Quantum coherence and conscious experience. Kybernetes 26, 265–276.

Ho, M.-W., Knight, D.P., 1998. The acupuncture system and the liquid crystalline collagen fibers of the connective tissues. Am. J. Chin. Med. 26 (3–4), 1–13.

Huijing, P.A., Hollander, P., Findley, T.W., Schleip, R. (Eds.), 2009. Fascia Research, Basic Science and Implications for Conventional and Complementary Health Care. Elsevier, Munich.

Hush, N.S., 2003. An overview of the first half-century of molecular electronics. Ann. N. Y. Acad. Sci. 1006, 1–20.

Hyman, J.M., McLaughlin, D.W., Scott, A.C., 1981. On Davydov's alpha-helix solitons. Physica 3D(1&2), 23–44.

Hynes, R.O., Naba, A., 2011. Overview of the matrisome—an inventory of extracellular matrix constituents and functions. In: Hynes, R.O., Yamada, K.M. (Eds.), Extracellular Matrix Biology. Cold Spring Harbor Perspectives in Biology. Cold Spring Harbor Laboratory Press, Cold Spring Harbor, NY.

Ingber, D.E., 1993a. The riddle of morphogenesis: a question of solution chemistry or molecular cell engineering? Cell 75, 1249–1252.

Ingber, D.E., 1993b. Cellular tensegrity: defining new rules of biological design that govern the cytoskeleton. J. Cell Sci. 104, 613–627.

Ingber, D.E., 1998. The architecture of life. Sci. Am. 278 (1), 48–57.

Libbin, R.M., Person, P., Papierman, S., Shah, D., Nevid, D., Grob, H., 1979. Partial regeneration of the above-elbow amputated rat forelimb. II. Electrical and mechanical facilitation. J Morphol. Mar;159 (3), 439–52.

Levin, S.M., 1981. The icosahedron as a biologic support system. In: Proceedings, 34th Annual Conference on Engineering in Medicine and Biology, Huston.

Levin, S.M., 1986. The icosahedron as the three-dimensional finite element in biomechanical support. In: Proceedings of the Society of General Systems Research Symposium on Mental Images, Values and Reality G14-26 Society of General Systems Research, St. Louis, MO.

Levin, S.M., 1990. The primordial structure. In: Banathy, B.H., Banathy, B.B. (Eds.), Proceedings of the 34th Annual Meeting of The International Society for the Systems Sciences. pp. 716–720, Portland, OR, vol. II.

Levin, S.M., 1995. The importance of soft tissues for structural support of the body. In: Dorman, T. (Ed.), In: Spine: State of the Art Reviews, 9 (2), Hanley and Belfus, Philadelphia, PA.

Levin, S.M., 1997. Putting the shoulder to the wheel: a new biomechanical model for the shoulder girdle. Biomed. Sci. Instrum. 33, 412–417.

Levine, J., 1985. The man who says yes. Johns Hopkins Mag. 36 (1 and 2), 34.

Mele, G., Sessions, S., 2014. Stem cells aid heart regeneration in salamanders. Abstract FASEB, Experimental Biology FASEB Journal 28 (1) Supplement.

Mitchell, P., 1976. Vectorial chemistry and the molecular mechanics of chemiosmotic coupling: power transmission by proticity. Biochem. Soc. Trans. 4, 399–430.

Oschman, J.L., 1994. A biophysical basis for acupuncture. In: Proceedings of the First Symposium of the Committee for Acupuncture Research, Winston Salem, NC.

Oschman, J.L., 1996. The nuclear, cytoskeletal, and extracellular matrices: a continuous communication network. Poster presentation for 'the cytoskeleton: mechanical, physical and biological interactions', a workshop sponsored by the Center for Advanced Studies in the Space Life Science at the Marine Biological Laboratory, Woods Hole, MA, November 15–17, 1996.

Oschman, J.L., 2003. Energy Medicine in Therapeutics and Human Performance. Butterworth Heinemann, Edinburgh.

Oschman, J.L., Oschman, N.H., 1988. Book Review and Commentary [on]: Biological Coherence and Response to External Stimuli. Fröhlich, H. (Ed.), Springer-Verlag, Berlin, NORA Press, Dover, NH.

Oschman, J.L., Oschman, N.H., 1995. Physiological and emotional effects of acupuncture needle insertion. In: Proceedings of the Second Symposium of the Society for Acupuncture Research, held in Washington DC on Sept 17–18, 1994. Society for Acupuncture Research, Winston Salem, NC.

Paoletti, S., 2006. The Fasciae: Anatomy, Dysfunction & Treatment. Eastland Press, Seattle, WA, 151–161.

Pienta, K.J., Coffey, D.S., 1991. Cellular harmonic information transfer through a tissue tensegrity–matrix system. Med. Hypotheses 34, 88–95.

Pischinger, A., 2004. Das System der Grundregulation. Karl F. Haug Verlag, Stutgart.

Pischinger, A., 2007. Matrix and Matrix Regulation: Basis for a Holistic Theory in Medicine. North Atlantic Books, Berkeley, CA.

Pugh, A., 1976. An Introduction to Tensegrity. University of California Press, Berkeley, CA.

Rosenberg, F., Postow, E., 1969. Semiconduction in proteins and lipids—its possible biological import. Ann. N. Y. Acad. Sci. 158, 161–190.

Sarpeshkar, R., 2010. Ultra Low Power Bioelectronics: Fundamentals, Biomedical Applications, and Bio-inspired Systems. Cambridge University Press, Cambridge, UK, 907 pp.

Sherrington, C.S., 1951. Man on his nature. Doubleday Anchor, Garden City, NY.

Szent-Györgyi, A., 1941. Towards a new biochemistry? Science 93, 609–611 (Also published in 1941 as: the study of energy levels in biochemistry. Nature 148:157–159).

Szent-Györgyi, A., 1988. To see what everyone has seen, to think what no one has thought. Biol. Bull. 175, 191–240 (This symposium volume contains a complete listing of publications of Szent-Györgyi 1913–1987.).

Virchow, R.C., 1871. Die Cellularpathologie in ihrer Begründung auf physiologische und pathologische Gewebelehre. Verlag von August Hirschwald, Berlin.

Wang, J.Y., Butler, J.P., Ingber, D.E., 1993. Mechanotransduction across the cell surface and through the cytoskeleton. Science 260, 1124–1127.

Wiener, N., 1965. Cybernetics, second ed. The MIT Press, Cambridge, MA, 212 pps.

CHAPTER 12

Energy Medicine and the Sciences of the Subconscious and Intuition

We must recollect that all of our provisional ideas in psychology will presumably one day be based on an organic substructure.

Freud (1914)

Chapter Summary

The living matrix and ground regulation concepts have been valuable for explaining a wide range of previously inexplicable phenomena that take place in complementary and alternative medicine, the martial arts, and in peak athletic and artistic performances. The matrix is viewed as a continuous energetic substrate for communications taking place throughout the human body. It is thought to be the fabric that is damaged by physical or emotional traumas and the place to begin treatments for resolving traumas of all types. Because its molecular, and cellular and tissue components have been so widely studied, the living matrix provides an ideal academic model for understanding holistic interventions of all kinds. Indeed, the matrix may be a component of the 'organic substructure' referred to by Freud in 1914. This chapter summarizes what we know about the living matrix in relation to conscious and subconscious processes. Understanding the nature of intuition and the science of the subjective can help us understand how therapists come to 'know' what is going on in the patient before them.

Introduction

Speculations on the nature of mind and brain have been going on for a very long time. An early image is shown in Figure 12.1. In the modern era, no respectable scientist would write about consciousness or the subconscious[1] and expect to remain respectable. These subjects were considered by many to be too subjective and too elusive for scientific study – something to be left for the philosophers to ponder. Some in the field of psychology even suggested that the subconscious does not exist. Fortunately, this situation has changed dramatically. One turning point for consciousness studies came when Sir Francis Crick, a distinguished 'thought leader' and co-discoverer with James D. Watson of the double helical structure of DNA, stated that it was time to set aside the philosophical dilemmas and get on with the neuroscience that would reveal the mechanisms involved in the different aspects of consciousness (e.g., pain, visual awareness, self-consciousness) (Kandel, 1999). Since then, consciousness has become a respectable topic for scientific study, as exemplified by the emergence in 1994 of a peer-reviewed *Journal of Consciousness Studies* and, the same year, a series of biennial interdisciplinary international conferences, *Toward a Science of Consciousness,* sponsored by the University of Arizona. These meetings have explored the whole spectrum of approaches from philosophy of

---

[1]In this chapter, no distinction will be made between the terms *subconscious* and *unconscious*.

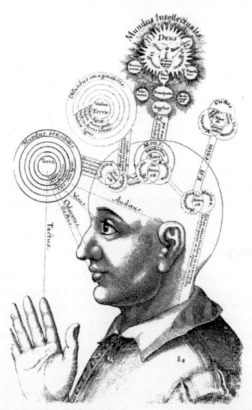

Figure 12.1 Robert Fludd (1574–1637) was a prominent English physician and student of Paracelsus (1493–1541). This diagram of the mental faculties is from Fludd's Utriusque Cosmi, an encyclopaedic masterwork in which he attempted to illustrate and synthesize all of medieval science and mystical philosophy. It is based in part on 'ventricular' theory. There are three internal cavities, each consisting of two faculties. The first cavity couples the five senses to the imaginary world, which is the shadow of the sensible world. The second cavity is "cogitative" and deals with reason, intellect and mind, through which the brain communicates with God. The third cavity is the place of memory and "motivation" which commands movements through the spinal cord.

mind and cognitive science, to neurobiology, pharmacology, molecular dynamics, phenomenological accounts, physics and quantum physics. The aim is to lay a sound scientific foundation for consciousness research.

The significance of studies of consciousness and the subconscious is that a barrier to wider acceptance of complementary and alternative medicine and energy medicine exists because the practice of these methods involves a number of anomalies that seem to defy analysis with conventional thinking. For example, intention is a key concept in many therapies. This suggests some kind of connection between consciousness and therapeutic outcomes. Homeopathy appears to provide another dramatic example of a seemingly anomalous phenomenon.

Beyond its disciplined reliance upon constructive iteration of sound experimental data with incisive theoretical models, good science is characterized by thorough and respectful cognizance of relevant past and present work by others, humility in the face of empirical evidence, and openness of mind to new topics, new approaches, new ideas, and new scholars ... anomalies demand immediate attention to discriminate between artifacts of flawed experimentation or theoretical logic, and the entry of genuine new phenomena onto the scientific stage. Error in this discrimination can divert or extend science along false scholarly trails, while proper identification and assimilation of real anomalies can open more penetrating paths than those previously followed … Unfortunately, such intellectual respect for the role of anomalies has tended to be more honored in the abstract than in actual practice.

JAHN AND DUNNE (1997)

The Study of the Subconscious Mind

Progress in the study of the subconscious was summarized recently at a gathering of leading neuroscientists, including Eric Kandel, Patricia Churchland, Stanislas Dehaene, Timothy Wilson, and Nicholas Schiff (Rose, 2011).

*In the next century, biology is likely to make deep contributions to the understanding of mental processes by delineating the biological basis for the various unconscious mental processes, for psychic determinism, for the role of unconscious mental processes in psychopathology, and for the therapeutic effect of psychoanalysis. Now, biology will not immediately enlighten these deep mysteries at their core. **These issues represent, together with the nature of consciousness, the most difficult problems confronting all of biology—in fact, all of science.***

ERIC KANDEL, NOBEL PRIZE IN PHYSIOLOGY OR MEDICINE (2000)

An expanded summary of some of the main points raised during the discussion referenced above:

- Freud pointed out that a lot of our mental state is unconscious. We are functioning unconsciously most of the time. Consciousness is the tip of the iceberg (sometimes referred to as the brainberg, Figure 12.2.)

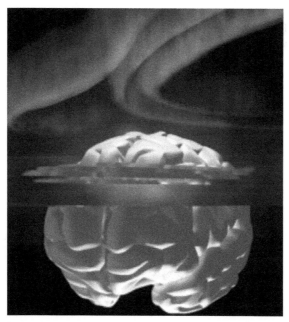

Figure 12.2   The brainberg. Logo for a conference "Toward a Science of Consciousness, Brain, Mind, Reality", Stockholm Sweden, May 2-8, 2011.

- Freud understood that the language of the unconscious is different from the language of consciousness, but didn't appreciate that under many circumstances unconscious processes can be very much faster and efficient at integrating sensory inputs and interpreting events than conscious processes.
- The conscious mind can only focus on one item at a time. The unconscious mind can deal with several items simultaneously. If you have to make a decision between two alternatives, consciousness is the way to go. However, if you have to make a decision between many alternatives, the unconscious often leads to more satisfactory solutions. Such solutions may emerge as sudden flashes of insight or in dreams.
- Helmholtz studied perception and realized that a lot of non-conscious processing is not just dumb automatic reflexes but is adaptive and creative. The subconscious assembles basic bits of information from the sensory systems and makes sophisticated decisions.
- The subconscious delivers to consciousness images that integrate a lot of current information and also brings in stored information (memories, traumatic memories, archetypes, personality structure) (Brown, 1977, 2015.)
- In his early years, Freud was an aphasiologist – he studied linguistic problems caused by brain damage. He noticed that we don't consciously pick the words that we're going to use. We don't consciously form the grammatical structure. All of that is done for us non-consciously, and we just speak. We know the gist of what we are going to say but we don't know precisely what we are going say until we say it. This involves some very complex processing and exemplifies the remarkable feats the subconscious is capable of accomplishing.
- Until the 1980s, the nature of consciousness and the subconscious seemed to be an intractable problem. At that time, Bernard Baars and others recognized that neuroscience actually has a variety of tools that can be applied to the problem. Baars developed a global workspace theory that suggests that consciousness arises from highly coordinated widespread activities in the brain (Baars, 1986, 1988, 1997). When sensory signals are localized in specific brain areas, sensations are not consciously perceived. When sensory signals spread to a wider network of neurons across much of the cortex, termed the *global workspace*, we become conscious of the sensations. The ways these diverse representations and sensations are integrated into a coherent conscious moment is known as the binding problem (Von der Malsburg, 1995).

The global workspace is a 'momentarily active, subjectively experienced' event in working memory – the inner domain where we can rehearse to ourselves phrases that people have said to us or that we want to say to someone, telephone numbers, and carry on the narrative of our lives. It is usually thought to include inner speech and visual imagery. It involves a fleeting memory lasting only a few seconds. Its contents are thought to correspond to what we are conscious of. Memories are broadcast from the global workspace to a multitude of unconscious cognitive brain processes, called receiving processes. Other unconscious processes, operating in parallel and with limited communication between them, can form temporary coalitions that can act as input processes to the global workspace. Since globally broadcast messages can evoke actions in receiving processes throughout the brain, the global workspace can exercise executive control to perform voluntary actions. Individual as well as allied processes compete for access to the global workspace, striving to disseminate their messages to all other processes in an effort to recruit more cohorts and thereby increase the likelihood of achieving specific goals.

Memory and Consciousness

Before proceeding to the next section, it is important to point out that the mechanisms of memory, consciousness, and the subconscious are by no means understood. As Eric Kandel pointed out in the quotation provided above, 'These issues represent … the most difficult problems confronting all of biology — in fact, all of science.' Likewise, as we look for Freud's *organic substructure* for

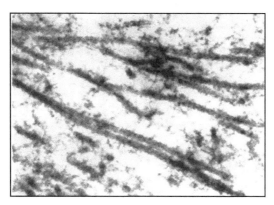

Figure 12.3   Neurotubules: There are close to a billion miles of these semiconducting fibres in the brain.

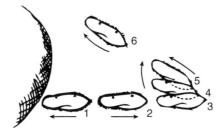

Figure 12.4   A single-celled paramecium swims gracefully, avoids predators, finds food, mates, and has sex, all without a single synapse. 'Of nerve there is no trace. But the cell framework, the cytoskeleton might serve'. (Sir Charles Sherrington, 1951)

consciousness, the subconscious, and psychology in general, we need to be open to new ideas and approaches. One such idea is presented next in Figures 12.3 and 12.4.

Conventional approaches to memory focus on synaptic switching (roughly 10^{11} brain neurons, 10^3 synapses/neuron, switching in the millisecond range of 10^3 operations per second) and predict about 10^{17} bit states per second for a human brain (Moravec, 1987). Stuart Hameroff and others have done extensive work on the role of a major component of the cytoskeleton, the microtubule, which they view as a self-organizing quantum computer capable of storing vast amounts of information, i.e., memory. Hameroff pointed out that the cells in the brain contain many miles of microtubules. Living cells typically each contain approximately 10^7 tubulin molecules (Yu and Baas, 1994). A tiny neuron, a thousandth of an inch in diameter, has about 9 feet of cytoskeleton. Hence, there are close to a billion miles of semiconducting fibres in the brain. In the next section, we will suggest that these microtubules, together with other semiconducting cytoskeletal structures, form a sophisticated electronic communication network extending throughout the nervous system and throughout the whole body. Nanosecond switching in microtubules predicts roughly 10^{16} operations per second, per neuron. This capacity could account for the adaptive behaviours of single-cell organisms like paramecium, for example, who elegantly swim, avoid obstacles, and find food and mates without benefit of a nervous system or synapses. Because the human brain contains about 10^{11} neurons, nanosecond microtubule automata offer about 10^{27} brain operations per second. This is 10 orders of magnitude more operations than can be achieved by synaptic switching. This means that the on-off switches known as synapses, which are obviously important components of neural networks, may not be the only place where memories are stored and processed. The neural model of memory was developed by Sir John Eccles, for which he received the

Nobel Prize in 1963, and ruled neuroscience research for an entire generation, but was rejected as inadequate by Eccles himself in 1992 (Pribram and Eccles, 1992).

Another perspective on this topic came from Francis O. Schmitt, a professor at MIT and founder of a very distinguished group of neuroscientists called The Neuroscience Research Programme.

> *Contrary to widespread belief, the problems of memory and consciousness are not likely to be resolved by further elaboration of electrophysiological techniques, however detailed.... Much of the higher activity of the brain eludes detection by conventional electrophysiological methods ... remembering, learning, and thinking may be sub-served by phenomena that are electrically silent to those instruments. Memory will be found in giant macromolecular polymers such as proteins, RNA and DNA. Only in giant macromolecular polymers is the diversity possible that is required for the specificity manifested in fundamental life phenomena. A polymer composed of 1000 monomers of 4 monomer species (e.g., RNA) could have 4^{1000} variants; with 20 monomer species (protein) there could be 20^{1000} variants!*

SCHMITT (1961)

The Living Matrix

During the 1980s and 1990s there emerged the scientific basis for another theory to explain aspects of memory, consciousness, and the subconscious. It is only with the writing of this chapter that we realize that the background for these concepts was emerging at about the same time that Crick and Baars and others were making strides in understanding consciousness.

This theory was founded on discoveries in cell biology and biophysics revealing that organisms have a continuous *living matrix* (Oschman and Oschman, 1993) or ground regulation system (Pischinger, 2007) that reaches into every part of the body, including every cell and nucleus.

Two discoveries provided the basis for this concept. The first was the discovery of important molecules called integrins that connect the extracellular matrix (connective tissue and fascia) with the cytoskeletons within every cell (Bretscher, 1971), and additional molecules that span the nuclear envelope, connecting the cytoskeleton with the nuclear matrix (Figure 12.5) (Berezney and Coffey, 1977) and DNA (Oschman, 1983).

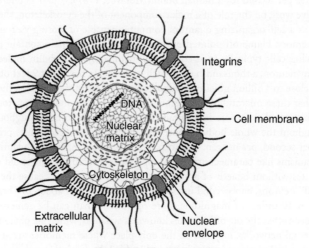

Figure 12.5   The living matrix.

The second discovery was that this pervasive global matrix is composed of semiconductor molecules capable of forming a body-wide electronic circuit. Since organic molecules are being used in the electronics industry to manufacture microscopic molecular circuits, it is not a big leap to suggest that a molecular electronic network within the organism is capable of communicating, storing, and processing information and making the kinds of rapid decisions or interpretations that are recognized as attributes of the subconscious. Important but rarely mentioned research of Albert Szent-Györgyi and materials scientists around the world led to the development of new fields of submolecular and electronic biology (Szent-Györgyi, 1960, 1968). The ability of the living matrix to support vibrational communications was eloquently spelled out by Pienta and Coffey as was described in the last chapter.

Faster than Neurons

The ability of organisms to carry out very rapid and sophisticated regulations, cognitions, and movements without conscious processing was the topic of a book entitled *Energy Medicine in Therapeutics and Human Performance* (Oschman, 1993). This book included a discussion of phenomenal athletic and artistic performances as well as therapeutic insights that are often observed but rarely discussed in terms of mechanisms. It was proposed that the living matrix provides very high-speed electronic and electromagnetic processing of sensory data and sophisticated decision-making and movements that are far quicker than can be accomplished by slow-moving nerve impulses and chemical signaling. The martial arts provide remarkable examples of this system in operation. This ultrafast biology is only explainable by electronic information transfer and processing and other high-speed processes.

It was also proposed that sensory information reaching the various receptors is split into two pathways, one to the nervous system and the other to the living matrix (Figure 12.6). The neural system gives rise to conscious awareness and decision-making, and the matrix system provides much more thorough analysis of the kind that takes place in fields such as applied kinesiology, the martial arts, Continuum movement, peak athletic and artistic performances, and profound therapeutic encounters. The result of these analog processes has been termed *authentic action*, in contrast to thoughtful actions produced by digital neural processing.

In an article entitled "An Anatomical, Biochemical, Biophysical, and Quantum Basis for the Unconscious Mind" Oschman and Pressman (2013) describe the living matrix as one of several pervasive high speed, faster than neuronal communication networks in the human body. The

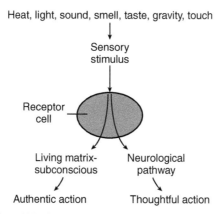

Figure 12.6   Proposed bifurcation of sensory pathways.

extracellular part of the living matrix, often referred to as fascia, forms a continuous head-to-toe network surrounding and permeating all tissues and organs (Langevin, 2006). This semiconductor network probably functions in concert with the "wetware" or cellular biochemical signal processing systems described by Dennis Bray (2009). As described in Chapter 9, Ahmed Zewail has estimated the velocity of movement of metabolites in cells at 1000 meters/second, almost ten times faster than the fastest neurons. Various authors have also proposed ultra-weak light signaling between molecules. The scheme is illustrated in Figure 3.11. Researchers in Germany have shown that individual molecules can act as transmitting and receiving antennas, efficiently communicating from molecule to molecule via single photons (Figure 3.12). In 2012, Polycarpou and colleagues measured the shape of individual photons for the first time. Pulses of light can have almost any shape in space and time, depending on the amplitudes and phases of the pulse's frequency components. Data can thus be encoded by modulating the amplitude or phase of the light. Evidence for speed-of-light messaging has been obtained from the study of cell to cell communication under chemically separated but optically coupled in vitro conditions (Albrecht-Buehler, 1992; Shen, 1994). These concepts are important for the therapists who have an intuition that their work involves light in some manner.

Another potentially extremely rapid system that is just beginning to be explored is quantum coherence of water molecules, in which "spins" are coupled (see Figure 11.4). In a breakthrough article entitled "Quantum Coherence and Conscious Experience", Mae-Wan Ho (1997) gave evidence for large-scale spatiotemporal coherence of brain activities that cannot be satisfactorily explained by neural/synaptic mechanisms. "The brain functions, not as a collection of specialized brain cells, but as a coherent whole. Moreover, how the brain functions as a coherent whole is inseparable from the question of how the organism functions as a coherent whole. Quantum Coherence effectively frees the organism from thermodynamic constraints so that it is poised for rapid, specific intercommunication, enabling it to function as a coherent whole. In the ideal, the organism is a quantum superposition of coherent activities, with instantaneous (nonlocal) noiseless intercommunication throughout." This rapid intercommunication corresponds to the process that has been termed 'systemic cooperation' by Oschman (2003) and 'Gestaltbildung' by Popp and Beloussov (2003).

The next chapter will summarize evidence that the fabric of the body consists of tensegrity systems, which can readily conduct vibrational energy, including both sound and light. Taken together, these studies open new vistas for understanding links between physiology and biophotons. Every molecule in the body is a potential biophoton emitter and receiver.

Technologies are emerging that could test these profound concepts. Raman and infrared spectroscopic techniques are now enabling rapid and sensitive chemical characterization of samples based on the vibrational signatures of the molecules present in a sample. When applied to biological systems, the techniques provide highly complex spectra that document changes taking place in the entire genome, proteome and metabolome. Real time in-vivo applications are possible. The January 2013 issue of the Journal of Photonics documents recent developments (Krafft and Bird, 2013).

References

Albrecht-Buehler, G., 1992. Rudimentary form of cellular "vision". Proc. Natl. Acad. Sci. 89 (17), 8288–8292.

Baars, B., 1986. The Cognitive Revolution in Psychology. Guilford Press, New York, NY.

Baars, B., 1988. A Cognitive Theory of Consciousness. Cambridge University Press, New York, NY.

Baars, B., 1997. In the Theater of Consciousness: The Workspace of the Mind. Oxford University Press, New York, NY.

Berezney, R., Coffey, D.S., 1977. Isolation and characterization of a framework structure from rat liver nuclei. J. Cell Biol. 73, 616–637.

Bray, D., 2009. Wetware: A computer in every cell. Yale University Press, New Haven, CT.

Bretscher, M.S., 1971. A major protein which spans the human erythrocyte membrane. J. Mol. Biol. 59, 351–357.

Bretscher, M.S., 1971. Major human erythrocyte glycoprotein spans the cell membrane. Nat. New Biol. 231, 229–232.

Brown, J.W., 1977. Mind, Brain, and Consciousness: The Neuropsychology of Cognition. In: Academic Press, New York, NY.

Brown, J.W., 2015. Microgenetic Theory and Process Thought. Imprint Academic, Exeter, UK.

Freud, S., 1914. On narcissism: an introduction, In: Complete Psychological Works, standard edition, vol. 14. Hogarth Press, London, 1957, pp. 67–102.

Ho, M.-W., 1997. Quantum coherence and conscious experience. Kybernetes 26, 265–276.

Jahn, R.G., Dunne, B.J., 1997. Science of the subjective. J. Sci. Explor. 11 (2), 201–224.

Kandel, E.R., 1999. Biology and the future of psychoanalysis: a new intellectual framework for psychiatry revisited. Am. J. Psychiatry 156, 505–524.

Krafft, C., Bird, B. (Eds.), 2013. Vibrational Spectroscopy in Medicine. Journal of Photonics 6 (1).

Langevin, H.M., 2006. Connective tissue: a body-wide signaling network? Med Hypotheses 66 (6), 1074–1077.

Moravec, H.P., 1987. Mind Children. University Press, San Francisco, CA.

Oschman, J.L., 1983. Structure and properties of ground substances. Am. Zool. 24 (1), 199–215.

Oschman, J.L., 1993. Energy Medicine in Therapeutics and Human Performance. Churchill Livingstone/Harcourt Brace, Edinburgh.

Oschman, J.L., Oschman, N.H., 1993. Matter, energy, and the living matrix. October, 1993 issue of Rolf Lines, the news magazine for the Rolf Institute, Boulder, CO, 21(3), 55–64.

Oschman, J.L., Pressman, M., 2013. An Anatomical, Biochemical, Biophysical, and Quantum Basis for the Unconscious Mind. Energy Psychology 5 (1), 1–15.

Pienta, K.J., Coffey, D., 1991. Cellular harmonic information transfer through a tissue tensegrity-matrix system. Med. Hypotheses 34, 88–95.

Pischinger, A., 2007. The Extracellular Matrix and Ground Regulation: Basis for a Holistic Biological Medicine. North Atlantic Books, Berkeley, CA.

Polycarpou, C., Cassemiro, K.N., Venturi, G., Zavatta, A., Bellini, M., 2012. Adaptive Detection of Arbitrarily Shaped Ultrashort Quantum Light States. Phys. Rev. Lett. 109, 053602 – Published 3 August 2012.

Popp, F.-A., Beloussov, L.V., 2003. Integrative Biophysics: Biophotonics. Springer, Berlin pp. 401–402.

Pribram, K.H., Eccles, J.C., 1992. Rethinking Neural Networks. Appalachian Conference on Behavioral Neurodynamics. Lawrence Erlbaum Associates, Inc., Mahwah, NJ.

Rose, C. Charlie Rose Brain Series, Year 2, December 6, 2011, PBS and Bloomberg Television, New York, NY.

Schmitt, F.O., 1961. Molecule-cell, component-system reciprocal control as exemplified in psychophysical research. The Robert A. Welch Foundation Conferences on Chemical Research. V. Molecular Structure and Biochemical Reactions, Houston, Texas, December vol. V, Chapter III, pp. 33–37.

Shen, X., Mei, W., Xu, X., 1994. Activation of neutrophils by a chemically separated but optically coupled neutrophil population undergoing respiratory burst. Experientia 50, 963–968.

Sherrington, C.S., 1951. Man on his nature. Doubleday Anchor, New York, NY.

Szent-Györgyi, A., 1960. Introduction to a Submolecular Biology. Academic Press, New York, NY.

Szent-Györgyi, A., 1968. Bioelectronics. Academic Press, New York, NY.

Von der Malsburg, C., 1995. Binding in models of perception and brain function. Curr. Opin. Neurobiol. 5, 520–526.

Yu, W., Baas, P.W., 1994. Changes in microtubule number and length during axon differentiation. J. Neurosci. 14 (5), 2818–2829.

CHAPTER 13

The Energetic Blueprint of Life and Health

Blueprint: a detailed architectural plan.

What maintains vitality and aliveness in an organism are not linear sequences of chemical reactions, messages, or physiological events, but the ways they are dynamically regulated and integrated. The human body contains a vast network of intricate processes – proliferations, specializations, movements, differentiations, de-differentiations, metabolic syntheses, enzymatic breakdowns, cross-linkages, feed-forwards, and feedbacks – of startling complexity and diversity, all directed at growing then maintaining and restoring the *orderly pattern of the whole* described in this chapter.

Chapter Summary

This chapter focuses on the processes and forces that determine the form or architecture of the body as a whole as well as of its component parts. While much research has been done on this subject, we still do not know the source of the plan that enables the body to grow into its adult form and that restores tissues to normal after injury or disease. Because we are discussing a problem that has not been solved, the reader is asked to suspend judgment until a variety of hypotheses have been presented.

Introduction

Physicians and other therapists have daily and intimate encounters with the intricate and sophisticated forces that shape the human body. They therefore engage in a personal relationship with the greatest unsolved mystery of biology and medicine. This is the process that is unveiled when a single cell develops into a mature organism and that is unveiled every time order must be restored after injury or disease. A pressing issue of our times, cancer, is a part of the same mystery.

The healing of an injury must reference the original blueprint of the organism – the plan that enabled the body to grow into its adult form. This simple fact brings embryology, developmental biology, wound healing, and cancer research together at the forefront of medical theory and practice. The effectiveness of any science-based medical system is vitally dependent on a detailed and accurate understanding of these phenomena. The thesis of this book is that adding an energetic perspective to existing understandings can open new avenues for research and clinical practice. In addition to exploring the energetic picture, we must look at what has already been discovered and the questions that have been raised through other approaches such as physiology, biochemistry, embryology, developmental biology, and so on. This is challenging for both the student and the researcher because recent progress has rendered many standard texts on these subjects seriously outdated.

This chapter focuses on the processes and forces that determine the form or architecture of the body as a whole as well as of its component parts. A starting point is locating the blueprint of the body and the processes by which this global plan gives rise to living structures and puts them into operation. This is a challenging endeavour because most of us have been taught that DNA is the blueprint of life, and we can therefore regard this as a solved problem. The only difficulty is that DNA is only a part of the story. Because of this we must look at a variety of hypotheses and keep an open mind about all of them, even the ones that may seem preposterous. As Sherlock Holmes said to Watson, 'How often have I said to you that when you have eliminated the impossible, whatever remains, however improbable, must be the truth?' (Doyle, 1890).

This approach to inquiry was strongly reinforced by T.C. Chamberlin in a famous paper first published in 1890 and reprinted in *Science* in 1965. Chamberlin wrote *The Method of Multiple Working Hypotheses*. His philosophy was designed to avoid the dangers of what he called 'parental affection' for a favourite theory (Chamberlin, 1965).

> *The effort is to bring up into view every rational explanation of new phenomena, and to develop every tenable hypothesis respecting their cause and history. The investigator thus becomes the parent of a family of hypotheses: and, by his parental relation to all, he is forbidden to fasten his affections unduly upon any one. The total outcome is greater care in ascertaining the facts, and greater discrimination and caution in drawing conclusions.*
>
> CHAMBERLIN (1890)

Before describing the principles or rules involved in 'reading' the blueprint and assembling parts according to its plan, we begin with a summary of what these rules are *not* and the reasons we know this:

1. DNA is *not* the blueprint of the organism.
2. Ontogeny (morphogenesis or the developmental history of an organism) does *not* recapitulate (repeat) phylogeny (the evolutionary history of a species).
3. The growth of an organism is *not* brought about by a set of linear cause and effect events like the construction of an automobile on an assembly line.
4. It is no longer believed that differentiation is a one-way street, that once a cell has been 'committed' to become, say, an intestinal cell, it cannot revert to the undifferentiated state.
5. The organism does not, in fact, develop.

Having listed what the blueprint is *not* and the mechanisms that are *not* involved in growing living structures, there is an obligation to state what the rules really are. This chapter will not provide a final answer. Indeed, some of the most interesting perspectives documented here conflict with each other, and this is a good thing. The conflicts are worthy disagreements and can ultimately lead us towards more clarity. The presentation will document some of the pieces of the puzzle of development including the actual purpose of DNA, tensegrity, twins, morphic fields, the role of immediate early genes, epigenetics, Humpty-Dumpty, the origin of life, spontaneous self-assembly, emergent properties, complex adaptive systems, and chaos theory.

Stating the Problem

A New Image of Man in Medicine contains a presentation by embryologist Paul Weiss, followed by an article on general systems theory by Ludwig von Bertalanffy. Weiss (1977) wrote *The System of Nature and the Nature of Systems: Empirical Holism and Practical Reductionism Harmonized*.

Like other perceptive biologists (e.g., Strohman, 1993; Wilson, 1994), Weiss reiterates the basic fact that we simply do not know how an organism develops from a single cell or how a seed grows into a mature plant. There is an illusion prevalent in the halls of science that this is a solved problem, an answered question. It is not. The incomplete answer goes like this: Chemical processes, directed by DNA in the chromosomes, build up the various molecules, cells, tissues, organs, and functions that comprise the adult organism. The inherited genetic material is a complete blueprint for the form and function of the adult body and supervises its growth and activities. All of life obeys the laws of chemistry and physics, and life is therefore reducible to a sequence of linear machine-like processes, an 'assembly line', involving reading the DNA blueprint, translating it into structures (proteins), and then animating those structures. Life is therefore the inevitable outcome of a sequence of linear cause-effect events. Likewise, disease and disorder can be traced to individual defects that can be repaired to produce healing. The chemist, and particularly the molecular biologist, will therefore eventually be able to provide all of the answers to our questions about the nature of life. 'Life is biochemistry and molecular biology'.

There are simple and profoundly significant flaws in all of this reasoning and in the ways it is applied in our medicine. It is true that physical and chemical processes are taking place in living systems. But the laws of physics and chemistry do not include concepts *of the living plan and form*. In a physics book you can find details of the four states of matter: solid, liquid, gas, and plasma. Gerald Pollack has described a fourth phase of water, solid, liquid, gas, and exclusion zone water (see Figure 3.14). You will not, however, find in a physics book a description of *the living state*.

To say that cells obey the laws of chemistry and physics is largely irrelevant and may be incorrect. As mentioned in the Preface, chemistry and physics are based on studies on non-living matter. It might be argued that organic chemistry and biochemistry deal with living material, but we will soon see that this is not the case. Organic chemistry and biochemistry are limited because they do not include the most significant attributes of 'aliveness'. Many of our medical problems, and their high cost in terms of human suffering and money, persist because we think we have already answered fundamental questions, when we have, in truth, not even asked them. One of the profound contributions of energy medicine is to bring up these fundamental questions and to see if an energetic perspective can give rise to new hypotheses that can be verified or refuted.

Yes, the DNA does contain the hereditary code for the assembly of protein molecules such as enzymes, collagen, haemoglobin, and neuropeptides. The mechanisms by which this code is conveyed from generation to generation and the ways the code is read and translated into new proteins are among the most important discoveries of recent science.

There is, however, a profound illusion that arises from careful observation of life at this microscopic molecular level. In this fragment of the whole, one observes parts (proteins) being precisely and repeatedly created from existing patterns of order (base sequences in the DNA). The fundamental formula, the central dogma of molecular biology, is that DNA *replicates* itself to pass genetic information from one cell to another and from one generation to the next; DNA *transcribes* its information into another molecule, RNA, that can migrate out of the cell nucleus; the RNA *translates* the information to form specific proteins.

So impressive is the regularity and predictability and reproducibility of protein synthesis that it seems obvious that the same mechanism must operate at, and thereby create, all levels of size and complexity. The logical mind has a natural tendency to grasp processes occurring at one level and assume they operate similarly at other scales. It was therefore logical for molecular biologists to predict that we would soon be able to understand how the entire plan of the organism is carried within the DNA and where the plan goes wrong to cause disease. The specific model is as follows (Kevles and Hood, 1992):

DNA → RNA → protein → everything else, including diseases.

An optimistic point of view was expressed by James D. Watson, co-discoverer with Francis Crick of the double helical structure of DNA:

> *These successes (in understanding heredity) have created a firm belief that the current extension of our understanding of biological phenomena to the molecular level (molecular biology) will soon enable us to understand all the basic features of the living state.*

WATSON (1970)

Vast sums, many careers, university departments and institutes, and a giant pharmaceutical industry have been devoted to finding ways to treat the symptoms that arise when the body fails to adjust, adapt, and repair itself. Much continues to be learned in this process, and some interesting ideas are being tested. However the 'master plan' and the 'causes' of major diseases remain elusive.

To solve challenging biological and medical problems, we must examine the basic aspects of life that mainstream biomedicine has traditionally been reluctant to examine. Viewed whole, the living organism displays properties that cannot be accounted for as a synthesis of the behaviours of parts. These 'whole systems' properties cannot be studied by taking things apart. Sadly, holistic thinking has long been dismissed in many modern academic circles as some new-age nonsense. In fact, biology began with whole systems approaches and is now returning to that perspective.

The Genes Are Not on Top, They Are on Tap

In the words of Strohman (1993), the genes are important but not on top – just on tap! Genes are undoubtedly involved at every step of development, but this does not mean they deserve all of the credit for establishing structures and functions at every level of scale. The most spectacular example to prove the point is provided by identical twins – two individuals arising from a single egg, endowed with identical complements of genes. If genetic determinism is the rule, identical twins should always develop into identical adults. Sometimes this happens, and sometimes it does not. 'Identical' twins can look so different that it is hard to recognize that they are members of the same family.

Scientists from around the world are now researching the nature of the whole systems processes that direct the formation of structures and their functional integration. Vitalism and vitality are being put back into living matter after centuries of being 'anti-establishment' and politically incorrect and therefore banished from consideration. The fascinating story that is emerging is slowly making its way into textbooks and medical curricula. It is a slow process because it requires multidisciplinary thinking – it is based on discoveries in a variety of areas of investigation, and our challenge is to fit the pieces together into logically consistent pictures and testable hypotheses.

Epigenetics

The term epigenetics refers to changes in phenotype (appearance) or gene expression caused by mechanisms other than changes in the underlying DNA sequence, hence the name epi- (Greek: over; above) genetics. The basic discovery is that non-genetic factors can cause an organism's genes to behave (or 'express themselves') differently.

Possibly the most significant recent breakthrough in genetic research is the discovery of a phenomenon that a few years ago was regarded as preposterous. For a long time we have thought that our genes control our structures, functions, our lives, and even our psychology and happiness. Recent research summarized in countless scientific reports and popular/scientific books by Church (2009), Lipton (2008), Feinstein et al. (2005), and others paints an entirely different picture.

In his brilliant and engaging lectures on epigenetics, Dr. Dawson Church often begins with the example of the Tesauro twins (Figure 13.1). Josephine Tesauro never thought she would live so long. At 92, she is straight backed, firm jawed, and vibrantly healthy, living alone in an immaculate brick ranch house high on a hill near McKeesport, a Pittsburgh suburb. She works part time in a hospital gift shop and drives her 1995 white Oldsmobile Cutlass Ciera to meetings of her four bridge groups, to church, and to the grocery store.

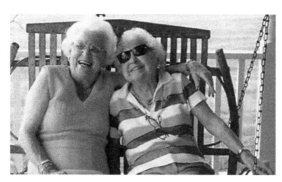

Figure 13.1   Ninety-two-year-old identical twins with exactly the same genome but completely different health outcomes. Josephine Tesauro (left) and her sister.

Mrs. Tesauro does, however, have a living sister, an identical twin. But she and her twin are not so identical anymore. Her sister is incontinent, she has had a hip replacement, and she has a degenerative disorder that destroyed most of her vision. She also has dementia. 'She just does not comprehend,' her sister says.

Researchers who study aging are fascinated by such stories. How could it be that two people with the same genes, growing up in the same family, living all their lives in the same place, could age so differently?

The study of epigenetics began with about five scientific reports published during the late 1950s and a few dozen in the 1960s and 1970s. Epigenetics has now become a major focus of scientific investigation with literally thousands of peer-reviewed articles per year. Of key importance is a family of genes known as immediate early genes (Figure 13.2). These genes respond quickly to the events in our lives and to cues from our environment – some being activated within seconds to minutes. Some of these genes activate other genes, which provide code for the proteins that regulate the behaviour of cells in all of the body's systems.

As can be seen from Figure 13.2, by 2002 about 100 immediate early genes had been identified. These genes influence virtually every aspect of physiology and behaviour. This research is accelerating, with over 25,000 scientific reports already published on epigenetics.

The outcome of this line of investigation: Genetic research has paved the way for genetic therapies that we can actually use on ourselves, once we know a little bit about them. This is one of the major revolutions in healthcare being ushered in under the academic umbrella of energy medicine. We are learning that we are doing genetic engineering on ourselves all the time.

In the space of one generation, we have discovered, or rediscovered, techniques that can make us happier, less stressed, and much more physically healthy – safely, quickly, and without side effects. Techniques from Energy Medicine and Energy Psychology can alleviate chronic diseases, shift autoimmune conditions, and eliminate psychological traumas with efficiency and speed that conventional treatments can scarcely touch. The implications of these techniques for human happiness, for social conflicts, and for political change promise a radical positive disruption in the human condition, one that goes far beyond healthcare. They have the promise of affecting society as profoundly as the rediscovery of mathematical and experimental principles during the Renaissance changed the course of medieval civilization. And they are at the cutting edge of science, as experimental evidence stacks up to provide objective demonstration of their effectiveness.

Church (2009)

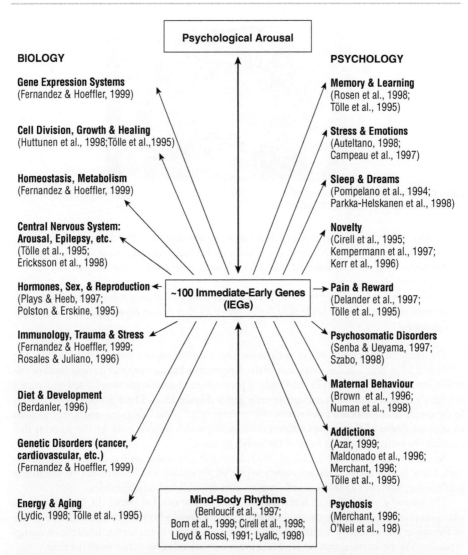

Figure 13.2   Immediate early genes play a vital role in regulating a great many psychological and physiological functions. *(From Rossi, 2002. The Psychobiology of Gene Expression: Neuroscience and Neurogenesis in Hypnosis and the Healing Arts. Used with permission of W.W. Norton & Company.)*

Scientists are describing the pathways by which our experiences, thoughts, feelings, and spoken words can cause profound shifts in our physiology, neurology, biochemistry, and in the expression of our genetic material. While some of these pathways are biochemical and neurological, others are energetic, involving the living matrix, which reaches into every part of the genome in every cell in the body (see Figure 10.7A). The exciting inquiry into these phenomena is bringing the technical details from generations of genetic research into the mainstream of human affairs (Rossi, 2002). Energy psychology is an emergent aspect of energy medicine.

Weiss on the Development of the Organism

In his essay, *The System of Nature and the Nature of Systems: Empirical Holism and Practical Reductionism Harmonized*, Weiss recounts the way the deep mystery of life presents itself in the development of the mature organism. He does so from the perspective of a lifetime of careful and distinguished laboratory investigation. The vital questions he raised are profound.

The same generative processes that give rise to the mature organism continue to operate in the adult for the constant 'turnover' or replacement of parts. Many energy therapies encourage and enhance the flows of energy, information, and new materials into the structures of the organism. These processes continue while the organism continues its dynamic activities. The flows of energy, information, and matter permit patients to reconstruct or renew or regenerate themselves along the ideal line or pattern or blueprint that is their birthright. That such a regeneration can and does take place, on a large scale, is at the same time the marvel of energy medicine and what is urgently needed in our health system.

To illustrate the central problem of biology in a simple manner, Weiss presents a diagram showing a chick embryo that has been removed from its egg and suspended in a test tube in a balanced salt solution. The chick is homogenized into mush, a uniform suspension of its parts. These parts are then separated or fractionated by centrifugation. The enhanced gravity field in the centrifuge forces the heavier components to the bottom of the tube, while the lighter and dissolved components stay on top.

The process just described is one of the basic techniques used in modern biochemistry for the study of reactions taking place in tissues or organs. Here the method is being used on a whole organism. The solution at the top of the last tube is still 'alive' in the sense that it contains functional enzymes capable of carrying out chemical reactions essential to living matter. By studying these reactions in the test tube, free of annoying and distracting structures, biochemists have been able to map out the metabolic pathways that convert sugars into energy and amino acids into proteins, the vital processes that lead to the construction of living matter. Hence, if some sugar is added to the top of the tube containing the dissolved proteins from the embryo, one can trace its stepwise and energy-producing breakdown into pyruvate, a process called glycolysis that is described in any biochemistry text. Likewise, molecular biologists have been able to isolate the parts of the cell responsible for replicating the DNA as well as transcribing and translating it for the manufacture of specific proteins.

Next Weiss poses the question, 'Can we reverse the process just described? Can we 'synthesize' the chick from the mush?' The problem is similar to the question of the origin of life. One popular theory is that living complexity originally arose from a nutrient-rich 'primordial ooze' by the more or less chance combination of molecules into structures that could reproduce themselves.

The question Weiss poses may seem absurd, but we could say, 'Why not?' For the tube containing the dissolved chick embryo contains the same molecules as the intact embryo. All we need to know is how to assemble the scrambled parts in the proper order. And, since this information is thought to be available in the DNA blueprint, and since the tube contains both the DNA and the enzymatic equipment to read the code and assemble proteins, we have all of the essentials to mesh the parts back together into a fully alive chick.

However, the process just described cannot be reversed to restore the original living chick. Like Humpty-Dumpty, all of the great scientists and all of the great engineers cannot put the chick back together again. What is revealed by stating the question in this way is the central problem of biology and a major puzzle for biomedicine: While we understand much about how the component parts are made, we do not have a complete understanding of how these pieces assemble into larger structures and into the organism as a whole, with its myriad functions.

We might ask, 'If we wait long enough, or if we perturb the tube containing the dissolved chick embryo in some appropriate manner, might we trigger a process that spontaneously allows our hapless chick to reassemble itself?' Perhaps we should expose the tube to electrical sparks. This idea comes from recalling the famous Miller–Urey experiment published in 1953, in which a mixture of water, methane, ammonia, and hydrogen was exposed to sparks to simulate lightning in the prebiotic atmosphere. At the end of one week, Miller and Urey observed that some of the carbon within the system was now in the form of organic compounds including amino acids that are used to make proteins in living cells. Sugars, lipids, and some of the building blocks for nucleic acids were formed as well (Miller, 1953). Perhaps the appropriate conditions would permit our chick to spontaneously reassemble itself.

Self-Organization

Molecular and developmental biologists have devised a simple concept to explain how the parts of the organism come together. Once the molecules of life are formed, they spontaneously or automatically *self-assemble*, much like the way atoms join together to form a crystal. What we refer to as 'life' somehow arises in the process.

Spontaneous self-assembly has a simple appeal, and many examples can be found in the biological literature. The biochemist can describe the various processes and the energetics involved in the manufacture of a molecule and ways this molecule can combine with others to produce larger structures. At the molecular level, self-assembly involves structures with certain charge distributions that are attracted to other structures with complementary charge distributions (Figure 13.3). They mesh together, sort of like the bumpy surface of a key fits with a corresponding surface inside of a lock. Because of the way the charges are distributed along one molecule, it will be attracted to and fit with another molecule with a complementary pattern of charges. In other words, self-assembly is an energetic process involving attraction and alignment between patterns of charge.

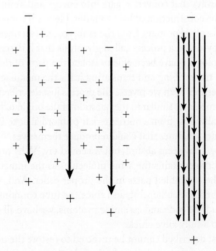

Figure 13.3 An array of tropocollagen dipoles (left) forming a collagen fibril (right). Tropocollagens are staggered or off-set from each other. Polarities of the individual molecules add together, giving the fibril as a whole an electrical polarity. The bulk of the collagen fibrils in the vertebrate body are oriented vertically, so the organism as a whole has an overall electrical polarity, with the head negative with respect to the tail or feet (Athenstaedt, 1974).

What happens in connective tissue involves very long tropocollagen molecules with an intricate distribution of charges that causes these molecules to assemble with their characteristic offset alignment, as shown in Figure 13.3. Water molecules also 'spontaneously' enmesh themselves in very precise ways into the forming liquid crystal (see Figures 3.4 and 11.9).

Ways for order to emerge from the chaotic mixture produced by homogenizing the chick embryo have been the subject of modern theories of chaos and self-organization and complex adaptive systems:

As a first approximation, organisms can be defined by the complement of cell types that they possess. Each cell type is defined by its specific collection of signal transduction pathways. While many pathways are common to most cell types (e.g. glycolysis), others are specific to a particular cell type and serve to characterize that cell. Many diseases, including cancer, are characterized by aberrations in general and specific signal-transduction pathways. These pathways are generally intricate and not easily modeled. The formalism of complex adaptive system theory, however, provides the tools by which these pathways can be investigated. By modeling signal-transduction pathways from the viewpoint of complex adaptive systems, a deeper understanding of their intricacies may result. This could eventually lead to novel methods of therapeutic intervention in diseases that arise from aberrant signal transduction.

SCHWAB AND PIENTA (1997)

Figure 13.4 provides an example of a model of a complex adaptive system.

It is a simple signal transduction pathway that links structure to function. The structure is the three-dimensional environment of the cell, and the function is mitosis. The pathway contains a detector with two properties, the capability to make decisions based on available information and an effector that relays the signal or carries out some action. These three attributes are present, to some extent, in all nodes of signaling pathways. Assume the cell has only two requirements to undergo mitosis. It needs an adequate supply of energy to duplicate its DNA, and space must be available for the new cell. On the periphery of the cell is a network of 'pressure transducers' (i.e. detectors) that provide the cell with information about its extracellular environment; they measure deformation of the cytoskeleton. This network will answer the question 'Is there room to grow?' In the cytoplasm there is an energy meter that indicates how much energy is available to the cellular machinery. For the cell to divide, two criteria must be met. First, the cell must not be completely surrounded. Second, the meter must read at least 75% full.

Schwab and Pienta (1997)

Emergent Properties

At each level of complexity, new properties emerge that are not possessed by the parts. A science has been developed to explore these important 'emergent' properties, which have been referred to as synergistic, cooperative, or collective properties. Some features arise because dissimilar materials combine to form composites. Some properties only emerge when the assembly reaches a certain size.

As mentioned above, an oversimplified answer to the problem of morphogenesis is that the molecular structure, transcribed from the DNA blueprint, includes features that cause the molecules to 'spontaneously' align and order themselves in particular ways. Another answer is that the DNA specifies the manufacture of specific proteins and enzymes that serve as the 'hands' and 'tools' of the genetic material, carrying out DNA's instructions by guiding the assembly process and gluing things together. Self-assembly is complemented with directed assembly. Weiss pointed out the problems with this concept.

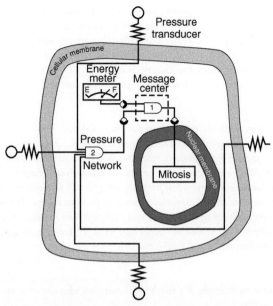

Figure 13.4 A model of a complex adaptive system. *(From Schwab and Pienta, 1997. Modeling signal transduction in normal and cancer cells using complex adaptive systems. Med. Hypotheses 48, 111–123.)*

The Organism Does Not, in Fact, Assemble

Weiss has a surprising perspective on all of this. He tells us that the organism does not, in fact, assemble.

> The basic premise that embryonic development is an assembly process is false. The orderly patterns with an organism, and its integrated behaviours, are not products of an assembly process in the usual sense of a set of linear cause-effect chains.

> *Weiss (1977)*

This perspective demolishes Watson's ambitious plan for molecular biology to solve all of the riddles of nature. It also explains why a major national research focus, the Human Genome Project, did not, as initially advertised, lead to cures for a vast number of diseases.

> We can watch an automobile being put together on the linear assembly line. A large number of orderly steps result in a complete, functional car. The organism, however, is not the sum, the 'outcome' of a comparable linear sequence of steps. In essence, the automobile is finished when it comes off the assembly line, and it deteriorates thereafter. In living systems the 'assembly line' and the flow of components never ceases. The organism possesses properties that the automobile lacks: It continually renews itself, and it can repair itself when necessary; it can change its structural organization, or adapt, according to the ways it is used; it has consciousness, whatever that is.

In contrast to the automobile that wears out, the body always has the possibility of regenerating and even *improving* its structural and functional integration. To see this process in action, watch an athlete or other performer practicing. Watch the gradual changes taking place in his or her structure, movement patterns, and emotional state as the body and psyche perfect themselves in preparation for an important contest or performance.

We have learned much about the mechanics and scheduling of the various processes taking place during embryonic development, but this is not the whole picture. That something is missing is revealed by careful study of the behaviour of cells in the growing organism. Embryologists have long recognized that there are specific regions within the early embryo that are earmarked as forerunners of the various organs: heart, liver, kidney, brain, etc. The embryo is a busy place, with cells wandering about until they settle down and form stable relationships with other cells to create specific tissues and organs. This process has been so thoroughly studied that there is no doubt that cells undergo profound changes when they switch from an early indeterminate or undifferentiated, wandering state, with the capacity to form *any* organ in the body (called 'totipotent'), to a determinate, differentiated or *committed* state.

There has been a biological 'law' about this process: Differentiation is a one-way street. The process is irreversible. Cells cannot resume their totipotent condition once they have become 'committed' to form a particular kind of tissue.

Like any statement of an 'absolute' in biology or medicine, there are annoying exceptions that ruin the lovely law. For example, Gurdon (1968) showed that even highly differentiated intestinal epithelial cells in frogs retain sufficient genetic information to produce the whole animal. He demonstrated this by transplanting nuclei from the highly differentiated intestinal cells into frog eggs that had had their nuclei removed. These eggs developed into normal embryos and adults capable of reproducing. The conclusion of this and similar experiments is that differentiation does not change the genome in a permanent way, but instead alters the *expression* of the genes, so that only those needed in a particular tissue are active. De-differentiation can and does occur. This phenomenon is extremely relevant to the important goal of regeneration of missing parts and to the abilities of various therapies to encourage restoration of traumatized tissues.

Morphogenesis

Now we return to the embryological assembly process. If we follow individual cells from one stage to the next, we find that they take different paths in different individuals. While the overall outcome is two adults with a similar set of similarly structured organs, the formative processes do not correspond to each other. Determination of an individual cell is a response to *its position in the orderly pattern of the future whole*, rather than a result of an orderly and precisely directed assembly process.

Two complementary interpretations emerge from this discovery. First, there is far more order in the whole than would be expected from the seemingly capricious behaviours of the cells as they assemble. And, therefore, the ordered state in the adult cannot be the outcome of a defined sequence of microscopic cause-effect chain reactions in the embryo. Some other 'whole systems' processes are operating.

Defining 'System'

A system is an entity, a whole, whose configuration and functioning are achieved and maintained. The form is not conserved because of a rigid linking together of constituents. In fact, the opposite is the case. The components are not tightly interlocked, except where structural stability and rigidity are required for functioning. But even the most rigid components, such as bones and cartilage, are held together with bonds that can be readily broken to facilitate the constant turnover of components without compromising structures or functions.

A system is a complex unit in space and time so constituted that its parts, by 'systemic coopera-tion' (Oschman, 2003), attain a certain configuration and a certain set of dynamic functions and preserve these in spite of constant changes in the environment. The parts, despite their ability to change shape and position, are coordinated by being enmeshed in a living fabric – the continuum that was introduced in Chapter 10. The pattern of the whole is a joint property of the inter-linked components. As explained by Szent-Györgyi (1963), 'Whenever we separate two things, we lose something, something which may have been the most essential feature'. It is the loss of this essential 'something', the loss of 'systemic cooperation', that prevents the reassembly of the chick from the mush as described in the "thought experiment" posed by Weiss and mentioned above. Intractable diseases may not really have 'causes' in the usual sense, but may instead be the consequence of a loss of the properties that give rise to 'systemic cooperation'. Our emerging un-derstanding of the restoration of Szent-Györgyi's 'something essential' and Oschman's 'systemic cooperation' to the whole organism is one of the emerging miracles of CAM therapies. The valid-ity of this statement is documented by the successes of energy medicine approaches in treating acute injury and supporting sustained peak performances in competitions.

A simple revelation emerges: Holism and reductionism are analytical procedures that are not separable. Neither can describe nature completely, and they are therefore complementary rather than contradictory representations. Again, 'complementarity' is used in the same sense that Niels Bohr reconciled the wave–particle duality in physics. Matter can be viewed as a wave or as a particle, and the phenomena are very different conceptually. Yet the two views complement each other in that the nature of an object cannot be fully understood without considering both of its aspects. Similarly, holism and reductionism are two complementary perspectives on human struc-ture and function.

Notice the evolution of our conceptualization of how nature works. For the physicists, the sequence of discovery involved particles, waves, their incompatibility, and the resolution of the dilemma by complementarity. For biologists the microscope and molecular biology revealed the fundamental 'particles' of living matter, leading to a highly reductionist picture of life that was argued to be superior to superficial views of the whole. Energy medicine and quantum entangle-ment unite all of these parts and the wholes into a fascinating continuum.

There are signs of another step in this intellectual process, because of a breakdown in the fun-damental truth that the wave and particle views cannot be reconciled. Experiments have shown that atoms *can* have wave-like and particle-like behaviour at the same time (reviewed by Gribbin, 1995). The point is that complementarity is a useful point of view that, like most of our views, is giving way to a more comprehensive perspective. The irreconcilable is being reconciled.

If we analyze the whole by focusing on its parts (which in themselves are also wholes of a smaller order), we acquire a certain microscopic precision in our descriptions. But this precision is obtained at the expense of losing the information or rules or Szent-Györgyi's 'beautiful vistas' or the 'something essential' or the 'systemic cooperation' that enables the higher levels of what we call *organization* to exist, as demonstrated by higher levels of health and performance.

Weiss illustrated this (Figure 13.5). The drawing has been modified to include the degree of 'organization' in relation to precision and information. Also added is a notation of the part of this scheme that is the focus of several body-centred therapies (see Chapter 7). By introducing information and organization to the whole system, significant results are obtained that extend to the cellular and subcellular levels, without the necessity of knowing about the microscopic details.

Stated differently, in physics and biology and human lives, the transition from randomness to order is most remarkable and most visible at the level of the whole. Yet all parts of the continuum participate. If the focus of a therapy is on the whole organism, the parts will, in a sense, take care of themselves. This is a predictable aspect, perhaps even a 'law' of the natural living continuum. It is dramatically illustrated by structural bodywork procedures such as osteopathy, chiropractic, structural integration, Rolfing, the Trager approach, the Duggan/French approach, and so on.

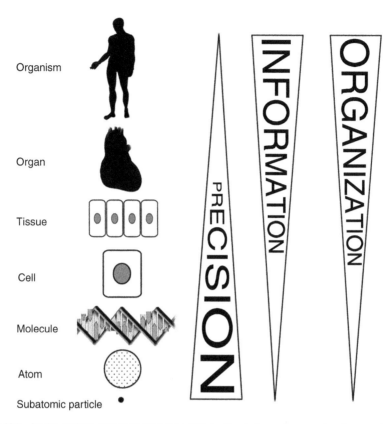

Figure 13.5 As the analysis descends from the whole to its smaller parts, we gain microscopic *precision* and detailed knowledge, but we lose the essential information that governs the structure and function of the whole, which we can refer to as *organization*.

For example, when breathing is enhanced by increasing the flexibility at the places where the ribs insert into the vertebrae, enabling the diaphragm to move more freely, the oxygen supply to every cell in the body is enhanced and metabolism is everywhere facilitated. When the musculoskeletal system is balanced, other systems will inevitably adjust accordingly, i.e., they will become balanced as well. Different systems move toward balance at different rates, depending on the rates at which metabolic turnover takes place in the different systems. It is inevitable, though, that balance and flexibility will be contagious. If the focus is exclusively on the parts, as in conventional medicine, the whole may or may not respond in the manner desired. Surgery, for example, may correct a local issue, but the procedure will be followed by scarring and compensations that can create problems in parts of the body that are distant from the site of intervention. In this sense, cause and effect are actually more predictably linked in complementary holistic approaches.

Wound Healing

Wound healing and recovery from disease are among the most important and remarkable of living processes, involving the integrated and cooperative activities of many regulatory systems throughout the body. Level upon level of intricate control systems and feedback loops join together to accelerate and inhibit myriad activities, on a moment-to-moment basis. Even the smallest pin-prick alters the behaviour of millions of cells, billions of molecules, trillions of atoms, and untold numbers of subatomic particles. While biology and medicine are aware of some aspects of this continuum, what is truly remarkable is that 'hands-on' therapists are able to interact with all of it in profoundly significant ways that await thorough scientific investigation. Often intuition and intention guide the hands, without analysis of the details. And we would like to know how intuition and intention have the remarkable effects they have. The following summarizes technical details of the invisible dynamic that lies under the physician's or other therapist's fingertips and whose functioning is enhanced when structural, energetic, and kinetic balance are restored to the living system:

> *Any trauma sets off an intricate cascade of physiological activities and adjustments. If the injury is severe, both local and systemic responses are initiated, and all of the systems in the body can be involved.*
>
> *An injury or disease triggers the migration of a variety of kinds of cells toward the site of the problem. Platelets release clotting factors; waves of white cells move in to fight infection and to resorb fragments of damaged cells and "non-self" materials; epithelial cells, fibroblasts, and osteoblasts crawl into position to replace damaged bones and soft tissues and to form scar tissue. These processes are triggered and regulated by a variety of messages that radiate from a site of disorder. A wide range of stimulating and inhibiting factors activate and integrate wound repair or tumor absorption, and then wind down the processes when healing is complete.*
>
> *Cells migrating into a wound or a tumor must be replaced by cell division. If the problem is extensive, clotting, inflammatory reactions, or tumor resorption consume cells which must be replaced by proliferation of stem cells in distant organs, such as the lymph nodes, bone marrow, or liver. Healing therefore involves an array of dynamic interactions between local and systemic processes. Fever, allergic reactions, and the "fight or flight" response are all examples of life-saving systemic regulations.*
>
> *Many physiological responses are nonlinear because of the intricate web of whole-body feedback and feed-forward regulatory pathways that are involved. Some activities persist for weeks after an injury. Vital living processes must be maintained during repair. This may require temporary shifting of functions to other parts or systems or pathways. Redundancy is the hallmark of vital functions.*

Assembly Rules for Whole Systems

The topics discussed in this section may represent the most important and underappreciated subject in all of medicine because the way the human body forms and re-forms is key to injury repair and regeneration. As mentioned above, an ability to regenerate damaged or missing body parts would be of extreme value to medicine and is a topic worthy of sustained study. Certainly a Nobel Prize should be waiting for the person who is able to accomplish regeneration in humans.

Some whole systems rules for the assembly of the human body have been worked out from a remarkable series of studies conducted by Erich Blechschmidt at the Anatomical Institute of the University of Göttingen between 1942 and 1972. The project examined some 200,000 serial sections and resulted in 64 enlarged total reconstructions of embryos. Careful study of the Blechschmidt Collection of Human Embryos has provided new understandings of human differentiation and development. Previous investigations had focused on molecular approaches applied to animals other than humans, and the conclusions had not been tested on humans. Blechschmidt's work focused mainly on the first 8 weeks after conception, and he wrote more than 120 scientific papers and a number of books on the way form and functions develop. Older interpretations based mainly on phylogenetic and molecular studies had to be re-evaluated on the basis of these observations.

Much of Blechschmidt's work was published in German (e.g., Blechschmidt, 1973), but two translations have made this important research available in English (Blechschmidt, 2004; Blechschmidt and Gasser, 2012). Study of this work requires that one be willing to forget preconceptions of anatomy and embryology and begin over again. Those who have not been steeped in traditional embryology and developmental biology will therefore have an advantage when looking at Blechschmidt's work and conclusions. Note that Blechschmidt takes a humble and open-minded approach. He raises many issues as important topics for discussion and contemplation and makes no claim that his answers are the last word on the subjects. For example, he states at the beginning that the body is not composed of systems:

... concepts such as body 'systems' (e.g., the cardiovascular system, the nervous system, etc.) are quite artificial; their only use is for the convenience of dividing the subject matter into sections or chapters. Body systems do not exist in reality—it is always impossible to define where one system ends and the next starts. The body functions as a whole and it is only as a whole that we should attempt to comprehend it.

Blechschmidt (2004)

A second concept that Blechschmidt dismisses at the beginning is the idea that structures develop to serve a purpose. One could argue that the human hand, the claw of a cat, or the scales of fish are produced to serve particular functions, and this functionality drives the developmental process. A close look at this logic reveals that the functions of a part of the body actually provide absolutely no information on the processes involved in their formation. A more scientific perspective is that it is the growth process that gives rise to the final form. A second principle, then, is that growth functions precede all higher functions. 'The achievements of the embryo are always the precursors of all subsequent accomplishments' (Bleichschmidt, 2004).

Notice that this perspective of Blechschmidt seems to contrast with the statement of Weiss that determination of an individual cell is a response to its position in the orderly pattern of the future whole (see above in the section Morphogenesis). This seeming contradiction points to a fascinating and absolutely vital issue. After half a century of looking into this question, Szent-Györgyi (1974) concluded that living matter has a 'drive to perfect itself'. The real nature of this drive, if it really exists, provides an unanswered and even untouched question for the biologist (and also for the philosopher). Where, how, and when this drive arose during evolution is an even greater mystery, but one that is worthy of exploration. The search, after taking many directions, is beginning to focus on the most natural strategies for bringing forth natural wisdom and order and systemic cooperation within the natural continuum.

Tensegrity

Before summarizing the modern rules governing morphogenesis, it is essential to describe two relatively new architectural principles. The first of these is the tensegrity concept originally developed by the sculptor, Kenneth Snelson (Heartney, 2009), applied to living systems by Fuller and Marks (1960), and specifically applied to cell behaviour by Donald Ingber and his colleagues (Ingber, 1998). See the earlier discussion of tensegrity in Chapter 11, especially Figure 11.15. The second principle is the morphogenetic field concept developed by Rupert Sheldrake.

Figure 13.6 shows the tensegrity scaffolding under the skin, based on skilled high-resolution video imaging accomplished by the French plastic surgeon, Dr. Jean-Claude Guimberteau. Of this arrangement, Guimberteau states:

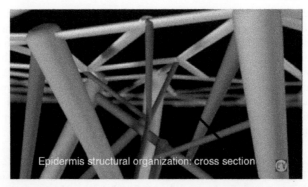

Figure 13.6 Tensegrity scaffolding under the skin. *(From Guimberteau (2012), used by permission of Dr. Guimberteau.)*

From the DNA helix to the cytoskeleton, including the links to the integrins and neighboring cells, everything is in continuity, everything is connected, everything moves to fit, and everything moves and always comes back.

GUIMBERTEAU (2012)

Tensegrity structures obey versatile architectural principles identified by Buckminster Fuller (Figure 13.7). In particular, tensegrity systems stabilize themselves by dynamically redistributing and balancing tensions and compressions. Simple mechanical rules operating at different levels of scale can govern cell behaviour, including movements and shape changes, and thereby partly explain how tissues and organs develop. Tensegrity provides a universal set of building rules that guide the design of organic structures from simple carbon compounds to complex cells and tissues (Ingber, 1998). Tensegrity is a valuable design principle for living bodies because:

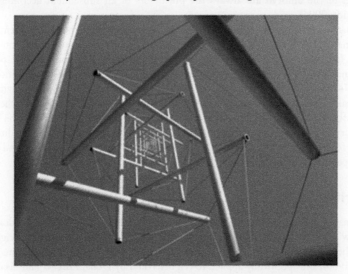

Figure 13.7 Photograph of Kenneth Snelson's Needle Tower (1968), currently housed at the Hirshhorn Museum and Sculpture Garden in Washington, DC. This image illustrates the discontinuous compression member property of tensegrity structures; this property is considered to be the distinguishing and representative feature of a large proportion of Kenneth Snelson's body of work. Illustrating this work contributes to understanding of tensegrity structures and the significance of Snelson's work in twentieth-century sculpture and biology.

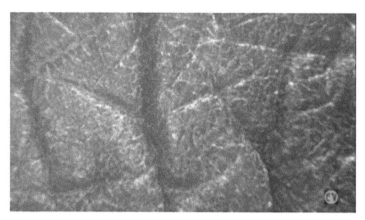

Figure 13.8   Polygonal structures at the skin surface. *(Guimberteau, J.-C., 2012. Interior Architectures: DVD from Endo Vivo production, www.endovivo.com)*

- A tensegrity system becomes stronger and more stable when it is loaded, i.e., when weight is being supported.
- A tensegrity system readily absorbs impacts by conducting the energy through the structure. Places where tensegrity is compromised, such as by contact between struts, are vulnerable and are the places where injuries can take place.
- A tensegrity system readily conducts vibrational energy, such as by plucking one of the tendons or by introducing other forms of vibration, such as sound, light, or pressure.
- A tensegrity system composed of proteins such as collagen is also an aqueous system with water molecules associated and aligned with every part. This gives rise to liquid crystallinity and quantum coherence.

Note the polygonal geometry under the skin and inside of cells (Figure 13.6). These polygonal aspects are also found at the skin surface (Figure 13.8).

These polygonal geometries may have profound significance in relation to the mechanism of morphic resonance and the morphogenic field, to be described next.

The Morphogenetic Field

Given our lack of understanding of the nature of the 'blueprint of life' as discussed above, it is important to look carefully at new ideas when they emerge. The morphic field and morphogenetic resonance are concepts developed many years ago by Oxford biologist, Rupert Sheldrake (Sheldrake, 1995a,b). This concept was met with complete and immediate rejection and even scorn by the scientific community:

In 1981, Sir John Maddox wrote a famous article, 'A Book for Burning?', in *Nature* about Sheldrake's first book, *A New Science of Life*. This was followed by a series of further hostile reviews in *Nature* and in British newspapers. He wrote 'This infuriating tract ... is the best candidate for burning there has been for many years'. In an interview broadcast on BBC television in 1994, he said: 'Sheldrake is putting forward magic instead of science, and that can be condemned in exactly the language that the Pope used to condemn Galileo, and for the same reason. It is heresy.'

When a new scientific concept is put forward and encounters such violent rejection, it is often a sign that something important has happened. Albert Einstein stated that, 'If at first the idea is not absurd, then there is no hope for it'. And, 'Condemnation without investigation is the height of ignorance'. And, 'Great spirits have always encountered violent opposition from mediocre minds'.

Sheldrake's dreaded hypothesis can be summarized as follows:

- Morphogenetic fields give rise to all forms.
- Matter assumes form when it resonates with a field.
- The fields involved are not classical electromagnetic fields.
- Morphogenetic fields are derived from a body's own past actions and from the structures and actions of ancestors.
- Fields act across space and time.

Sheldrake also pointed out that leading philosophers have generally agreed that memory and consciousness are not in the brain (Sheldrake, 2013). This idea goes strongly counter to conventional thinking, in spite of the fact that prominent investigators from diverse fields agree on this matter. At the time of the publication of Sheldrake's book, there was little understanding of the energetic structure of space and the interactions of space with matter. However, we now know that space has a spiral grain (Ginzburg, 1996) and that space is filled with scalar waves, spin waves, or torsion waves (Kozyrev, 2005; Swanson, 2011; Meyl, 2003; Panov, 1997).

Sheldrake's critics are very vocal, but more reasoned opinions can be found in the reviews of his latest book. For example:

Science is often portrayed as a paragon of intellectual freedom. It's a quaint idea, but it's not true. Some key concepts in science have hardened into unshakeable, unquestioned dogma. Science Set Free *exposes ten of the key dogmas of modern times. If even one is slightly off, then the scientific world is in for a shock, and the aftershocks will have huge impacts on technology, medicine, and religion. Rupert Sheldrake skillfully examines each dogma and argues, with evidence, that all ten dogmas are wrong. After reading this book I am persuaded that he's right. If you agree that science must be freed from the shackles of antiquated beliefs, then read this book. If you don't agree, then read it twice.*

DEAN RADIN, PH.D., AUTHOR OF *THE CONSCIOUS UNIVERSE*

Guimberteau's images (Figures 13.9E and 13.8) show geometrical patterns in the surface and under the skin. Veltheim and Oschman (2013) have pointed out the similarities between the geometric patterns found in models of space, the surface of the skin, the tissues under the skin, and geometric elements in cells (Figure 13.9).

A number of scientists have suggested that memory is an inherent property of all objects found in nature (e.g., Sheldrake, 1995a,b, 2009; Sheldrake et al., 2001; Schwartz and Russek, 2006). These concepts have been met with a vast amount of skepticism, but the method of multiple working hypotheses requires that we give them equal weight, especially considering the fact that we are dealing with extremely important but unsolved problems.

Regeneration Versus Prosthetics

The present thrust of clinical investigation in orthopedic surgery is towards the replacement of missing or damaged skeletal parts with metallic or plastic implants. One can only agree that major advances have recently been made in this direction, and at this time such procedures are frequently the best method of therapy for many pathological conditions of the skeletal systems. Despite their popularity and demonstrated efficiency, the use of such devices fails to take into consideration two basic facts: First, the human skeletal system is capable of considerable self-repair; second, no inorganic implant has the capacity of growth and remodeling and can only decline in mechanical strength with the passage of time. The statement that the best replacement for a damaged femoral head would be a new structure regenerated by the individual himself still remains unchallenged.

Becker (1972)

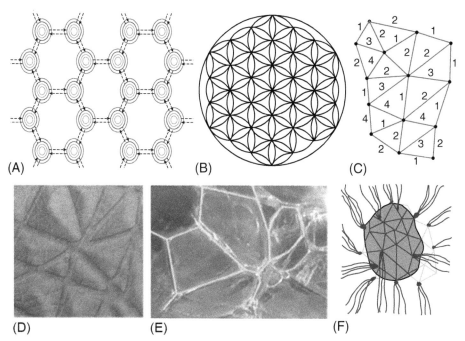

Figure 13.9   (A–C) Geometric fabric of space as suggested by Milo Wolff (A), sacred geometry (B), and Roger Penrose (C). Geometric fabric on the skin surface (D) and under the skin (E) *(Guimberteau, J.-C., 2012. Interior Architectures: DVD from Endo Vivo production, www.endovivo.com)* (F) the nuclear geodome described by Lazarides and Revel (1979). *(Lazarides E, Revel JP: The molecular basis of cell movement, Sci Am 1979 Mar;240(5), 100–113)*

Robert O. Becker pointed out repeatedly that regeneration of damaged or missing body parts is a far more natural and effective medical technology than the use of prosthetic devices or transplants (see box). Much research has been focused on mechanical substitutes for hearts and other organs and transplantation of organs, rather than determining how to induce the body to form its own replacements.

Becker has shown that very low levels of electrical stimulation can cause cultures of so-called differentiated cells to de-differentiate into totipotent cells capable of forming all of the tissues needed to replace a lost or damaged part. His fascinating description of this breakthrough research can be found in his book (Becker and Sheldon, 1985).

The key to Becker's demonstration was reducing the strength of electrical stimulation. Following the usual way scientists tend to look at such matters, he assumed a large current would be more effective than a small one. The opposite was correct. In the experiments on frog red blood cells, conducted with a student named Frederick Brown, the test current was reduced, a step at a time, until they reached the lowest current the apparatus could produce, with the intensity control turned to zero, about half a billionth of an ampere. This stimulation produced a dramatic de-differentiation. Note that red blood cells in frogs have nuclei, unlike human red cells.

The reason for mentioning these experiments is that they have profound medical implications, yet they have been given little attention by biomedical researchers. Moreover, the extremely low levels of stimulation required to produce dedifferentiation and regeneration are comparable to the levels present in the human energy field. This topic was discussed earlier in Chapter 2, Figure 2.9 when we looked at the very low levels of stimulation produced by electromagnetic healing devices that facilitate the repair of bone fractures and healing in a variety of other tissues. Hence it is not surprising to find accounts of acupuncture and other complementary approaches stimulating repair and even regeneration of tissue. This is an example of an important line of medical inquiry that fascinates many in the CAM community.

These discoveries relate to our health crisis. Biomedicine continues to emphasize the most difficult, painful, and expensive methods, such as artificial organs and organ transplants, instead of examining the more natural approach of regeneration:

> *...all of the circuitry and machinery is there; the problem is simply to discover how to turn on the right switches to activate the process.*
>
> WEIL (1995)

New Rules

We have seen that what maintains vitality and aliveness in an organism is not linear sequences of chemical reactions, messages, or physiological events, but the ways they are regulated and integrated. We are dealing with a vast network of processes – proliferations, specializations, movements, differentiations, de-differentiations, interactions, cross-linkages, feed-forwards, and feed-backs of startling complexity and diversity – all directed at maintaining and restoring the *orderly pattern of the whole* described in this chapter.

Having explained in detail what the rules of growth and morphogenesis are *not*, we can now begin a list of what they really are.

1. DNA acts as a stable reference.
2. Tensegrity provides a connection between cell shape and metabolism.
3. Identical twins can show very different characteristics as they age.
4. Morphic fields provide an alternative to DNA as the blueprint, with the morphic blueprint actually referencing the evolutionary history of an organism.
5. Immediate early genes are quickly and profoundly influenced by environmental changes.
6. Epigenetics is the study of the effects of the environment on gene expression.
7. Humpty-Dumpty and disintegrated organisms cannot spontaneously reassemble.
8. Experiments on the origin of life have shown how electric fields provided by 'sparks' can cause the spontaneous formation of amino acids, sugars, lipids, and some of the building blocks for nucleic acids (Miller, 1953; Miller and Urey, 1959).
9. Spontaneous self-assembly can take place when proteins with particular distributions of surface charge mate with proteins with complementary charge profiles.
10. Emergent properties are new properties that arise from combinations of identical components.
11. Chaos theory, popularly known as the butterfly effect, mathematically models how subtle interventions in a dynamical system can lead to large changes such as the shift from chaos to order.

Conclusions

At this point, we can be specific about the importance of thinking about these ideas. The outcome of this line of inquiry will profoundly affect the future of all of us. This is so because our most debilitating, painful, and costly medical problems are breakdowns at the level of whole systems, which then lead to observable problems with the parts.

The future of mainstream medicine depends on willingness to look at and explore and research the deep significance of complementary medical practices and the natural wisdoms of the body they reveal. Ultimately patients will judge the entire biomedical enterprise by its ability to uncover methods that lead to improvements in curing, caring for, and comforting patients. Practical innovations are bound to emerge from both conventional and unconventional sources, and from their integration.

We can get even more specific about the reasons for making these statements. Our serious, costly, and painful health problems arise when our inherent whole-system mechanisms for defence and repair are compromised. One of the accomplishments of energy medicine and energy psychology is to slow or reverse the accumulation of subtle traumas, disorders, and imbalances that compromise our immune defences and repair systems. Structural and movement approaches stimulate the body's repair systems to repair themselves, restoring 'systemic cooperation', with many beneficial consequences. It is much easier to prevent than to cure, and prevention is definitely not a cure given in advance.

References

Athenstaedt, H., 1974. Pyroelectric and piezoelectric properties of vertebrates. Ann. N.Y. Acad. Sci. 238, 68–94.

Becker, R.O., 1972. Augmentation of regenerative healing in man. A possible alternative to prosthetic implantation. Clin. Orthop. Relat. Res. 83, 255–262.

Becker, R.O., Sheldon, G., 1985. The Body Electric. Electromagnetism and the Foundation of Life. William Morrow and Company, Inc., New York, NY.

Blechschmidt, E., 1973. Die pränatalen Organsysteme des Menschen. Hippokrates, Stuttgart.

Blechschmidt, E., Freeman, B., 2004. The Ontogenetic Basis of Human Anatomy: A Biodynamic Approach to Development from Conception to Birth. North Atlantic Books, Berkeley, CA.

Blechschmidt, E., Gasser, R.F., 2012. Biokinetics and Biodynamics of Human Differentiation: Principles and Applications. North Atlantic Books, Berkeley, CA.

Chamberlin, T.C., 1890. The method of multiple working hypotheses. With this method the dangers of parental affection for a favorite theory can be circumvented. Science 15, 92–97.

Chamberlin, T.C., 1965. The method of multiple working hypotheses. With this method the dangers of parental affection for a favorite theory can be circumvented. Science 148, 754–759.

Church, D., 2009. The Genie in Your Genes. Epigenetic Medicine and the New Biology of Intention, second ed. Energy Psychology Press, Santa Rosa, CA.

Doyle, A.C., 1890. The Sign of the Four. The Penguin Complete Sherlock Holmes (1981), Chap. 6, p. 111.

Feinstein, D., Eden, D., Craig, G., Bowen, M., 2005. The Promise of Energy Psychology: Revolutionary Tools for Dramatic Personal Change. Jeremy P. Tarcher/The Penguin Group, New York, NY.

Fuller, R.B., Marks, R., 1960. The Dymaxion World of Buckminster Fuller. Anchor Books, Garden City, NY, 1973 (originally published in 1960 by So. Ill. Univ. Press).

Ginzburg, V.B., 1996. Spiral Grain of the Universe: In Search of the Archimedes File. Univ Editions, Huntington, WV.

Gribbin, J., 1995. Schrödinger's Kittens and the Search for Reality. Little, Brown, Boston, MA.

Guimberteau, J.-C., 2012. Interior Architectures: DVD from Endo Vivo production, www.endovivo.com.

Gurdon, J.B., 1968. Transplanted nuclei and cell differentiation. The nucleus of a cell from a frog's intestine is transplanted into a frog's egg and gives rise to a normal frog. Such experiments aid the study of how genes are controlled during embryonic development. Sci. Am. 219 (6), 24–35.

Heartney, E., 2009. Kenneth Snelson: forces made visible. Hard Press Editions, Lenox, MA.

Ingber, D.E., 1998. The architecture of life. Sci. Am. 278 (1), 48–57.

Kevles, D., Hood, L. (Eds.), 1992. The Code of Codes: Scientific and Social Issues in the Human Genome Project. Harvard University Press, Cambridge, MA.

Kozyrev, N.A., 2005. Sources of Stellar Energy and the Theory of the Internal Constitution of Stars. Prog. Phys. 3, 61–99.

Lazarides, E., Revel, J.P., 1979. The molecular basis of cell movement. Sci. Am. 240, 100–113.

Lipton, B.H., 2008. The Biology of Belief: Unleashing the Power of Consciousness, Matter, & Miracles. Hay House, New York, NY.

Meyl, K., 2003. Scalar Waves. Indel GmbH.

Miller, S.L., 1953. Production of amino acids under possible primitive earth conditions. Science 117, 528.

Miller, S.L., Urey, H.C., 1959. Organic compound synthesis on the primitive earth. Science 130 (3370), 245–251.

Panov, V.F., Kichigin, V.I., Khaldeev, G.V., Klyuev, A.V., Testov, B.V., et al., 1997. Torsion Fields and Experiments. Journal of New Energy, Vol. 2 (3,4):29-39, Emerging Energy Marketing Firm, Inc., Salt Lake City, UT.

Rossi, E., 2002. The Psychobiology of Gene Expression. Norton, New York, NY, p. 237.

Schwab, E.D., Pienta, K.J., 1997. Modeling signal transduction in normal and cancer cells using complex adaptive systems. Med. Hypotheses 48, 111–123.

Schwartz, G.E., Russek, L.G., 2006. The Living Energy Universe: A Fundamental Discovery that Transforms Science and Medicine. Hampton Roads Publishing, Charlottesville, VA.

Sheldrake, R., 1995a. A New Science of Life. Park Street Press, Rochester, VT.

Sheldrake, R., 1995b. The Presence of the Past: Morphic Resonance and the Habits of Nature. Park Street Press, Rochester, VT.

Sheldrake, R., 2009. Morphic Resonance: The Nature of Formative Causation. Park Street Press, Rochester, VT.

Sheldrake, R., 2013. Science Set Free: 10 Paths to New Discovery. Deepak Chopra, Carlsbad, CA.

Sheldrake, R., McKenna, T., Abraham, R., Houston, J., 2001. Chaos, Creativity, and Cosmic Consciousness. Park Street Press, Rochester, VT.

Strohman, R.C., 1993. Ancient genomes, wise bodies, unhealthy people: limits of a genetic paradigm in biology and medicine. Perspect. Biol. Med. 37 (1), 112–145.

Swanson, C., 2011. Life Force, the Scientific Basis. Volume II of the Synchronized Universe Series. Poseidia Press, Tucson, AZ.

Szent-Györgyi, A., 1963. Lost in the Twentieth Century. Annu. Rev. Biochem. 32, 1–14.

Szent-Györgyi, A., 1974. Drive in living matter to perfect itself. Synthesis I, 14–26.

Veltheim, J., Oschman, J.L., 2013. The biophysical mind. PaRama LLC, Sarasota, FL.

Watson, J.D., 1970. Molecular Biology of the Gene, second ed. W.A. Benjamin, Inc., New York, NY.

Weil, A., 1995. Spontaneous Healing. How to Discover and Enhance Your Body's Natural Ability to Maintain and Heal Itself. Alfred A. Knopf, New York, NY.

Weiss, P.A., 1973. In: The system of nature and the nature of systems: Empirical holism and practical reductionism harmonized. Conference on Man Centered Physiological Science and Medicine, Herdecke, Germany September 24-28. A New Image of Man in Medicine, vol. I.

Wilson, E.O., 1994. Naturalist. Island Press/Shearwater Books, Washington, DC.

CHAPTER 14

Acupuncture, Acupressure, Shiatsu, and Related Therapies

Chapter Summary

After decades of neglect, modern medical researchers and other academic scientists have begun serious and very revealing studies of the acupuncture meridian systems and points and the ways they relate to various structures, functions, and pathophysiologies. A growing number of physicians are adding acupuncture to their clinical practices. Enough new work has been done that a thorough review would fill a book much larger than this one. This chapter presents some highlights and directs the interested reader to some sources of recent information. The current status of acupuncture research will emerge from a look at the work of the following investigators and their colleagues: Helene Langevin, Steven and Donna Finando, Stanley Rosenberg, Joie P. Jones, and Kwang-Sup Soh (Figure 14.1).

An understanding of acupuncture theory and practice has become a major topic for a wide range of therapeutic approaches far beyond acupuncture (e.g., Micozzi, 2010) and is also important for the growing number of people who wish to use the methods on themselves and others to maintain health and vitality. Centuries of clinical experience have shown that acupuncture points, or acupoints, can be stimulated by needling, herbs, pressure, light (including laser light), or heat to resolve clinical problems. For a long time, there appeared to be no anatomical basis for meridians, and this made acupuncture an easy target for skeptics. Others tried to fit the meridians with known structures such as nerves, muscles, or lymphatic vessels. This situation has changed dramatically. Acupuncture research is pointing toward the connective tissue and fascia as the location of the meridians. The research of Joie P. Jones and colleagues, using sophisticated techniques including functional magnetic resonance imaging (fMRI) and quantitative ultrasonic imaging, has developed three-dimensional images of acupoints. They have also followed the day-to-day migrations of the points and shown how points rotate when needled. This research brings acupuncture into important relationships with virtually all other forms of energy medicine as well as with the various manual therapies. The concepts of the living matrix and the ground regulation system, discussed in Chapters 10 and 11, provide a possible explanation of the systemic effects of Oriental medicine.

Research in Asia has revealed a new and novel circulatory system that also seems to have correspondences with the acupuncture meridians. For many years this was known as the Bonghan system (BHS), named after the North Korean surgeon who discovered it in 1963. In 2010, a group of Korean scholars chose, with good reasons, to give the BHS a new name, the primo vascular system (PVS). A key breakthrough was the discovery of a specific dye, trypan blue, which selectively stains this system, thereby enabling detailed study of its anatomy, histology, physiology, and roles in pathophysiology. The fluid from the ducts has also been analyzed. The discovery of this system is opening up new areas of medical research.

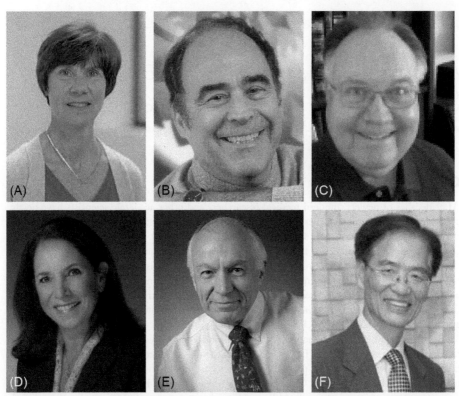

Figure 14.1 (A) Dr. Helene Langevin, Department of Neurology, University of Vermont School of Medicine. Currently Director of the Osher Center for Integrative Medicine at Harvard Medical School and Brigham and Women's Hospital, Boston, MA. (B) Stanley Rosenberg, Stanley Rosenberg Institute, Copenhagen, Denmark. (C) Dr. Joie Pierce Jones (1941–2013), formerly Professor of Radiological Sciences at UC Irvine. (D, E) Donna Finando, M.S. L.Ac., L.M.T, and Steve Finando, Ph.D., L.Ac., practicing acupuncturists at Heights Healthcare, Roslyn Heights, NY. (F) Dr. Kwang-Sup Soh, Seoul National University, Korea, and Editor-in-Chief, *Journal of Acupuncture & Meridian Studies*.

Introduction

Selected Recent Texts on Acupuncture Research

Energy Medicine East and West: A Natural History of Qi (Mayor and Micozzi, 2011)
  Acupuncture and the Chakra Energy System: Treating the Cause of Disease (Cross, 2008)
  Electroacupuncture: A Practical Manual and Resource (Mayor, 2006)
  Quantum Acupuncture (Henry, 2011)
  Quantum Shiatsu (Stefanani, 2011)
  Acupuncture: Theories and Evidence (Hong, 2013)
Acupuncture Research: Strategies for Establishing an Evidence Base (MacPherson, Hammerschlag, Lewith and Schnyer, 2007)

Recent texts have described advances in acupuncture research (see box). *The Journal of Alternative and Complementary Medicine*, the *Journal of Bodywork and Movement Therapies*, and the various societies related to acupuncture and Oriental medicine have articles on aspects of acupuncture. A variety of theories on the identity of the meridians have been proposed. Here are a few:

- An early model by Walthard and Tchicaloff (1971) was based on the fact that the skin over a muscle motor point has low resistance to electrical stimulation. Therefore, the acupuncture points might correspond to the relatively fixed patterns of motor lines.
- Yang (2008a,b) suggested that the traditional acupuncture meridians are zones in loose connective tissue containing rich intercellular fluid, enabling them to be passages with lower resistance for diffusion of meridian-signal carriers, that these signal carriers ought to be histamine, and that the meridian biological signal amplifier ought to be mast cells.
- Longhurst (2010) suggested a 'neural hypothesis', in which the clinical influence of acupuncture is transmitted primarily through stimulation of sensory nerves that provide signals to the brain, which processes this information and then causes clinical changes associated with treatment.
- Robert O. Becker suggested that the system of acupuncture points and meridians are solid state structures that serve as input channels for the global direct current perineural system described in Chapters 9 and 11 and Figure 11.13. He regarded the meridians as electrical transmission lines (Reichmanis et al., 1975).
- The fascia acupuncture hypothesis described by Finando and Finando (2011, 2012) and others.
- The Bonghan system (BHS) recently renamed the primo vascular system or PVS.
- The Bonghan-fascia model (Lee and Soh, 2009) revealed by vital staining with Trypan blue, which showed the Bonghan networks within and from the fascial system.

Meridians and Fascia

Two thoughtful essays by Finando and Finando (2011, 2012) present a number of important issues related to acupuncture, meridians, and research. The Finando report is of interest to acupuncturists and to others involved in fascial manipulation. It has implications for osteopaths and chiropractors for whom somato-visceral and viscero-somatic reflexes are important. The following summarizes some of their discussion, along with the evidence supporting the points they raise. The Finandos describe correspondences between the location of meridians and particular lines of fascia (Figure 14.2).

The Finandos' call for a return to the traditional palpation techniques that were eliminated from the trainings to standardize and streamline acupuncture teaching and recent research on point location with ultrasound supports this suggestion. They point out that 'Traditional Chinese Medicine' (TCM) as it is currently referred to by many practitioners and the lay public, and that is the most commonly used acupuncture practice among Western practitioners, represents an acupuncture that is primarily the result of political, social, and economic influences. It is a specific product of the Cultural Revolution rather than the ancient traditions of classical Chinese medicine. Birch and Felt (1999) refer to TCM as 'modern' acupuncture because it is a specific creation of the People's Republic of China, beginning sometime around 1950. TCM was a development of a new political structure that faced a major health crisis and needed healthcare for a massive population. TCM had to be amenable to large classroom training, rather than by traditional apprenticeship, since there was a need for rapid, uniform training. Careful training in palpation was virtually eliminated, diagnoses were connected to Western-defined diseases, and textbooks began to provide treatments for arthritis, gastritis, and other such Western-defined pathologies (Finando and Finando, 2012).

TCM is the most commonly employed approach in acupuncture clinical research. Most of what is known scientifically about the clinical effects of acupuncture is based upon study of TCM, rather than the palpation approaches that are still used by a minority of practitioners. TCM marks a significant movement away from an acupuncture that was based upon careful attention to the body toward the use of a more formulaic approach with charted acupuncture points. 'It has replaced attention to the "terrain" with a prescribed use of the "map"' (Finando and Finando, 2012).

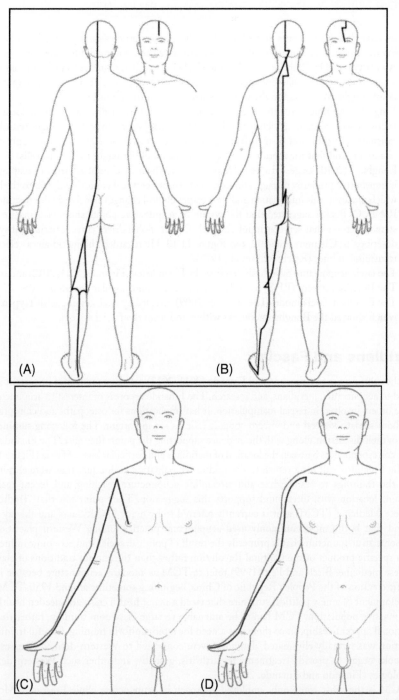

Figure 14.2 Correspondences between the location of meridians and particular lines of fascia based on Finando and Finando (2011, 2012). Left: Comparison of superficial back line (A) and Bladder channel (B). Right: Comparison of deep front arm line (C) and Lung channel (D). *((A) and (C) Redrawn from Myers, T., 2001. Anatomy Trains: Myofascial Meridians for Manual and Movement Therapists. Churchill Livingstone, London; (B) & (D) Redrawn from Finando, S., Finando, D., 2011. Fascia and the mechanism of acupuncture. J. Bodyw. Mov. Ther. 15, 168–176 and Finando, S., Finando, D., 2012. Qi, acupuncture and the fascia: a reconsideration of the fundamental principles of acupuncture. J. Altern. Complement. Med. 18 (9), 880–886.)*

Research supporting a major role of fascia in acupuncture has been done by the investigators and clinicians shown in Figure 14.1.

The Finando (fascia) hypothesis is summarized by three ideas (see box).

The (Fascia) Hypothesis: Summarized by Three Ideas

1. Needle manipulation of the superficial fascia stimulates activity within the fascia.
2. There is extensive anatomical correlation between the classical locations of the acupuncture channels and points with fascial planes and septa.
3. Recent fascia research has demonstrated numerous similarities between the functions of acupuncture channels and the functions of the fascia.

1. Needle manipulation of the superficial fascia stimulates activity within the fascia.

The effects of needle manipulation on superficial fascia were demonstrated by Langevin et al. (2001b). Specifically, acupuncturists commonly notice that the tissue seems to tighten around an inserted needle, particularly when the needle is twisted. This is called 'needle grasp'. Moreover, when the therapist pulls out the needle, it feels like it is stuck, and the skin is lifted. This is called 'tenting' (Langevin et al., 2001a,b). A measurable force is required to pull the needle out. Langevin and colleagues actually measured the force required to pull needles out. They compared unidirectional needle twisting (UNI) with bidirectional twisting (BI) and no twisting (NO), and they also compared acupuncture points with non-points. They found 167% and 52% increases in mean pullout force with UNI and BI, respectively, compared with NO ($P<0.001$). Pullout force was on average 18% greater at acupuncture points than at control points ($P<0.001$). Needle grasp is therefore a measurable biomechanical phenomenon associated with acupuncture needle manipulation and also with acupoints compared to non-points.

Langevin and colleagues also observed that when a needle is rotated, collagen fibres stick to it and become wrapped around it. If the needle is removed and examined under the microscope, strands of collagen are still attached to it. Needle rotation creates tension in the fascial layer that causes fibroblast cells to become deformed. This deformation is thought to trigger metabolic changes in the cells (Chen et al., 1997; Chicurel et al., 1998; Chiquet et al., 2003). Ultrasonic imaging shows spiral deformation, a vortex, in the tissue during needling with rotation. Histology of the same tissue shows the tensional pattern or vortex created by needle rotation.

Julias Edgar Buettner and Schreiber (2008) obtained similar results using collagen gels *in vitro* (Figure 14.3A). The vortical pattern in the gel produced by needle rotation was monitored by cross-polarized optics, which showed the development of birefringence (Figure 14.3B).

    2. There is extensive anatomical correlation between the classical locations of the acupuncture channels and points with fascial planes and septa.

Langevin and Yandow (2002) explored the relationship between acupuncture points and meridians and connective tissue planes (Figure 14.4). The illustration shows ultrasound imaging of acupuncture (AP) and control (CP) points. Ultrasound imaging revealed a connective tissue intramuscular cleavage plane at acupuncture points but not at control points. (Langevin and Yandow, 2002).

These imaging studies were confirmed by Stanley Rosenberg, on the basis of palpation, as shown in the box.

The acupoints feel like depressions that enable me to contact several fascial layers at once. It feels like putting your finger into a cone. Initially there is more tension in the tissue when you try to twist in one direction compared to the opposite direction. After the tissue has released, the resistance to twisting is the same in both directions.

Stanley Rosenberg, Copenhagen

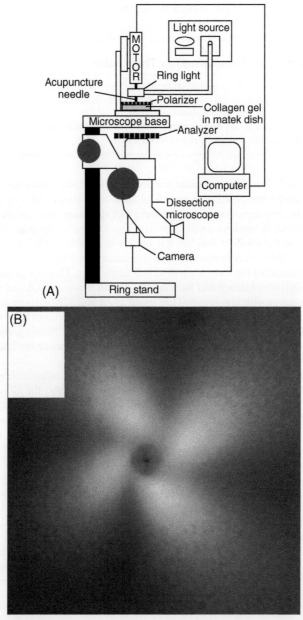

Figure 14.3 (A) Apparatus used to insert and rotate an acupuncture needle in a collagen gel. (B) Polarized light microscope image of a collagen gel showing a characteristic 'four-leaf clover' pattern of birefringence that increases in size as the gel becomes increasingly aligned due to winding around the needle. *(Julias M, Edgar LT, Buettner HM, et al: An in vitro assay of collagen fiber alignment by acupuncture needle rotation, Biomed Eng Online 2008 July 7;7:19.)*

Again, Finando and Finando (2011) illustrated the correspondences between the fascial planes as described by Myers (2001) and specific meridians (the Bladder channel and the Lung channel, Figure 14.2).

3. Recent fascia research has demonstrated numerous similarities between the functions of acupuncture channels and the functions of the fascia.

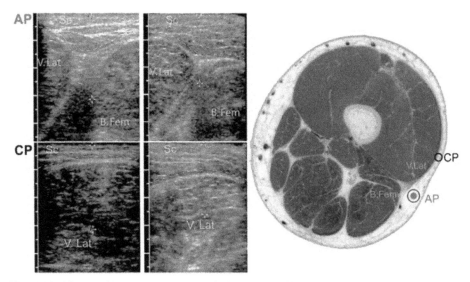

Figure 14.4 Ultrasound imaging of acupuncture (AP) and control (CP) points. Acupuncture point GB32 was located by palpation in two normal human volunteers, as well as a control point located 3 cm away from the acupuncture point. After marking both points with a skin marker, ultrasound imaging was performed with an Acuson ultrasound machine equipped with a 7 MHz linear probe. A visible connective tissue intramuscular cleavage plane can be seen at acupuncture points but not at control points. V. Lat, vastus lateralis; B. Fem, biceps femoris; Sc, subcutaneous tissue *(From Langevin HM, Yandow JA: Relationship of acupuncture points and meridians to connective tissue planes, Anat Rec 2002 Dec 15; 269(6):257–265).*

The fascia and extracellular matrix (ECM) are the environment of every cell, and therefore affect immune function, metabolism, circulation, organ function, and virtually every aspect of human physiology.

The extracellular matrix (ECM) is the environment that is most immediate to the human cell. Its functions include nutrient transfer, nerve signal transduction, regulation of intercellular communication, and transmission of mechanical stresses exerted on the cytoskeleton. Oschman (2007) states: 'Every function and every process of the living body involves the matrix in one way or the other. The reason for this is that every cell in the body is nourished via the matrix, and all waste products of cellular metabolism likewise pass through the ground substance, which is the actual milieu. The matrix is also the terrain in which all immune responses and tissue repair processes take place.' The ECM is a fundamental component of the fascia.

FINANDO AND FINANDO (2012)

Additional work by Langevin et al. (2004) using a combination of histochemistry, immunohistochemistry, confocal scanning laser microscopy (confocal microscopy), and electron microscopy revealed that fibroblasts in subcutaneous and interstitial connective tissues form a reticular web throughout the tissue (Figures 14.5 and 14.6). Connexin 43 immunoreactivity was present at apparent points of cell-to-cell contact. It appears that soft tissue fibroblasts form an extensively interconnected cellular network extending throughout the skin (Figure 14.6B). When you touch the skin in one place, you are, in a sense, touching the whole skin. A similar reticulum occurs in bone (Figure 14.6C).

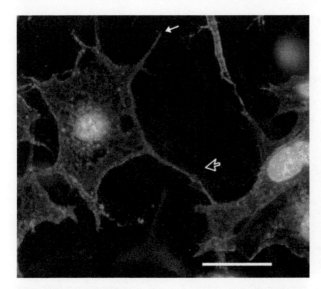

Figure 14.5 Fibroblasts in subcutaneous and interstitial connective tissues form a reticular web throughout the tissue. Connexin 43 immunoreactivity was present at apparent points of cell-to-cell contact (arrows). *(From Langevin, H.M., Cornbrooks, C.J., Taatjes, D.J., 2004. Fibroblasts form a body-wide cellular network, Histochem Cell Biol July 122 (1), 7–15.)*

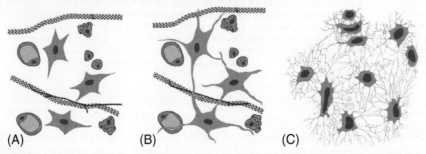

(A)   (B)   (C)

Figure 14.6 (A) Conventional view of the distribution of fibroblasts scattered through loose connective tissue. (B) Revised view with fibroblasts forming a reticular web, possibly extending throughout the tissue. (C) Comparable arrangement of osteoblasts in bone. This is called a syncytium.

Medical Imaging Approaches of Joie P. Jones and Colleagues

Joie P. Jones and his colleagues (Cho et al., 1998) used medical imaging techniques such as functional magnetic resonance imaging (fMRI) and quantitative ultrasonic microscopy to study signal transmission through the meridians and to determine the microscopic structure of the points. Their early work demonstrated that needling specific acupoints on the foot along the Urinary Bladder meridian increases blood flow in certain parts of the visual cortex. These are the same areas that are activated by flashes of light into the eyes. When nearby non-acupuncture points were needled, no such effects were obtained. The fact that these responses were obtained at specific acupoints along a specific meridian, and not nearby, gave support to the meridian concept. Moreover, the points stimulated along the Urinary Bladder meridian were those described in ancient acupuncture texts for treatment of eye disorders. A similar relationship was confirmed between auditory-related acupoints and the auditory cortex (Cho et al., 2000).

Next, Jones (1999) stimulated the same vision-related acupoint (Bladder 67, located on the lateral side of the small toe about 3 mm proximal to the corner of the nail; Figure 14.7) with

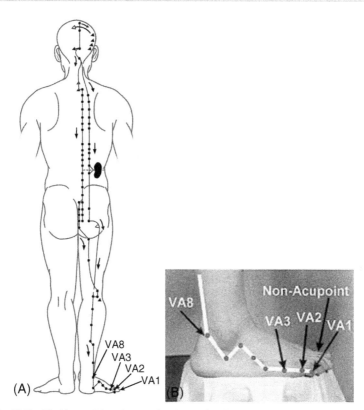

Figure 14.7 (A) The Bladder meridian showing the vision-related acupoints VA1, VA2, VA3, and VA8. These points are known in the oriental acupuncture literature as BL-67 (VA1), BL-66 (VA2, BL-65 (VA3), and BL-60 (VA8), respectively. (B) Location of the vision-related points on the foot.

pulses of ultrasound and monitored the brain activity with fMRI. For a wide range of ultrasound parameters, the fMRI effects on the occipital lobes were indistinguishable from those produced by conventional acupuncture needles. Ultrasonic stimulation of an acupoint required higher energy levels than those used for conventional ultrasonic imaging. Again, there was a close correlation between direct stimulation of the eye using light and stimulation of the vision-related acupoint using either a needle or pulses of ultrasonic energy (Figure 14.8).

The use of fMRI for characterizing brain responses to acupuncture has become widespread, to the point that a literature review has been performed on 779 papers, from the earliest until September 2009. This was literature in English, Chinese, Korean, and Japanese databases. Thirty-four of these papers were eligible for meta-analysis, which showed that acupuncture can modulate the activity within specific brain areas, including somatosensory cortices, the limbic system, basal ganglia, the brain stem, and the cerebellum (Huang et al., 2012).

The next step was to obtain actual images of the acupoints. Conventional ultrasonic imaging used to determine the best placement of the acupuncture needle did not reveal any details of point structure. However, after some experimentation, a method was developed that produced a detailed image. Technical aspects are introduced in the box. A further detailed presentation of the technical aspects was published by Jones et al. (2012). Acupoints correspond to regions of enhanced elasticity (increased ultrasonic attenuation). A challenge was overcoming perhaps the most well-known issue in acoustics: reflection of a plane acoustical wave from a planar boundary. Earlier work had concluded that reflection from a discontinuity in absorption could not occur

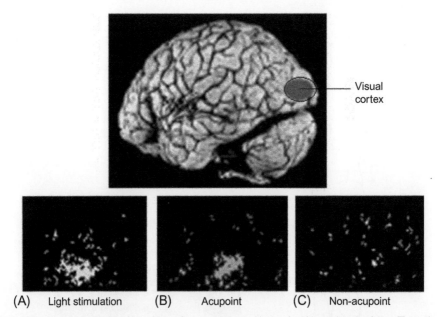

(A)   Light stimulation   (B)   Acupoint   (C)   Non-acupoint

Figure 14.8 Non-acupoint stimulation (control) in comparison with visual and acupoint stimulation. The activation maps of the visual cortex (the shaded area in upper figure) resulting from visual stimulation of the eye (A), acupuncture stimulation at VA1 (B), and non-acupoint stimulation (C), respectively (volunteer 1).

(Linsay, 1960). However, Jones and his colleagues determined that there was an error in Linsay's calculations, and Nolan (1988) reported the analysis in a thesis.

A more detailed or higher resolution ultrasound image requires a higher frequency scanner. Since these were not available, Jones and colleagues switched to a simple pulse-echo data acquisition system using a 50 MHz hand-held transducer. Holding the small (1 mm diameter) transducer on the surface of the skin, a short (30 ns) ultrasound pulse was transmitted into the tissue. The reflected signal, known as an A-mode trace, was recorded and stored in a standard PC. Power levels were well below those required to stimulate the point. The transducer could be moved step by step along a rectangular grid, leading to a series of A-lines. The points proved to be local regions of enhanced attenuation and elasticity. Further technical details are available from Jones and Bae (2004) and Jones et al. (2011).

The technical achievement of imaging the acupoints with ultrasound led to the following discoveries:

- Even in the same person, a given acupoint changed in size, shape, and location over time (Figure 14.9). This led to the realization that acupuncturists who follow the textbook formulas for locating points may mislocate the points about 50% of the time. Ultrasonic localization of acupoints could be used to ensure that the stimulation was applied at the correct location, with the correct amplitude, for the desired effect, all of which would be unknown to the patient. These discoveries reinforce the suggestion of Finando and Finando that acupuncture training include the traditional palpation techniques that were eliminated from the teachings to standardize and streamline acupuncture education.
- Standard acupuncture texts (e.g., Ellis et al., 1991) suggest that an acupoint should be located precisely in relation to anatomical landmarks. However, in the real world, the discerning practitioner typically searches for the acupoint around the standard location, assuming that

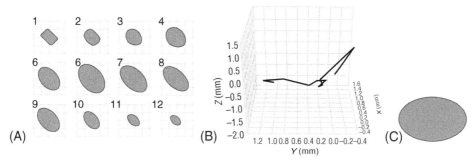

Figure 14.9 (A) Changes in size and shape of acupoint BL-67 over a 12-day period. (B) Changes in relative locations of the center of acupoint BL-67 over a 12-day period. (C) Size of acupoint followed in (B).

the location may be different in each person and may change in time (Miyawaki, 1994). The studies of Jones and colleagues support this approach, as advocated by Finando and Finando.

■ Comparing the point location data with textbook anatomical cross-sections shows that all of the points imaged in the Jones et al. (2004) study were located within the connective tissue. This finding agrees with the observations of Langevin and Yandow described above, and with the proposal of the Finandos that the meridians are in the fascia.

■ Advances in ultrasonic microscopy by Jones and colleagues enabled more detailed images of the acupoints (Figure 14.10). The point appears to have a polyhedral shape.

■ In an ingenious experiment, Jones was able to observe the acupoint while needling it. Remarkably, the points rotate when they are needled. And the top half rotates in the opposite direction compared to the lower half. An interpretation is that the two halves pull on different fascial planes (Figure 14.11).

■ In another ingenious experiment, Jones was able to observe the first five points along the Bladder meridian. The points rotated in sequence, with a few seconds delay between the rotation of each point (Figure 14.12).

■ Using an ultrasonic pulse to stimulate the acupoint enabled Jones to make precise measurements of the time between stimulation and nerve firing in the occipital cortex. Three different velocities were observed. One was extremely fast, on the order of 7 µs, making it the fastest biological process ever measured. The time delay was within the limit of resolution of the fMRI technique, meaning that it is impossible to know how fast it was. It could have been speed of light or instantaneous. More research on this fascinating topic is needed (Figure 14.12).

The BHS, Renamed the PVS

Research in Asia has revealed a new and novel circulatory system thought to correspond to the acupuncture meridians. For many years this was known as the BHS, Bonghan corpuscles, or Bonghan ducts, named after the North Korean surgeon, Bong Han Kim, who discovered it (Kim, 1963). In 2010, a group of scholars chose, with good reasons, to give the BHS a new name, the primo vascular system (PVS).

There was great interest in this system for nearly 40 years, but it was impossible to confirm its existence because Bong Han Kim never described his methods. A prominent Soviet cytologist condemned it (without evidence) as a fraud (Alexandrov, 1993). A real breakthrough took place with the discovery of a BHS-specific dye, trypan blue (Lee et al., 2009) (Figure 14.13). With this technique, the BHS in adipose tissue became traceable, and the BHS was discovered on the fascia surrounding tumors.

Modern research on the PVS is being done by about 10 groups in Korea and various others around the world. For example, a collaboration between Korean investigators and Bulgarian

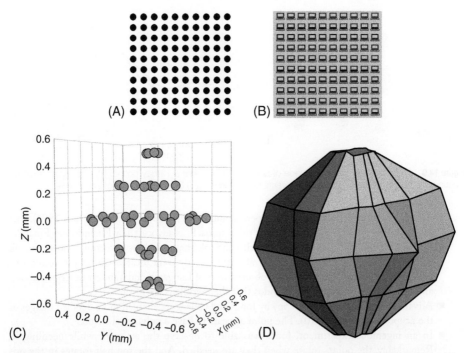

Figure 14.10 (A) Jones and colleagues assembled a 10 × 10 array of transducers, each connected to a 5 GB laptop computer (B). This enabled them to record the three-dimensional shape of BL-67 (C). The transducer operated at 50 MHz. The reflected A-line trace was digitized at 200 Hz. A Two-dimensional grid of A-lines was recorded over the acupoint. Attenuation was calculated along each A-line. (D) Reconstructed attenuation image of an acupoint.

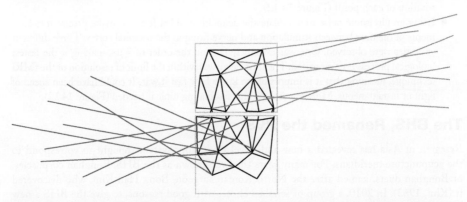

Figure 14.11 Ultrasonic imaging showed that the point (BL-67) rotates during needle insertion. Also, the upper half of the point rotates in the opposite direction to the lower half. One interpretation is that the two halves of the point are connected to different levels or planes in the fascia (see Figure 14.4) and the twisting puts tension on both fascial planes.

scientists resulted in the schemes shown in Figure 14.3 (Stefanov et al., 2013). Many superb illustrations of the system have been published in the *Journal of Acupuncture and Meridian Studies* (JAMS) that was launched in 2008 and published bimonthly since then. There is now little doubt of the existence of this system, and its further study will undoubtedly be very rewarding for every aspect of biomedicine.

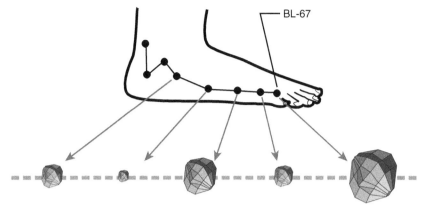

Figure 14.12 Ultrasonic microscopy showed that the points along the Bladder meridian rotated in sequence, with a few seconds delay between each point.

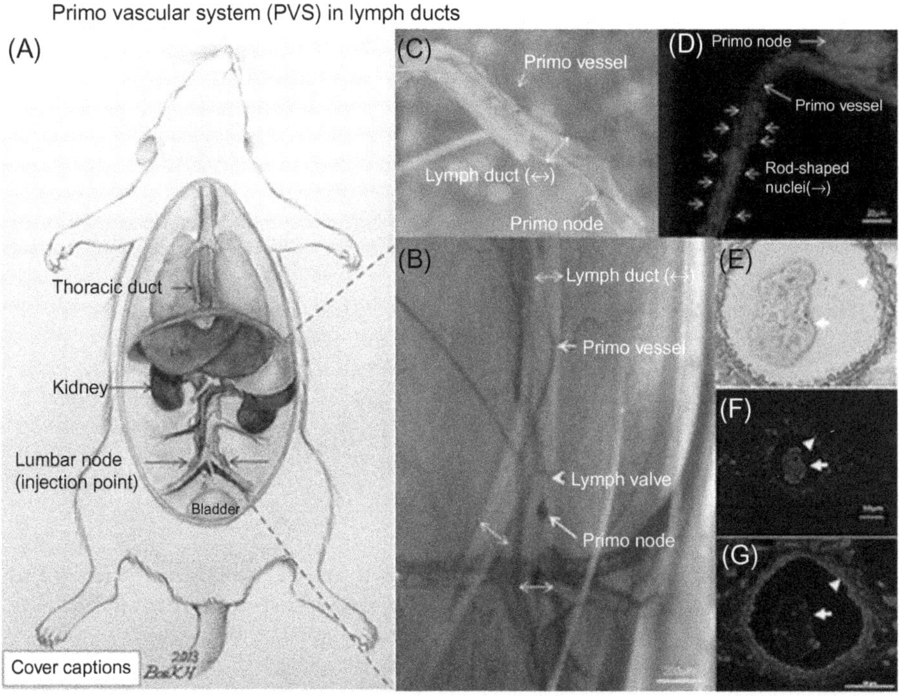

Primo vascular system (PVS) in lymph ducts

Figure 14.13 (A) The thoracic duct and the lymph ducts (both labelled) around the vena cava in the abdomen of a rat. (B) Stereomicroscopic image of the lymph ducts in the area of (A) indicated by dotted lines. The dark thread-like structures inside the lymph ducts are primo vessels, which become blue by absorbing Alcian blue, which was injected into the lumbar lymph node. Note the branching of the primo vessel at the branching of the lymph duct. The primo node is the corpuscle-like body dangling from the primo vessel. (C) Isolated primo vessel in a lymph duct on a slide. (D) Confocal laser scanning microscope image of DAPI-stained rod shaped nuclei of the endothelial cells in a primo vessel. (DAPI is a fluorescent stain). The nuclei are aligned along the primo vessel's direction. Notice that the primo node is packed with other types of nuclei. (E) Cross-section of a primo node (arrow) in a lymph vessel (arrow head). Gordon and Sweet's silver staining shows the argyrophil fibres in the primo node. (F) EMP-3 immunohistochemical stained image of a cross-section showing the epithelial cells. (G) Dil-stained cross-section. The boundary of the primo node (arrow) shows a positive signal. The primo node is covered with a membrane, which shows that it is not an aggregate of tissue debris or cells. Dil is a lipophilic membrane stain.

Some modern physiologists have put forward a 'neural hypothesis'. They suggest that the clinical influence of acupuncture is transmitted primarily through stimulation of sensory nerves that provide signals to the brain, which processes this information and then causes clinical changes associated with treatment. This is natural, given the tendency of modern biomedicine to attribute just about everything to the nervous system. That the PVS is different from nerves is apparent from the many quality studies done in Korea. Strengthening the foundations of acupuncture meridian theory are specific relationships between acupoints and target organs as demonstrated by the fact that stimulating different acupoints on the body surface can help deal with many different diseases, including visceral issues. Connections between acupoints at the body surface and visceral functions have been elaborated by thousands of years of clinical experience and reinforced recently through extensive research.

Quantum Shiatsu

Patrizia Stefanini is a shiatsu practitioner and quantum physicist. She has looked at her clinical practice through the lens of quantum mechanics, following a direction given to her by her teacher, Pauline Sasaki, who studied closely with Shitzuto Masunaga. Stefanini finds that acupuncture points and meridians, like electrons, are not precisely localized as they are described in texts – they have variable nature and depth. Moreover, their information content is not always related to the present condition of the individual. The movement of meridians agrees with the results of Joie Jones, who found that the location of points changes from day to day (Figure 14.9). Moreover, Stefanini developed an appreciation for the way the wave/particle or energy/matter paradoxes are reflected in her work.

She cites her teachers from the distinguished Istituto Nazionale di Fisica Nucleare (INFN) in Milano (Del Giudice et al., 2009):

> In living systems, water takes part in the dynamics of life, not only because it accounts for 99% of all the biomolecules but also because it provides energy to living matter. Water has the ability to achieve an extended form of organization and provide an ensemble of different Coherence Domains which are phase locked, thus maximizing their ability to 'look for' energy from the environment. This 'coherence of coherences' of 'biological water' in living systems corresponds to a sort of higher organization. An efficient mechanism of energy transformation from Coherence Domains to biomolecules in living matter guarantees the transfer of biochemical energy necessary for the maintenance of life cycles.

This quote clarifies the concepts raised in Chapters 10 and 11 of this book. Stefanini also took inspiration from the work of Albert Szent-Györgyi, who wrote in 1957 that the inability of biologists to define animate versus inanimate matter depends on their neglect of the two most important ingredients of living matter: water and electromagnetic fields (and in particular the electromagnetic properties of water). He pointed out that excitation of the electron clouds of the biomolecule and their consequent chemical activation depend on the ordered, quasi-crystalline structure of layers of water, close to the cellular membranes and some hundreds of water molecules thick. The ordered structure of this 'interfacial' water was in turn the consequence of an electromagnetic field that was somehow trapped in the water layers.

We now know from the work of Gerald Pollack (Figure 14.14B) and Mae-Wan Ho that Szent-Györgyi's picture of ordered interfacial water (Figure 14.14A) and fields trapped in the water layers was accurate. Moreover, Pollack demonstrated how fields can accumulate in water layers (Figure 14.14C). These layers adjacent to hydrophilic surfaces form solute 'exclusion zones' as shown in Figure 14.13A.

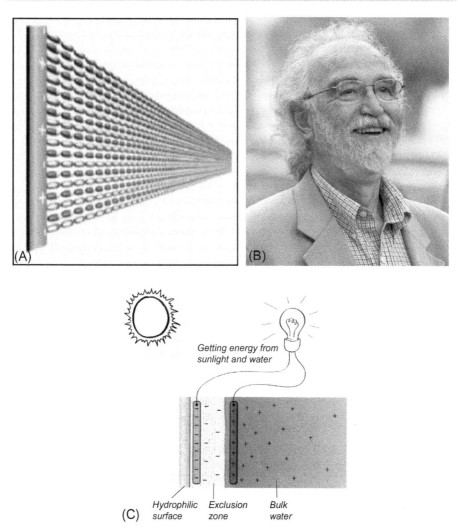

Figure 14.14 (A) The 'exclusion zone' or 'EZ water' at a hydrophilic (water-loving) surface such as a cell membrane or a molecule. (B) Gerald Pollack and his colleagues at the University of Washington in Seattle have made a series of remarkable discoveries about the structure and behaviour of water, described in his book, The Fourth phase of Water (2013) published by Ebner and Sons Publishers, Seattle, WA. One discovery, shown in (C), is that sunlight creates a charge separation between the EZ zone and the bulk phase away from the surface.

The X-Signal System of Manaka

A brilliant overview of biological information theory as it applies to acupuncture has been provided by a leading scientist/acupuncturist, Yoshio Manaka (Manaka et al., 1995). The work has significance for all therapeutic approaches. Manaka began to integrate modern scientific research and classical East Asian or Oriental medical theory with a system he refers to as the X-signal system. As a concept, the X-signal system acknowledges that there are unknown aspects of energy and information flow. (The term 'X' is often used in mathematics and physics to represent an unknown quantity. Solving an equation enables one to determine the actual value of the 'X' or unknown.)

In Manaka's X-signal system there are many unknown communication circuits and informational units. A formal mathematical representation of these unknowns is:

$$X_1, X_2, X_3, X_4, \ldots X_n$$

Manaka conceptualized the X-signal system to represent a 'primitive' regulatory system that is different from the classical nervous and hormonal systems. (See also Chapter 9.)

The X-signal system is primitive in the sense that it arose in evolution long before the nervous system. It is present in single-celled animals, which do not have nerves *per se*, but nonetheless react to external stimuli in order to avoid harm and to attract them to nourishment (Figure 12.5).

Manaka demonstrated that the X-signal system is separate from the nervous system by describing the various treatments used in Oriental medicine that profoundly affect the body without having any effect on the nervous system.

While ancient in terms of evolution, in comparison to the nervous/hormonal systems, the X-signal system is extremely important and potent in the human body because it regulates the communications and cellular migrations involved in defence against disease and wound healing.

In his writings, Manaka presented the X-signal system as a system that is well known from the clinical perspective of Oriental medicine, but that has no scientific basis. However, it is becoming more and more apparent that the energy systems in the living body being documented in this book are all components of Manaka's X-signal system. The energy fields of the body, the perineural system, and the living matrix are some of the substrates through which the X-signal system exerts its effects on cells and tissues. The living matrix, the energy fields, the acupuncture meridians, and the various biocircuits that energy therapists interact with during their therapy sessions are all related and are all components of Manaka's system.

Relation to Acupuncture

How does all of this fit with the theory of acupuncture? We can now show where the individual cell fits into the meridian scheme that is the basis of acupuncture (Figure 14.15). The cytoskeleton – which some biologists are now referring to as the nervous system of the cell – can be fitted into the scheme. The meridian system, which acupuncture theory visualizes as branching into every part of the organism, can be extended into the interiors of every cell in the body and even into the nuclei that contain the genetic material. The meridians are simply the main channels or transmission lines in the continuous molecular fabric of the body.

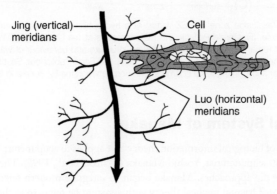

Figure 14.15   A vertical meridian or channel and its horizontal branches, which are envisioned to extend into every part of the body, including the surfaces and interiors of every organ, and even into the individual cells and organelles. *(Meridian drawing taken from Matsumoto and Birch (1988), used by kind permission of S. Birch and Paradigm Publications, Brookline, MA.)*

The molecular web is more than a mechanical anatomical structure. It is a continuous vibratory network. As such, it presents possibilities of profound biological and clinical significance.

A vertical meridian or channel, and its horizontal branches are envisioned to extend into every part of the body, including the surfaces and interiors of every organ, and even into the individual cells and organelles (Figure 14.15).

Hypothesis

Every part of the body, including all of the molecules so thoroughly studied by modern science as well as the acupuncture meridians of traditional East Asian or Oriental medicine, form a continuously interconnected semiconductor electronic network. Each component of the organism, even the smallest part, is immersed in, and generates, a constant stream of vibratory information. This is information about all of the activities taking place everywhere in the body.

Complete health corresponds to total interconnection. Accumulated physical and/or emotional traumas impair the connections (Oschman and Oschman, 1995). When this happens, the body's defence and repair systems become impaired, and disease has a chance to take hold. Acupuncture and other energy therapies restore and balance the vibratory circuitry, with obvious and profound benefits. The body's defence and repair systems are able to repair themselves.

Many individuals, both scientists and therapists, have contributed valuable insights to this emerging picture of how the body functions in health and disease. Phenomena that previously seemed disconnected and unrelated are now complementing one another, giving us a more complete understanding than we could have obtained by any single approach.

References

Alexandrov, V.Y., 1993. The Difficult Years of Soviet Biology: Contemporary Notes. Science, St. Petersburg. Available at: http://vivovoco.rsl.ru/VV/BOOKS/ALEXANDROV/CONTENT.HTM; 1993 (accessed 6.05.13) (in Russian).

Birch, S., Felt, R., 1999. Understanding Acupuncture. Churchill Livingstone, London.

Chen, C.S., Mrksich, M., Huang, S., Whitesides, G.M., Ingber, D.E., 1997. Geometric control of cell life and death. Science 276, 1425–1428.

Chicurel, M.E., Singer, R.H., Meyer, C.J., Ingber, D.E., 1998. Integrin binding and mechanical tension induce movement of mRNA and ribosomes to focal adhesions. Nature 392, 730–733.

Chiquet, M., Renedo, A.S., Huber, F., Fluck, M., 2003. How do fibroblasts translate mechanical signals into changes in extracellular matrix production? Matrix Biol. 22, 73–80.

Cho, Z.H., Chung, S.C., Jones, J.P., Park, J.B., Park, H.J., Lee, H.J., Wong, E.K., Min, B.I., 1998. New findings of the correlation between acupoints and corresponding brain cortices using functional MRI. Proc. Natl. Acad. Sci. U.S.A. 95, 2670–2673.

Cho, Z.H., Na, C.S., Wong, E.K., Lee, S.H., Hong, I.K., 2000. Investigation of acupuncture using brain functional magnetic resonance imaging. In: Lischer, G., Cho, Z.H. (Eds.), Computer Controlled Acupuncture. Pabst Science Publishers, Lengerich, Germany, pp. 45–64.

Cross, J.R., 2008. Acupuncture and the Chakra Energy System: Treating the Cause of Disease. North Atlantic Books, Berkeley, CA, 208 pp.

Del Giudice, E., Puselli, R.M., Tiezzi, E., 2009. Thermodynamics of irreversible processes and quantum field theory: an interplay for the understanding of ecosystem dynamics. Ecol. Model. 220 (16), 1874–1879.

Ellis, A., Wiseman, N., Boss, K., 1991. Fundamentals of Chinese Acupuncture. Paradigm Publications, Brookline, MA.

Finando, S., Finando, D., 2011. Fascia and the mechanism of acupuncture. J. Bodyw. Mov. Ther. 15, 168–176.

Finando, S., Finando, D., 2012. Qi, acupuncture and the fascia: a reconsideration of the fundamental principles of acupuncture. J. Altern. Complement. Med. 18 (9), 880–886.

Henry, R., 2011. Quantum Acupuncture: The Next Level. CreateSpace Independent Publishing Platform, Seattle, WA, 240 pp.

Hong, H. (Ed.), Acupuncture: Theories and Evidence. 2013. World Scientific Publishing Company, Singapore.

Huang, W., Pach, D.D., Napaddow, V., Park, K., et al., 2012. Characterizing acupuncture stimuli using brain imaging with fMRI—a systematic review and meta-analysis of the literature. PLoS One 7 (4), 1–19.

Jones, J.P., 1999. Acupuncture stimulation using ultrasound. In: Proceedings of the International Workshop on New Directions in the Scientific Exploration of Acupuncture. Beckman Center, National Academies of Science and Engineering, Irvine, CA.

Jones, J.P., Leeman, S., Nolan, E., Lee, D., 2011. Reflection and scattering of acoustical waves from a discontinuity in absorption. In: André, M.P., Jones, J.P., Lee, H. (Eds.), Acoustical Imaging, vol. 30, Springer Science, Cham, Switzerland, pp. 279–283.

Jones, J.P., Bae, Y.K., 2004. Ultrasonic visualization and stimulation of classical oriental acupuncture points. Med. Acupunct. 15 (2), 24–26.

Jones, J.P., Bae, Y.K., Wilson, L., So, C.S., Kidney, D.D., 2004. Ultrasonic imaging and characterization of acupuncture points in classical oriental medicine. In: Arnold, W., Hirsekorn, S. (Eds.), Acoustical Imaging. Kluwer Academic Publishers, Dordrecht, the Netherlands, pp. 527–533.

Julias, M., Edgar, L.T., Buettner, H.M., Shreiber, D.I., 2008. An in vitro assay of collagen fiber alignment by acupuncture needle rotation. Biomed. Eng. Online 7, 19.

Kim, B.H., 1963. On the kyungrak system. J. Acad. Med. Sci. 10, 1–41.

Langevin, H.M., Yandow, J.A., 2002. Relationship of acupuncture points and meridians to connective tissue planes. Anat. Rec. 269 (6), 257–265.

Langevin, H.M., Churchill, D.L., Fox, J.R., Badger, G.J., Garra, B.S., Krag, M.H., 2001a. Biomechanical response to acupuncture needling in humans. J. Appl. Physiol. 91 (6), 2471–2478.

Langevin, H.M., Churchill, D.L., Cipolla, M.J., 2001b. Mechanical signaling through connective tissue: a mechanism for the therapeutic effect of acupuncture. FASEB J. 15 (12), 2275–2282.

Langevin, H.M., Cornbrooks, C.J., Taatjes, D.J., 2004. Fibroblasts form a body-wide cellular network. Histochem. Cell Biol. 122 (1), 7–15.

Lee, B.C., Kim, K.W., Soh, K.S., 2009. Visualizing the network of Bonghan ducts in the omentum and peritoneum by using Trypan blue. J. Acupunct. Meridian Stud. 2 (1), 66–70.

Lee, B.C., Soh, K.-S., 2009. A novel model for meridian: Bonghan system combined with fascia (Bonghan-Fascia Model). In Findley, T.W. (Ed.), Proceedings of the Second International Fascia Research Congress, October 27–30. Elsevier, Amsterdam, p. 144.

Linsay, R.B., 1960. Mechanical radiation. McGraw Hill, New York, NY, p. 77.

Longhurst, J.C., 2010. Defining meridians: a modern basis of understanding. J. Acupunct. Meridian Stud. 3(2), 67–74.

MacPherson, H., Hammerschlag, R., Lewith, G., Schnyer, R., 2007. Acupuncture Research: Strategies for Establishing an Evidence Base. Churchill Livingstone, Edinburgh.

Manaka, Y., Itaya, K., Birch, S., 1995. Chasing the Dragon's Tail: The theory and Practice of Acupuncture in the Work of Yoshio Manaka. Paradigm Publications, Brookline, MA.

Matsumoto, K., Birch, S., 1988. Hara Diagnosis: Reflections on the Sea. Paradigm, Brookline, MA, p 142.

Mayor, D., 2006. Electroacupuncture: A Practical Manual and Resource. Churchill Livingstone, Edinburgh.

Mayor, D.F., Micozzi, M.S. (Eds.), 2011. Energy Medicine East and West: A Natural History of Qi. Churchill Livingstone, Edinburgh, 420 pp.

Micozzi, M.S., 2010. Fundamentals of Complementary and Alternative Medicine (Fundamentals of Complementary and Integrative Medicine), fourth ed. Saunders, Philadelphia, PA, 524 pp.

Miyawaki, K., 1994. Comprehensive Extra Meridian Treatment. Ta Ni Ku Chi Pub., Tokyo, Japan.

Myers, T., 2001. Anatomy Trains: Myofascial Meridians for Manual and Movement Therapists. Churchill Livingstone, London.

Nolan, E., 1988. Reflection of acoustic waves from a discontinuity in absorption. MS Thesis, University of California Irvine.

Oschman, J.L., 2007. In: Pishinger, A. (Ed.), The Extracellular Matrix and Ground Regulation. Introduction to the English edition. North Atlantic Books, Berkeley, CA, p. xiii.

Oschman, J.L., Oschman, N.H., 1995. Physiological and emotional effects of acupuncture needle insertion. In: Proceedings of the Second Symposium of the Society for Acupuncture Research. SAR, Boston.

Reichmanis, M., Marino, A.A., Becker, R.O., 1975. Electrical correlates of acupuncture points. IEEE Trans. Biomed. Eng. 22, 533–535.

Stefanini, P., 2011. Ki in Shiatsu. In: Mayor, D.F., Micozzi, M.S. (Eds.), Energy Medicine East and West: A Natural History of Qi. Churchill Livingstone, Edinburgh, pp. 211–222, Chapter 16.

Stefanov, M., Potroz, M., Kim, J., Lim, J., Cha, R., Nam, M.-H., 2013. The primo vascular system as a new anatomical system. J. Acupunct. Meridian Stud. 6 (6), 331–338.

Walthard, K., Tchicaloff, M., 1971. Motor Points. In: Licht, S. (Ed.), Electro-diagnosis and Electromyography. third ed. Waverly Press, Baltimore, MD, pp. 153–170.

Yang, W., 2008. Investigation of the Lower Resistance Meridian III. Acta Sci. Nat. Univ. Pekin. 44 (2), 277–280.

CHAPTER 15

Silent Pulses and Rhythmic Entrainment

Let not wisdom scoff at strange notions or isolated facts. Let them be explored. For the strange notion is a new vision and the isolated fact a new clay, possible foundations of tomorrow's science.

Edward F. Adolph (Fregly and Fregly, 1982)

Silent Pulses

At all levels, nature is a composite of rhythms. The vast cycles of the heavens represent extremes of virtually unimaginable scales, with distances measured in light years. At the other limit are the minute oscillations of molecules, atoms, and subatomic particles, vibrations of millions to billions of times per second. Life is immersed in this spectrum and contributes its own unique set of rhythms. One long cycle is that between birth and death. Superimposed upon that rhythm are many cycles of replacement of the atoms and molecules comprising the body (Schoenheimer, 1942). Some tissues, such as bone and fascia, are completely replaced some 10–15 times during a lifetime, while others, such as skin and intestine, are replaced 10,000 times during the same period. Certain enzymes last only a few seconds before they are renewed (Ratner, 1979). And immediate early genes can be activated in seconds to minutes (Figure 13.2). Each organ has its own set of activity rhythms, such as the ovary, with its monthly cycle (Figure 5.18). Shorter yet are the rhythms of the cranio/sacral pulse, the breath, the heartbeat, and the brain waves, which average about one-tenth of a second in duration. Much faster are the vibrations of molecules, which spin, wiggle, and shake millions of times each second.

Medical Use of Electricity and Magnetism

Should you fracture a bone in an arm or leg, and it fails to heal in 3–6 months, there is a good chance that your orthopedic surgeon will prescribe an energy method called pulsed electromagnetic field (PEMF) therapy. Your prescription is for a small battery-powered pulse generator (Figure 15.1B) connected to a coil that you will place next to your injury for 8–10 h/day, or you will have an electrical stimulator implanted near the fracture (Figures 15.1C and 15.2). The PEMF device produces a magnetic field that induces currents to flow in nearby tissues.

The idea of jump-starting a healing process is familiar to anyone who has practiced energetic bodywork or movement therapies. It is fascinating to follow the saga of how the energetic approach to bone healing was discovered, accepted as a therapy, rejected, and reinstated by the medical community.

Modern use of energy fields to stimulate bone repair actually began shortly after the discovery of 'animal electricity' at the end of the eighteenth century. By the mid-1800s, the preferred method for treating slow-healing fractures was to pass electricity through needles surgically implanted in the fracture region (Figure 15.1A). The technique was banished from medical practice, along with unproven electrotherapies, early in the 1900s (see Chapter 4).

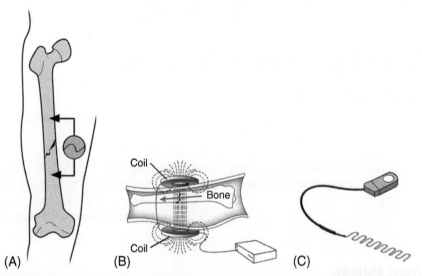

Figure 15.1 (A) In the 1800s, physicians in London discovered that passing an electric current through the fracture site in a broken bone that did not heal properly could jump-start the healing process. This became the method of choice for delayed union of fracture, referring to improper healing within 6 months; and fracture non-union, referring to improper healing after 6 months. (B) In the 1980s, it was discovered that weak magnetic fields could induce sufficient current flow through the fracture to start the healing process. (C) Currently, to get better compliance, orthopedic surgeons have gone back to electrical stimulation, using implanted stimulators.

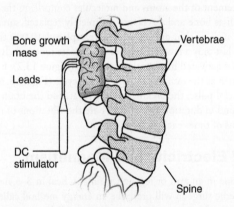

Figure 15.2 Implanted direct current stimulator being used to fuse a bone growth mass to two adjacent vertebrae of the spine. The illustration is from US Patent 5,441,527, dated August 15, 1995, for an implantable bone growth stimulator.

In the 1950s and 1960s, there was a resurgence of medical interest in electric and magnetic therapy. After considerable effort by scientists at a number of research centres (Bassett et al., 1982; Brighton et al., 1981), both electric and magnetic therapy for fracture 'non-unions' were granted the 'safe and effective' classification by the U.S. Food and Drug Administration. To obtain this status, many studies were done to document the success, lack of side effects, and mechanisms of energy field methods.

Not surprisingly, the scientific evidence is that PEMF therapy is effective because it conveys 'information' that triggers specific repair activities within the body. The currents induced in tissues by PEMF mimic the natural electrical activities created within bones during movements. Pulsing magnetic fields initiate a cascade of activities, from the cell membrane to the nucleus and on to the gene level, where specific changes take place (Bassett, 1995).

Magnetism and Soft Tissue Healing

After several decades of clinical success with the use of electric and magnetic fields to facilitate healing in hard tissues (bone), attention has turned to injuries of soft tissues, such as nerve, skin, muscle, and tendon, and the pain associated with such injuries.

Magnetic fields have advantages over electric fields because they are considered noninvasive and can be used for treating both soft and hard tissues simultaneously. Each tissue responds to a different frequency of pulsation.

Research employing electric and magnetic fields on soft tissues has been reviewed by Sisken and Walker (1995). The following effects have been observed:

- Enhancement of capillary formation
- Decreased necrosis
- Reduced swelling
- Diminished pain
- Faster functional recovery
- Reduction in depth, area, and pain in skin wounds
- Reduced muscle loss after ligament surgery (10 Hz optimum)
- Increased tensile strength of ligaments
- Acceleration of nerve regeneration and functional recovery.

A fascinating result was obtained in the research on nerve regeneration in rats. In the experiments, the sciatic nerve was damaged, and the entire animal was pulsed with a magnetic field. Nerve regeneration and functional recovery were accelerated. In some experiments, the animals were treated before the nerves were crushed. The pretreatment gave the same stimulation of nerve growth that was observed when the animals were treated after nerve damage. In other words, energy field therapy prior to injury enhanced the body's ability to respond to subsequent injury.

To be effective, PEMF pulses must be of low energy and extremely low frequency (ELF). Recent research shows that comparable fields emanate from the hands of practitioners of Therapeutic Touch and related methods.

Fields Projected from the Hands

Chapters 5 and 8 documented how the movements of electricity within the human body create biomagnetic fields in the surrounding space. Figure 2.6A showed the shape of the biomagnetic field around the body, as visualized in Polarity Therapy (see also Figure 15.3A). There are good reasons (given in the legend to that illustration) to suspect that this is an approximate representation of the overall biomagnetic field of the body, recognizing that there will be local variations in the field related to activities taking place within the various tissues. Figure 15.3B shows a representation of the detailed structure of the field around the head.

Because the biomagnetic field extends some distance from the body surface, the fields of two adjacent organisms will interact with each other. This general effect is illustrated in Figure 15.4A. Likewise, during non-contact Therapeutic Touch and related methods, as well as during manipulative techniques of all kinds, the biomagnetic field of the therapist will penetrate into the body of the patient. This is shown in Figure 15.4B, in which the lines of force of the biomagnetic field of the arm and hand have been superimposed upon an illustration from Leon Chaitow's book on soft-tissue manipulation (Chaitow, 1987).

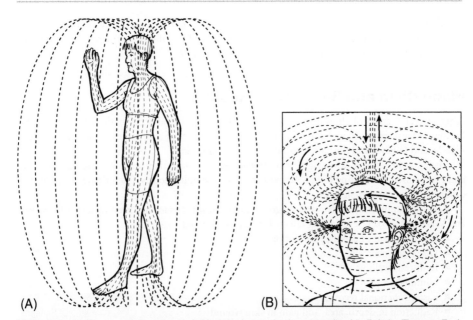

(A)   (B)

Figure 15.3 (A) The overall biomagnetic field of the human body as visualized in Polarity Therapy. Each organ and each tissue contributes to this pattern, which varies from moment to moment in relation to functional activities. The overall shape of the field results mainly from currents set up in the body by the heart, which produces the strongest biomagnetic field. The field is comparable in shape to that developed by the coil shown in Figures 2.8A and 15.1B. It is centred around the body axis because of the helical flow of heart electricity through a variety of tissues. The main flows are through the circulatory system, which is a good conductor because it is filled with a saline solution, plasma (Eyster et al., 1933). As with the coils shown in Figures 2.8 and 15.8, blood flow up and down through the aorta and major arteries is helical. Muscles are also good conductors of electricity, particularly along their longitudinal axes. There is resistance to current flow across the belly of a muscle. The musculature of the heart and arteries all the way down to the pre-capillaries is helically oriented (for references on helical flow and musculature in the circulatory system, see Marinelli et al., 1995). As the vascular system begins at the heart and extends into every nook and cranny of the body, it is ideally suited to distribute heart electricity to all of the tissues. (There are about 50,000 miles of blood vessels in the body). In addition, currents set up by the heart flow through the vertically oriented muscles associated with the vertebral column and backs of the legs – the erectors and hamstring system (Eyster et al., 1933). (B) Shows a representation of the field around the head in an etching drawn by Edwin D. Babbitt (1896), and is based on the patterns of light he observed around the body after spending some weeks in the dark, which greatly increased his visual sensitivity. A possible mechanism for sensing biomagnetic fields was discussed in Chapter 1 (see Figures 1.1 and 1.2). The pattern drawn by Babbitt corresponds primarily to the biomagnetic field expected from movements of nerve impulses through the corpus callosum connecting the two hemispheres of the brain.

Entrainment or Sync

All of these rhythms – from those taking place at the celestial scale to those in our organs, tissues, cells, and molecules – have significance for the healthy functioning of the human body. All of them are capable of entraining with each other. Rhythms in one person can entrain rhythms in another without touching (McCraty et al., 1998).

A very readable and classic book on this subject is *Sync: How Order Emerges from Chaos in the Universe, Nature and Daily Life*, by Steven Strogatz (2004):

- Synchronization (sync) pervades nature at every scale from the atomic nucleus to the cosmos.
- Our bodies are symphonies of molecular rhythms.
- Nature uses every available channel to allow its oscillators to talk to one another.

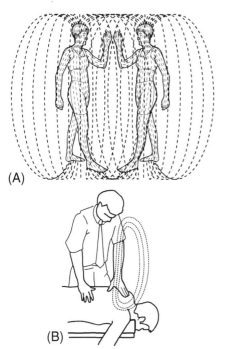

(A)

(B)

Figure 15.4 Biomagnetic field interactions between individuals. (A) The interactions of fields of nearby individuals. (B) Field interactions in the context of 'hands-on' bodywork. Superimposed on a diagram of a soft-tissue manipulation (thumb technique) is the pattern of biomagnetic emanations from the practitioner's hands. *(After Chaitow, 1987, Figure 13, p. 122, with kind permission from Dr. Leon Chaitow.)*

When considering the timing of any biological rhythm, the concept of entrainment is important. Physicists use this term to describe a situation in which two rhythms that have nearly the same frequency become coupled to each other, so that both have the same rhythm. Technically, entrainment means the 'mutual phase-locking of two (or more) oscillators'. For example, a number of pendulum clocks mounted on the same wall will eventually entrain, so that all of the pendulums swing in precise synchrony. For this to happen, the pendulums must have about the same period, which is determined by their length. What couples the pendulums are vibrations (elastic or sound waves) conducted through the structure of the wall.

Biologists have had a continuing fascination with the ways life is tied to the rhythms of nature, including the earliest astrological speculations, which far antedate the modern science of astronomy. Recent scientific explorations have replaced many early superstitions with accurate and repeatable observations and measurements. This exploration has had a pulse of its own as ideas of one generation give way to new truths, based on new data.

The exploration of biological rhythms has been confusing and controversial. There is an appropriate scientific style for presenting this story without adding to the confusion. Instead of listing interpretations and conclusions as facts about which we can argue, we present a series of hypotheses. These are tentative statements that can be tested and confirmed or refuted through systematic research and experience. We distinguish between findings and interpretations of findings.

Physicians are familiar with the electrical rhythms produced by the human body, and use them in diagnosis. These rhythms (Figure 15.5) include (a) the electroretinogram (Gotch, 1903; Holmgren, 1865), (b) the electrocardiogram (Einthoven, 1906), (c) the electroencephalogram (brain waves) (Berger, 1929), (d) electroencephalogram alpha (eyes closed or open) (Adrian and Bronk, 1929), and (e) the electromyogram, showing the oscillations produced during muscle contraction (Cram and Steger, 1983).

In terms of healing with signals applied to the body, important rhythms have been discovered by medical researchers who are employing magnetic pulses for 'jump-starting' the repair of a wide

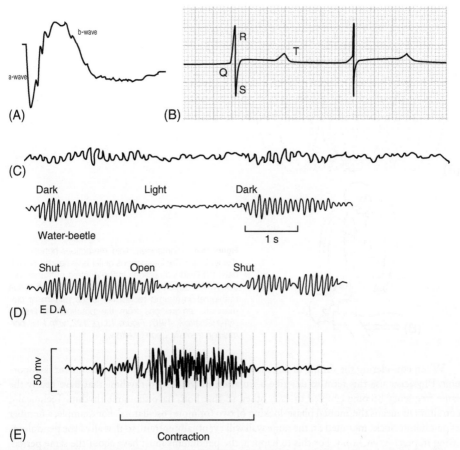

Figure 15.5 Electrical rhythms used in clinical medicine. (A) The electroretinogram (Gotch, 1903; Holmgren, 1865), (B) the electrocardiogram (Einthoven, 1906), (C) the electroencephalogram (brain waves) (Berger, 1929), (D) electroencephalogram alpha (eyes closed or open) (Adrian and Bronk, 1929), (EDA are the initials of Edgar Douglas Adrian) and (E) the electromyogram, showing the oscillations produced during muscle contraction.

spectrum of tissues and for treating diseases. While a variety of signals are being used, medical interest has especially focused on pulsing magnetic fields of low energy and ELF. The ELF range is arbitrarily defined as frequencies below 100 Hz. We shall see that there is evidence that similar frequencies emanate from the hands of practitioners of Therapeutic Touch and related methods. Moreover, the fields emitted by practitioners do not seem to be steady in frequency, but 'sweep' or 'scan' through the range of frequencies that medical researchers are finding effective in facilitating repair of various soft and hard tissues. This is a recent and profoundly exciting correlation worthy of a closer look.

As another example of the production of various frequencies in the body, the heart produces a variety of types and frequencies of energy that propagate through the circulatory system to every cell in the body (Figure 15.6). The fastest signal is an electromagnetic pulse (recorded with the electrocardiogram and the magnetocardiogram), followed by the heart sounds, a wave of pressure, and then a temperature change (infrared radiation). Russek and Schwartz (1996) refer to this as a dynamical energy system and describe its potential for communicating information throughout the body.

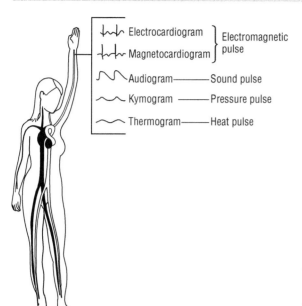

Figure 15.6 Heart pulses in the order of their velocities. The fastest signal is an electromagnetic pulse (recorded with the electrocardiogram and the magnetocardiogram), followed by a sound pulse, a pressure pulse, and then a temperature pulse (see Russek and Schwartz, 1996).

Frequency Windows of Specificity

Many frequencies have been tested in medical research laboratories. Many different types of tissues have been studied. Researchers have identified 'frequency windows of specificity', referring to specific frequencies that affect particular tissues (Table 15.1). References to the original reports are given in the review article by Sisken and Walker (1995). Since then, many frequencies have been tested for their effects on specific diseases. Some of these studies can be found in various U.S. patents (e.g., Liboff et al., 1993; Sandyk, 1995) and a report to NASA (Goodwin, 2003). Table 15.2 lists more frequencies from the scientific literature.

The Zimmerman Study

In the early 1980s, Dr. John Zimmerman (Figure 15.7) began a series of potentially ground-breaking studies on Therapeutic Touch with a SQUID (acronym for superconducting quantum interference device) magnetometer (see Chapter 8 and Figure 8.2) at the University of Colorado School of Medicine in Denver (Zimmerman, 1990). The experiments were done

TABLE 15.1 ■ **Healing Effects of Specific Frequencies (Frequency Windows of Specificity)**

Frequency	Effects
2 Hz	Nerve regeneration, neurite outgrowth from cultured ganglia
7 Hz	Bone growth
10 Hz	Ligament healing
15, 20, 72 Hz	Decreased skin necrosis, stimulation of capillary formation and fibroblast proliferation
25 and 50 Hz	Synergistic effects with nerve growth factor

From Sisken and Walker, 1995

TABLE 15.2 ■ **Frequency Sensitivities of Various Tissues Taken from the Scientific Literature**

1 Hz	Melatonin secretion (Lerchl et al., 1998)
2 Hz	Nerve regeneration, neurite outgrowth from cultured ganglia (Sisken and Walker, 1995)
5 Hz	Osteogenesis (Matsunaga et al., 1996)
6.4 Hz	Cartilage (Sakai et al., 1991)
7 H	Bone growth (Sisken and Walker, 1995)
10 Hz	Ligament healing (Lin et al., 1992; Sisken and Walker, 1995)
10 Hz	Cell growth (Miyagi et al., 2000)
10 Hz	Osteogenesis (Matsunaga et al., 1996)
10 Hz	Collagen production (Lin et al., 1993)
10 Hz	DNA synthesis (Takahashi et al., 1986)
15 Hz	Decreased skin necrosis, stimulation of angiogenesis and fibroblast proliferation (Sisken and Walker, 1995)
15 Hz	Osteoporosis (Takayama et al., 1990)
20 Hz	Decreased skin necrosis, stimulation of angiogenesis and fibroblast proliferation (Sisken and Walker, 1995)
20 Hz	Osteogenesis (Matsunaga et al., 1996)
25 Hz	Synergistic effect with nerve growth factor (Sisken and Walker, 1995)
40/116	Inflammation (Reilly et al., n.d.)
40/355	Inflammation (Reilly et al., n.d.)
50 Hz	Synergistic effect with nerve growth factor (Sisken and Walker, 1995)
50 Hz	Osteogenesis (Matsunaga et al., 1996)
50 Hz	Effects on mitosis and chromosomal aberrations in lymphocytes (Khalil and Qassem, 1991)
72 Hz	Decreased skin necrosis, stimulation of angiogenesis and fibroblast proliferation (Sisken and Walker, 1995)
100 Hz	Osteogenesis (Matsunaga et al., 1996)
100 Hz	Bony defect (Takano-Yamamoto et al., 1992)
100 Hz	DNA synthesis (Takahashi et al., 1986)
200 Hz	Osteogenesis (Matsunaga et al., 1996)

Notes:

1. The various devices and applications all are designed to produce/induce resonances within the body. These resonances can be disruptive to bacteria, parasites, or viruses, or they can stimulate normalization of function or repair in particular systems by activating particular types of cells or particular cellular activities.
2. There are many frequencies listed in non-scientific sources. For example, one extensive list (Stenulson) includes many Rife frequencies. These are not included here as they have not been validated in the peer-reviewed scientific literature.
3. One study (Peters, T.K., Koralewski, H.E., Zerbst, E., 1989 Apr. Search for optimal frequencies and amplitudes of therapeutic electrical carotid sinus nerve stimulation by application of the evolution strategy. Artif. Organs. 13 (2), 133–143) noted that the appropriate frequency for a particular patient must be determined individually. This is an important point, and validates the value of scanning the body with biofeedback to determine the frequency sensitivity profile for a particular patient.
4. One example is given in which two frequencies are used simultaneously.

with a SQUID detector of great sensitivity that had been designed to study some of the weakest of the human biomagnetic fields. These are called evoked fields; they are produced in the space around the head in response to external stimuli such as sounds or visual images (e.g., Reite and Zimmerman, 1978).

A Therapeutic Touch practitioner and his patient entered a magnetically shielded chamber containing a SQUID detector. The practitioner held his hand close to the patient, and a baseline recording was made with the SQUID. Then the therapist relaxed into the meditative or healing

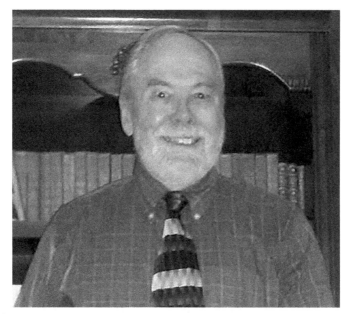

Figure 15.7   Dr. John Zimmerman, reproduced with his permission.

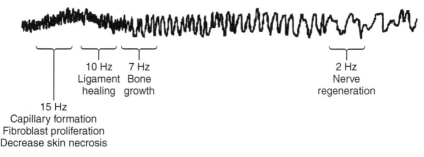

10 Hz	7 Hz	2 Hz
Ligament	Bone	Nerve
healing	growth	regeneration

15 Hz
Capillary formation
Fibroblast proliferation
Decrease skin necrosis

Figure 15.8   Signal recorded by Dr. John Zimmerman from the hand of a practitioner of Therapeutic Touch. The frequency was not steady, but varied from 0.3 to 30 Hz, with most of the activity in the range of 7–8 Hz. The wide brackets show portions of the 'sweep' that approximately correspond to some of the clinical results presented in Table 15.1. *(Reproduced with kind permission from Dr. Zimmerman.)*

state that is the focus of the Therapeutic Touch method. Immediately the SQUID detected a large biomagnetic field emanating from the practitioner's hand. The field was so strong that the amplifiers and recorder had to be readjusted so that a recording could be made. This was the strongest biomagnetic field Dr. Zimmerman had encountered in his years of medical research using the SQUID.

The Therapeutic Touch signal pulsed at a variable frequency, ranging from 0.3 to 30 Hz, with most of the activity in the range of 7–8 Hz. In other words, the signal emitted by the practitioner is not steady or constant, it 'sweeps' or 'scans' through a range of frequencies. One of the recordings is shown in Figure 15.8.

The pulsations are interesting in relation to the experiences of energy practitioners, who often report a sensation of vibration or tingling during the period when the technique seems to be particularly effective.

In Zimmerman's studies, non-practitioners were unable to produce the biomagnetic pulses. Recording sessions were repeated eight times and strong biomagnetic signals were recorded five times.

Zimmerman's observations represent a profoundly important but preliminary line of investigation into energy medicine. A problem was that the biomagnetic field produced during Therapeutic Touch was so strong that it was out of the calibrated range of the SQUID magnetometer. This meant that it was not possible to quantify the signal strength.

This difficulty was resolved in a study conducted in Japan: Seto et al. (1992) confirmed that an extraordinarily large biomagnetic field emanates from the hands of practitioners of a variety of healing and martial arts techniques, including QiGong, yoga, meditation, and Zen. The fields were measured with a simple magnetometer consisting of two 80,000-turn coils and a sensitive amplifier. The fields had a strength of about 10^{-3} gauss, which is about 1000 times stronger than the strongest human biomagnetic fields (from the heart), which are about 10^{-6} gauss, and about 1,000,000 times stronger than the fields produced by the brain. Figure 15.9 summarizes the Seto experiment and shows a typical recording. As in Zimmerman's study, the biomagnetic field pulsed with a variable frequency centred around 8–10 Hz.

The work of Zimmerman and Seto and colleagues could have profound implications in terms of correlating ancient concepts of energy medicine with modern science. Neither study documented that any clinical healing was taking place during the projection of energy, so further investigation is definitely needed. However, the evidence shows that practitioners can emit powerful pulsing biomagnetic fields in the same frequency range that biomedical researchers have identified for jump-starting healing of soft and hard tissue injuries. This implies that biomagnetism may be one form of the elusive Qi energy or life force. The projected fields are so strong that they can be detected with a relatively simple magnetometer, indicating that it is a robust effect that should be easy to study.

If the effect is so robust, why was it not discovered before? The answer is that it was described before. In 1779, Franz Anton Mesmer wrote his famous description of the magnet-like sensation he and his patients experienced while he held his hands near their bodies (Mesmer, 1948). When he invited physicians to witness his popular treatments of 'incurable' cases, the response was critical and hostile. Academic antagonism toward 'vitalism' hindered serious investigation of Mesmer's discoveries for more than 200 years. Attitudes are changing because, with a little training and practice,

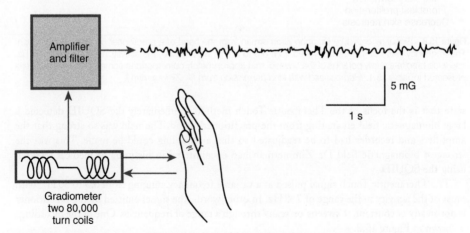

Figure 15.9 Biomagnetic field measurement during 'Qi emission' from the hand of a female subject in Tokyo. The double-coil magnetometer recording a pulsating magnetic field that averaged 2 mGauss, peak to peak, with a frequency of 8–10 Hz. *(After Seto et al., 1992 with kind permission from Acupuncture and Electro-Therapeutics Research International Journal and Cognizant Communications Corporation.)*

virtually anyone can experience the phenomenon Mesmer described. More and more people are having these experiences because of the increasing popularity of alternative medicine, including energy therapies.

Defining 'Healing Energy'

There is an obvious correlation between biomagnetic emanations from the hands of therapists and the 'frequency windows of specificity' found by biomedical researchers. While such correlations are exciting, they do not prove anything. More investigation is needed. Research begins with testable hypotheses that can be verified or refuted. We therefore present a hypothesis that is also a definition of healing energy, whether produced by a medical device or projected from the human hand (see Chapter 1, page 9).

Other Healing Frequencies

Medical experimentation is not confined to the ELF region of the energy spectrum. Popular devices such as the Diapulse machine emit 27 MHz (27 million pulses per second) and have been studied extensively. Clinical trials of the effects of the Diapulse on injuries have shown reduced swelling, acceleration of wound healing, stimulation of nerve regeneration, reduced pain, and faster functional recovery. References to this literature are given in the review by Sisken and Walker (1995).

The recording shown in Figure 15.8 shows only the ELF portion of the spectrum emitted from the hands of the Therapeutic Touch healer. Other frequencies and other forms of energy are undoubtedly present. These frequencies can be explained, in part, by the presence of the coherent Fröhlich oscillations mentioned in Chapters 11 and 17. For every frequency produced by the body, there are usually harmonics and subharmonics (i.e., signals that are exact multiples or fractions of the 'fundamental' frequency).

QiGong

The possible involvement of infrared radiation was mentioned above (see Figure 15.10). There is evidence that infrared radiation from the hands of QiGong practitioners can increase cell growth, DNA and protein synthesis, and cell respiration. There is also evidence that living systems emit microwaves (Enander and Larson, 1977) and light (Popp et al., 1992; Rattemeyer et al., 1981).

Research shows that masters of the QiGong technique can project measurable amounts of heat from their palms (so-called 'facilitating' Qi) that increases cell growth, DNA and protein synthesis, and cell respiration. Practitioners can also produce 'inhibiting' Qi, in which infrared energy is absorbed from the environment. This kind of Qi slows metabolism. References to more recent work on infrared and biomagnetic and QiGong effects can be found in an article from the Mount Sinai School of Medicine in New York (Muehsam et al., 1994). A description of healing effects of QiGong can be found in a series of articles published for physicians (Walker, 1994).

One explanation for facilitating and inhibiting Qi is based on the fact that the circulation to the skin is influenced by the autonomic nervous system. Years of research into biofeedback shows that anyone can learn to control autonomic parameters, including skin temperature. For example, biofeedback regulation of skin temperature has been used to treat migraine headache. Figure 15.10 shows how changes in circulation can alter skin temperature. The rates of chemical reactions and other processes are affected by ambient temperature, so a warm or a cool hand near another person can increase or decrease the rates of temperature-sensitive activities within their bodies.

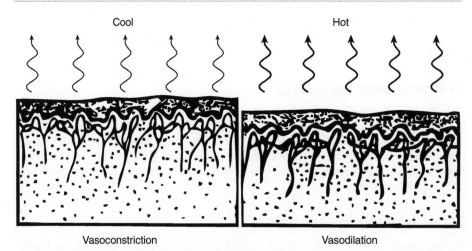

Figure 15.10 'Facilitating' and 'inhibiting' Qi may be produced by changes in the circulation to the skin mediated by the autonomic nervous system. Changes in circulation alter skin temperature. The rates of chemical reactions are proportional to ambient temperature, so a warm or a cool hand near another person can increase or decrease the rates of temperature-sensitive reactions within their bodies. *(Modified from Mackean, 1973, with kind permission from D.G. Mackean.)*

Mechanisms

Medical researchers have stated that energy field therapies are effective because they project 'information' into tissues. This triggers a cascade of activities, from the cell membrane to the nucleus and on to the gene level, where specific changes take place (see Bassett, 1995). The interpretation of these findings is that particular repair processes are triggered by the information contained in signals of specific frequencies.

While this is an interesting hypothesis, it leaves unanswered the question of why repair is not activated naturally. Why should it be necessary to trigger healing with an external signal, and precisely how does this signal trigger healing? The following describes some additional considerations.

The living matrix is one medium through which the cascade of activities takes place. Complete health corresponds to total interconnection through this matrix and its associated layers of water.

Suppose accumulated physical and/or emotional injury or trauma impairs continuity. The application of healing energy, whether from a medical device or from the hands of an energy therapist, would then open the network to the flow of energy and information. Once the whole network is functioning, natural biological communications could flow freely through the entire system, from the extracellular matrix, across the cell membrane, through the cytoskeleton, to the nucleus, and on to the gene level, and in the opposite direction as well (Oschman, 1993; Oschman and Oschman, 1994). In other words, activation of specific processes goes hand in hand with opening of the channels for the flow of energy and information.

A leading medical researcher has confirmed what alternative practitioners observe frequently: Application of therapeutic energy fields 'can convert a stalled healing process into active repair, even in patients unhealed for as long as 40 years (Bassett, 1995). The mechanism by which active repair is initiated probably involves both activation of specific cellular activities and the opening of the channels or circuitry for the natural biological communications required for initiating and coordinating injury repair.

Prevention

The free flow of messages and electronic excitation through tissues is essential for prevention and for simply 'feeling well'. An example of experimental evidence for preventive effects was given in Sisken and Walker (1995). Animals treated with magnetic fields prior to nerve injury experienced the same acceleration of nerve growth as animals treated after injury.

While the focus in this discussion is on the healing of wounds, energetic bodywork can be of profound significance to the organism even if no specific problem is present. A healthy individual will be both happier and less likely to have an injury or disease. If problems do arise, the person will recover more rapidly. Likewise, athletic, artistic, and intellectual performance is enhanced when all of the body's communication channels are open and balanced. This point is well understood in many complementary practices, in which regular maintenance treatments or 'tune-ups' are given. These treatments are not for specific ailments, but serve to reduce the future incidence of medical problems, to enhance performance of all kinds of activities, and generally to facilitate the progress of individuals in their personal evolution, or in the achievement of their personal goals or 'destiny'.

One mechanism of prevention comes from study of some of the effects of acupuncture: mild stimulation of tissues (as by insertion of an acupuncture needle, acupressure, shiatsu, Structural Integration, massage, etc.) can simulate an injury without actually injuring the tissue. By simulating an injury, the mild stimulus activates the cascade of repair processes through the living matrix. Mild stimulation of key points on a healthy individual is a sort of 'test run' or 'tune-up' of the repair channels (Oschman and Oschman, 1994).

After decades of being 'off limits' to academic science and Western medical practice, there is a resurgence of interest in energy medicine. Two areas of research are being extensively investigated: the study of magnetic fields produced by living things – biomagnetism – and the study of the effects of magnetic fields on living systems – magnetobiology.

Two techniques, representing opposite philosophies, are gaining popularity in hospitals and other clinical settings. The mainstream approach involves the use of artificial electric and magnetic fields to 'jump-start' healing processes. The traditional or complementary method is non-contact Therapeutic Touch, which is increasingly being used by hospital nurses and other practitioners (Krieger, 1975; Quinn, 1984, 1992, 1993). Closely related 'energy' methods, such as Healing Touch, Polarity Therapy, Reiki, Johrei, Aura Balancing, magnet therapy, and acupuncture, are also gaining in public acceptance.

Modern research is reconciling these superficially divergent approaches, both in terms of their remarkable effectiveness and in terms of the mechanisms by which they produce their effects. There are good reasons to believe that all the methods mentioned above involve similar cellular and molecular mechanisms.

Infrared Radiations

SQUID research has enhanced our understanding of 'the body magnetic', but this does not mean that biomagnetism is the whole story of healing energy. Several studies have implicated infrared signals (heat) in Therapeutic Touch (e.g., Chien et al., 1991; Schwartz et al., 1990). This is important because some practitioners of Therapeutic Touch and related methods do not experience Mesmer's magnet-like sensation, but rather a sensation of heat or warmth during their work.

IMPLICATIONS

If the ideas presented so far are valid, there are a number of obvious implications. First, on a practical level, manufacturers of medical devices might find it worthwhile to test the effects of stimulators that scan through a range of frequencies, rather than produce a single frequency (the Ondamed® system, Figure 15.11, is an example). It would obviously be worthwhile to try

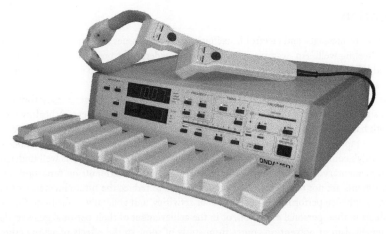

Figure 15.11 The Ondamed®, an example of a therapeutic device that produces a signal that sweeps through a large range of frequencies, from 0.5 to 32,000 Hz. *(Courtesy of ONDAMED, New Windsor, NY.)*

recording the natural emissions from the hands of a therapist and projecting the recorded signals into injured tissues.

Some research along this line has been done. A device has been developed that projects signals comparable to those produced by a QiGong practitioner (Niu et al., 1992; Walker, 1994). Interestingly, this device produces an ELF acoustic signal. Literature on this device and on other effects of QiGong can be accessed through a database (QiGong Institute, 1995) and a booklet (Lee, 1999).

Evolutionary biology leads to an additional perspective. The evidence presented so far suggests that an ability of organisms to project and respond to healing energy, as defined above, has evolved as a natural design feature of living systems. Our ancestors lived in a world fraught with hazards but had no hospitals or clinics to help them mend wounds of the flesh. A natural ability of individuals to facilitate injury repair in each other had obvious survival value in the earliest communities. Evolution by natural selection took care of the rest.

Hypothesis

An ability to project and respond to healing energy, as defined above, has evolved as a natural design feature of living systems.

If this hypothesis is valid, it points to a simple conclusion: No medical device, regardless of its sophistication, is likely to achieve the efficacy and safety obtainable by imposing a naturally generated signal to living tissue.

Biological Rhythms and Wound Healing

The next mechanistic questions concern the sources of the oscillating fields emitted by the hands of various energy therapists and the reason the signals scan or sweep through a range of frequencies. Research has led to detailed and rather remarkable answers to these questions. The focus is on biological rhythms and the ways they are regulated. Injury repair involves a wide spectrum of biological rhythms associated with the replacement of various tissue elements. How can these processes be coordinated? The problem can be stated as follows:

Wound healing is a remarkable and intricate process, involving the integrated and cooperative activities of a variety of systems. Each wound is different, and the body's response must be precisely appropriate if structure and function are to be fully restored. Dynamic interactions take place between local and systemic processes. A wide range of physiological activities are activated, and all must be down-regulated when repair is complete. Some repair processes persist for weeks, or even longer, after an injury.

Until recently, the medical approach has been almost exclusively molecular. Researchers have looked for, and found, a variety of chemicals that influence the repair of tissues. The clotting of blood involves a cascade of reactions involving many different substances. Fibroblast growth factors stimulate division of the cells that lay down collagen, a major structural protein used in healing wounds. Hence, healing can be promoted by adding natural growth factors, or genes for those growth factors, directly to a site of injury (e.g., Vogt et al., 1994).

It is easy to see how molecules can regulate the rates of cellular processes by activating or inactivating particular metabolic pathways. However, there is something missing from the picture. How can the ebbs and flows of regulatory substances provide a 'blueprint' for the restoration of elaborate architecture and functioning of cells and tissues and organs?

The Blueprint

Harold Saxton Burr was convinced that energy fields provide the blueprint for living systems (Chapter 13). Molecular biology can account for the manufacture of the parts, in appropriate quantities, but the forces exerted by living fields bring those parts together in meaningful ways to produce living structure and function.

The last entry in Table 15.1 supports Burr's hypothesis. Growth factors (molecules) stimulate the growth of nerves, but magnetic pulsations at 25 and 50 Hz synergize or enhance the effect. Therefore, another hypothesis:

Hypothesis

A complete description of the assembly and operation and repair of a living system requires an understanding of the regulatory effects both of molecules *and* of *energy fields*. The genes govern the manufacture of molecules in appropriate quantities, and patterns of forces exerted by energy fields bring molecules together to produce functional structures.

Hypothesis

A variety of electrical, electronic, magnetic, and other energetic phenomena take place within healthy tissue as a consequence of the communications needed to coordinate cellular activities. The resulting energy fields are radiated from the hands of the healthy individual. Whether caused by physical or emotional trauma, 'the wound that does not heal' is a wound that is not receiving the natural regulatory signals needed to initiate and coordinate repair processes. When healthy tissue is brought close to such a wound, essential information is transferred via the energy field, communication channels open and the healing process is 'jump-started'.

Sources of ELF Signals

The functioning of the heart, brain, and some other organs result in oscillations in the ELF range of the electromagnetic spectrum. The principal brain wave frequencies are shown in Figure 15.12.

Over the last half century, Robert O. Becker and others have done important research on the role of brain waves in healing. These studies have many implications for bodywork and movement therapies. Becker's work reveals one of the unknowns in the X-signal system of Manaka (see Chapter 11).

Modern neurophysiology focuses primarily on the activity of less than half of the cells in the brain (Becker, 1990a, 1991). The 'neuron doctrine' holds that all functions of the nervous system are the result of activities of the neurons. Integration of brain function is therefore regarded as arising from the massive interconnectivity of the neurons. This view is incomplete because it

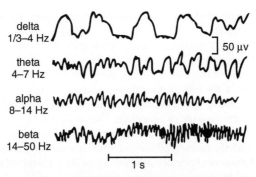

Figure 15.12 Brain waves. Dominant brainwave frequencies recorded with the electroencephalograph, with electrodes on the scalp. The frequency of brain waves is constantly changing. Delta activity occurs during deep sleep and in certain brain disorders. Theta activity occurs during various stages of sleep in normal adults and during emotional stresses, including disappointment and frustration. Alpha brain waves have been associated with a normal and alert state of mind. Beta waves are normally seen over the frontal portions of the brain during intense mental activity. Beta waves of higher frequencies (up to 50Hz) are associated with intense activation of the nervous system or tension. *(After Guyton, 1991, with kind permission from WB Saunders Company.)*

ignores an evolutionarily more ancient informational system residing in the perineural connective tissue cells that constitute more than half of the cells in the brain. Perineural cells (Figure 11.13) encase every nerve fibre, down to their finest terminations, throughout the body.

The perineural system is a direct current communication system reaching to every innervated tissue. The perineural system establishes a 'current of injury' that controls injury repair. Historically, the injury potential was discovered *before* the discovery of resting and action potentials of nerves (Davson, 1970). The current of injury is generated at the site of a wound and continues until repair is complete. One function of the current is to alert the rest of the body to the location and extent of an injury. The current also attracts the mobile skin cells, white blood cells, and fibroblasts that close and heal the wound. Finally, the injury current changes as the tissue heals, and therefore feeds back information on the progress of repair to surrounding tissues. Becker's research demonstrated that the current of injury is not an ionic current, but a semiconductor current that is sensitive to magnetic fields (the Hall effect). Semiconduction takes place in the perineural connective tissue and surrounding parts of the living matrix (Becker 1961).

Other tissues in the body are ensheathed in continuous layers of connective tissue: the vascular system is surrounded with perivascular connective tissue; the lymphatic system with perilymphatic connective tissue; the muscular system with myofascia; the bones with the periosteum. Conceptually, the living matrix encompasses all of these connective tissue systems, including the cellular and nuclear scaffolds within them (see Chapters 10–12 and Figures 10.7 and 12.6).

Oscillations of the brain's direct current field, the brain waves, are not confined to the brain. Instead, they propagate through the circulatory system, which is a good conductor, and along the peripheral nerves, following the perineural system, which reaches into every part of the body that is innervated. Similarly, oscillations of the heart's electrical activity are not confined to the heart muscle but are propagated through the vascular system, perivascular connective tissue, and living matrix to all parts of the body.

The measurable brain waves arise because of the rhythmic and synchronized spread of direct current through large populations of neurons in the brain. The field is relatively strong and partly coherent because it flows through massive numbers of parallel neurons in the vertically oriented pyramidal portion of the somatosensory cortex (see Kandel et al., 2012).

Becker's research shows that brain waves regulate the overall operation of the nervous system, including the state of consciousness. There is a neurophysiological basis for this concept.

The brain waves cause the local fields around individual neurons to vary rhythmically. The local field, in turn, determines the sensitivity of the neurons to stimulation. When the local field is such that the neuron is ready to send a signal (called the threshold for depolarization), a small stimulus will cause the nerve to fire. When the local field is far from the firing level (far from threshold), a much larger stimulus will be needed for the nerve to be excited. Hence there is a rhythm in the excitability of nerve cells throughout the body. Sophisticated research using microelectrodes has confirmed that the probability of a nerve firing in the brain changes rhythmically in relation to the electroencephalogram (Verzeano, 1970).

The Brain's Pacemaker

Brain waves are not constant in frequency, but vary from moment to moment. The 'pacemaker' or 'rhythm section' is located deep in the brain, specifically in the thalamus. The system is known as the thalamic rhythm generator or pacemaker (Andersen and Andersson, 1968).

Careful research is determining the cellular basis of the rhythms (Destexhe et al., 1993; Wallenstein, 1994). Calcium ions slowly leak into single thalamocortical neurons, which oscillate for 1.5–28 s, triggering and entraining the brain waves, which spread upward throughout the brain. Eventually, the thalamic oscillations cease because of the excess calcium built up in the thalamocortical neurons. During this 'silent phase', lasting from 5 to 25 s, the brain waves are said to 'free-run'. It is probably during this phase that the cortical brain waves are especially susceptible to entrainment by external fields, as will be discussed below. Eventually, the thalamic oscillations begin again, after the cells have restored their calcium levels to the point where they are once again able to oscillate.

The electroencephalographic waves spread not only throughout the brain, but throughout the nervous system (via the perineural system) and into every part of the organism. In this way, the brain waves regulate the overall sensitivity and activity of the entire nervous system (Becker, 1990a,b).

Entrainment of Biological Rhythms: More Controversy

This chapter leads toward a discussion of the possibility that external signals, including signals projected from the hands of an energy therapist, can entrain brain waves during the thalamic silent, or free-run, period. The reader should be aware that the entrainment of biological rhythms is a subject as controversial among biologists as the mechanism versus vitalism issue discussed in Chapter 4. The controversy is about whether biological rhythms are predominantly timed by 'internal clocks' or by 'external clocks'.

While there are good arguments on either side of this issue, the current consensus among scientists is that biological clocks are mostly set by internal pacemakers, such as the thalamus, and that organisms are, for the most part, independent of natural energy cycles, such as those discussed below. However, the history of science has repeatedly demonstrated that scientific consensuses have a rhythm of their own as ideas of one generation give way to new truths, based on new data.

Most scientists and non-scientists alike take a firm position on one side or the other of this question. For many, it is obvious that life is part of a larger fabric and that rhythms of the sun, moon, planets, and other celestial bodies must affect us (see, e.g., Leonard, 1978). For others, it is equally obvious that any such effects, if they do exist, are minimal. For many scientists, there is strong bias against any concept that might be taken as support for astrology, an endeavour that is widely frowned upon. There are good reasons to suspect that a person's point of view on this subject is based less on logical analysis and more on an individual emotional and personality structure.

Geomagnetic and Geoelectric Fields

Evidence will be presented that the 'free-run' periods, when the brain waves are not paced by the thalamus, allow the brain's field to be entrained by external electric and magnetic rhythms, either natural or man-made.

What is the source of natural electric and magnetic rhythms? The magnetic field of the Earth, called the geomagnetic field, causes the compass needle to point toward the North Pole. However, if you look carefully at a compass needle with a microscope, you will see that the needle is rarely still – it dances back and forth in a variety of rhythms. Some of these rhythms are diurnal (24-h), some are much slower, and others are quite fast (in the ELF range). The last are called geomagnetic micropulsations. They are caused by a unique geophysical mechanism known as the Schumann resonance.

An important geophysical phenomenon, the Schumann resonance provides a physical link between solar, lunar, planetary, and other celestial rhythms and human physiology.

In the 1950s, a German atmospheric physicist, W. O. Schumann, suggested that the space between the surface of the Earth and the ionosphere should act as a resonant cavity, somewhat like the chamber in a musical instrument.

What do we mean by a resonant cavity? Pressing the keys on a wind instrument changes the size of the air space or cavity, and therefore changes the frequency of the standing waves within that cavity. Standing waves are produced when waves travelling in the cavity are reflected from its boundaries. Each reflection gives rise to a wave travelling in the opposite direction. The reflected waves are superimposed on the original waves to produce what are called standing waves. Figure 15.13 shows what is meant by standing waves and resonant cavities in musical instruments and in the atmosphere. Organs use pipes of different sizes to produce standing waves of different frequencies. Pressing a guitar or violin string against the fret or fingerboard changes the effective length of the string and therefore the resonant frequency of the standing waves that can be produced.

Resonant tones are generated when the musician blows over an orifice or past a vibrating reed, or plucks or bows a string. Energy for the Schumann resonance is provided by cloud-to-ground lightning (Figure 15.13). While you may be experiencing calm weather where you are now, there are, on average, hundreds of lightning strikes taking place each second, some 40 million per day, scattered about the planet. To use the physics terminology, lightning pumps energy into the Earth–ionosphere cavity and causes it to vibrate or resonate at frequencies in the ELF range.

In a series of papers published between 1952 and 1957, Schumann gradually refined his resonance theory (see Sentman, 1995, for references). In 1954, Schumann and Konig detected the resonances (Schumann and Konig, 1954). After the initial reports, there followed a period of intense research (1965–1982), stimulated in part by the U.S. Navy, which was interested in studying the ELF band for use in communicating with submerged submarines. In the 1960s, Schumann's theory (1952) was confirmed (Balser and Wagner, 1960; Galejs, 1972).

Lightning creates electromagnetic standing waves that travel around the globe at the speed of light. These waves circumnavigate the entire planet on average 7.86 times per second. Hence, an observer at any point on the Earth's surface will experience both the high frequency electromagnetic signals from the lightning and the ELF pulsations generated by the atmospheric standing waves. The high frequency waves are reflected from the ionosphere, back to the Earth, back to the ionosphere, etc. (Figure 15.13). This 'skip' phenomenon has been widely studied, because it is the basis for long distance radio communication.

As electromagnetic waves, the low-frequency Schumann micropulsations can be detected either as electric or as magnetic fields. The average frequency is about 7–10 Hz, and this corresponds to the average frequency of brain waves in humans. This correlation is thought to have evolutionary and physiological significance (e.g., Becker, 1963, 1990a,b; Direnfeld, 1983). When the ionosphere gets higher – on the night side of the planet, for example – the cavity gets larger,

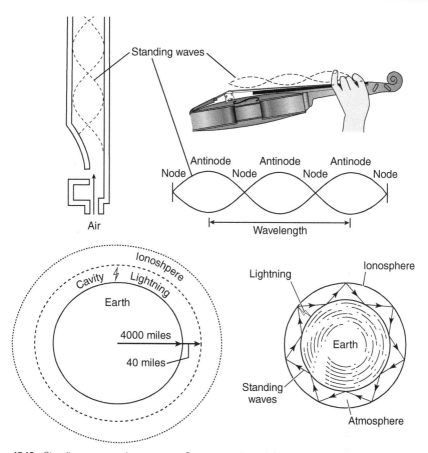

Figure 15.13 Standing waves and resonances. Organs use pipes of different sizes to produce different notes. Pressing a guitar or violin string against the fret or fingerboard changes the effective length of the string and therefore the resonant frequency of the standing waves that can be produced. Energy for the Schumann resonance is provided by cloud-to-ground lightning. The Schumann resonance is a unique electromagnetic phenomenon created by the sum of the lightning activity around the world. Electromagnetic pulses from lightning travel around the Earth, bouncing back and forth between the ionosphere and the Earth's surface. To use the physics terminology, lightning pumps energy into the Earth–ionosphere cavity, and causes it to vibrate or resonate at frequencies in the ELF range. Lightning creates electromagnetic standing waves that travel around the globe at the speed of light. These waves circumnavigate the entire planet on average 7.86 times per second. The high frequency waves are reflected from the ionosphere, back to the Earth, back to the ionosphere, etc. This 'skip' phenomenon has been widely studied, because it is the basis for long distance radio communication. At any given point on the Earth, the Schumann resonance shows up as electric and magnetic micropulsations in the range of 1–40 Hz. The frequency and strength of the signals depend on the distribution of global thunderstorm activity, local meteorological conditions and the conductivity of the Earth's surface at the point of observation. Bursts of Schumann pulses are easier to detect in fair weather, and occur more often during the day than at night. These terrestrial factors are, in turn, influenced by more distant extraterrestrial factors, such as solar and lunar position, sun spots, planetary positions, etc. (See Dubrov, 1978; Pressman, 1970.) *(Diagram at lower right is after Bentov, 1976, Figure 16, p. 145, with kind permission from Integral Publishing.)*

and the resonant frequency drops. Rhythms of terrestrial and extraterrestrial origin alter the height and other properties of the ionosphere, and thereby alter the Schumann frequency in the range of 1–40 Hz. There are also variations in the global lightning frequency. There are times when solar activity leads to magnetic storms that disrupt the ionosphere, and Schumann resonances cease completely. This can disturb long-distance radio communications.

To summarize, the Schumann resonance is created by terrestrial phenomena and is modified or modulated by extraterrestrial activities. A thorough and technical review of the literature on the Schumann resonance has been published by Sentman (1995).

VLF-Sferics

In addition to its role in 'pumping' energy into the atmosphere to maintain the Schumann resonance, lightning directly produces a variety of signals in the very low frequency (VLF) range (1-100 kHz). These are called VLF-atmospherics or VLF-sferics. Sferics are impulses that propagate at about the speed of light through the atmosphere. The signals gradually become dispersed and damped with distance, and higher and lower frequency components are lost, leaving a signal of about 10 kHz. At distances beyond 1000 km, the 10 kHz signal predominates (Schienle et al., 1998).

To summarize, the Schumann resonance is created by atmospheric events (lightning) and is modified or modulated by extraterrestrial activities. In radio terminology, the signals are frequency modulated.

Evidence for Entrainment by External Fields

The Schumann oscillations propagate for long distances and readily penetrate through the walls of buildings and into the human body. Schumann frequencies have considerable overlap with biomagnetic fields such as those produced by the heart and brain, but the Schumann resonance is thousands of times stronger. The similarity of a train of Schumann signals and an alpha brain wave are shown in Figure 15.14.

A number of biologists have concluded that the frequency overlap of Schumann resonances and biological fields is not accidental but is the culmination of a close interplay between geomagnetic and biomagnetic fields over evolutionary time (e.g., Direnfeld, 1983). Hence, researchers have examined interactions between external fields and biological rhythms.

Organisms are capable of sensing the intensity, polarity, and direction of the geomagnetic field (Gould, 1984). There is evidence that geomagnetic rhythms serve as a time cue in the organization of physiological rhythms (e.g., Cremer-Bartels et al., 1984; Gauguelin, 1974; Wever, 1968), although this continues to be controversial. A variety of behavioural disturbances in the human population are statistically related to disturbances in the Earth's electromagnetic field or to man-made interferences:

- Friedman et al. (1963, 1965) documented a relationship between increased geomagnetic activity and the rate of admission of patients to 35 psychiatric facilities.
- Venkatraman (1976) and Rajaram and Mitra (1981) reported an association between changes in the geomagnetic field due to magnetic storms and frequency of seizures in epileptic patients.

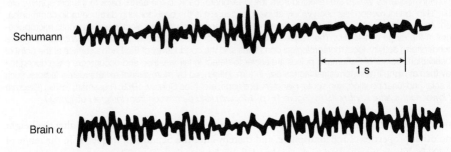

Figure 15.14 A Schumann signal and an alpha brain wave. *(After Konig, H.L., 1974. ELF and VLF signal properties: physical characteristics. In: Persinger, M.A. (Ed.), ELF and VLF Electromagnetic Field Effects. Plenum Press, New York, with permission.)*

- Perry et al. (1981) correlated suicide locations in the West Midlands, England, with high magnetic field strengths due to 50 Hz power lines.

Many studies have demonstrated the probable entrainment of brain waves by external rhythms of natural and artificial origin:

- Reiter (1953) measured reaction time, an important factor in traffic safety. Upon entering a cubicle at a traffic exhibition, visitors were asked to press a key. When a light came on, they were to release pressure on the key. Their reaction time (i.e., the time between 'light on' and 'key release') was recorded for many thousands of visitors over a 2-month period. At the same time, the ELF micropulsations (Schumann resonances) were monitored. The micropulsations slow when a thunderstorm is approaching, and Reiter found that the subjects were slower to respond during such periods. When the micropulsations speeded up, into the range of alpha brain wave activity, reaction times were faster.

- After the traffic exhibition, Reiter took his test cubicle to the University of Munich and lined the top and bottom with wire mesh connected to an electrical generator. He introduced artificial low-level, low-frequency signals similar to those of the Earth's field. Under these controlled conditions, the effects of the fields on reaction time were comparable to those obtained during the exhibition. Moreover, subjects in the laboratory experiments repeatedly complained about headaches, tightness in the chest, and sweating of the palms after several minutes of exposure to 3 cycle/second fields. When the headaches faded away, there was often a feeling of fatigue. These symptoms resemble the so-called 'weather sensitivity' complaints that some people have before the arrival of a thunderstorm.

- Hamer (1968, 1969) pulsed subjects with low-intensity artificial electric fields from metal plates on each side of their heads. Fields of 8-10 Hz speeded up reaction time, while slower oscillations of 2-3 Hz slowed down reaction times significantly. Similar results were reported by Friedman and colleagues in 1967.

- In 1977, Beatty reported studies on the practical significance of brain wave entrainment for people such as air traffic controllers, who need to maintain an alert state for long periods. Subjects monitored a simulated radar screen, watching for certain targets to appear. In agreement with the findings of Reiter and Hamer, slower brain waves were correlated with slower reaction times and poorer performance in the task.

- Over many years, Wever (1968) and colleagues at the Max Planck Institute in Germany observed hundreds of subjects who lived in two underground rooms that were shielded from external rhythms of light, temperature, sound, pressure, etc. One room also had an electromagnetic shield around it, consisting of a mesh of steel rods and plates that reduced the influence of geomagnetic rhythms by 99%. The rhythms of body temperature, sleep–waking, urinary excretion, and other physiological activities were monitored. All subjects developed longer and irregular or desynchronized or chaotic physiological rhythms. Those in the magnetically shielded room developed significantly longer and more irregular physiological rhythms. In some experiments, artificial electric and magnetic rhythms were pulsed into the shielding. Only one field had any effect: a very weak 10 Hz electric field. This field dramatically restored normal patterns to the biorhythm measurements.

Each of these important but seldom cited studies concluded that biological rhythms can be entrained with natural and artificial ELF electric fields. Entrainment of brain waves can set the overall speed of responsiveness of the nervous system to stimulation. This is called reaction time and is an easily measured parameter of consciousness. The results support Becker's contention that the pulsing DC electrical system (brain waves) set the tone of the entire nervous system.

These studies do not mean that when a thunderstorm approaches, everyone will get drowsy and react slowly and accidents will happen. Instead, they suggest that there is a statistically greater chance of slower reactions and more frequent accidents under these conditions. Geomagnetic pulsations do not affect everyone the same way. However, there is evidence that geomagnetic pulsations strongly entrain brain waves during meditation and other practices in which one 'quiets the mind' to allow the 'free-run' periods to be dominated by geophysical rhythms.

Mechanism of Entrainment

The pathways involved in the body's responses to external magnetic rhythms are shown in Figure 15.15. The pineal gland is the primary magnetoreceptor. Between 20% and 30% of pineal cells are magnetically sensitive. Exposure of animals to magnetic fields of various intensities alters

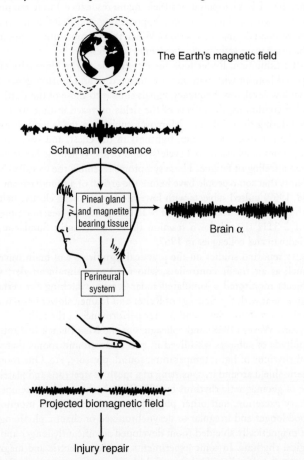

Figure 15.15 A summary of the proposed pathways involved in magnetoreception, the regulation of brain waves and therapeutic emissions from the hands of therapists. Micropulsations of the geomagnetic field, caused by the Schumann resonance, are detected by the pineal and magnetite-bearing tissues associated with the brain. During the 'free-run' period, when the brain waves are not being entrained by the thalamus, the Schumann resonance can take over as the pacemaker, particularly if the individual is in a relaxed or meditative state (Schumann signals are thousands of times stronger than brain waves). The brain waves regulate the overall tone of the nervous system and the state of consciousness. The electrical currents of the brain waves are conducted throughout the body by the perineural and vascular systems. The biomagnetic field projected from the hands can be much stronger than the brain waves (Seto et al., 1992), indicating that an amplification of at least 1000 times takes place somewhere in the body. Alternatively, the body may simply act as an effective antenna or channel for the Schumann micropulsations. The projected fields scan or sweep through the frequencies medical researchers are finding useful for 'jump-starting' injury repair in a variety of tissues (see Table 15.1). *(Portions of this illustration are after Becker, 1990b, reproduced with kind permission from Robert O. Becker, MD.)*

the secretion of melatonin, the electrical properties of pineal cells, and their microscopic structure (reviewed by Sandyk, 1995). In addition, various animal tissues contain particles of organic magnetite. Two separate research groups have now recorded magnetically influenced impulses in single neurons connecting magnetite-bearing tissues with the brain (reviewed by Kobayashi and Kirschvink, 1995).

The question of whether living systems are sensitive to the Earth's magnetic field has been bitterly controversial for more than a century. There are now a number of plausible and well-documented mechanisms for such interactions, and abundant evidence that they take place. Moreover, Becker's research has shown how geomagnetic entrainment of the brain waves can affect the entire nervous system at a very high level of control (i.e., the perineural DC system that extends throughout the body and has roles in regulating injury repair).

In terms of an energetic paradigm for bodywork and movement therapies, there is no need for us to hypothesize that geomagnetic fields, modified by terrestrial and extraterrestrial events, entrain brain waves. Scientists from around the world have already done so and continue to build solid supporting evidence.

An Attempt at Replicating the Zimmerman Study

The fascinating concept from the studies summarized here is that the human body may have a system, probably involving the magnetite-containing pineal gland, for sensing subtle variations in weak geophysical fields that are modulated by the movements and energies in the celestial environment (Figure 15.15). Baldwin et al. (2013) attempted to replicate the Zimmerman study described above, using a more sensitive magnetometer and a more completely shielded chamber at the Scripps Institute in La Jolla, CA. Their focus was on the electromagnetic fields radiated from the hands and hearts of Reiki masters. While the SQUID magnetometer detected fields related to the heartbeat, no signals > 3 pT were observed. However, the investigators pointed out that the strong magnetic shielding used in their study probably blocked the Schumann resonance. The shielding used in the original Zimmerman study, 2-inch thick aluminum, did not block the Schumann resonance. A superficial interpretation is that the Zimmerman results were not confirmed; a closer look supports the idea that the Schumann resonance could modulate the pineal gland and thence the overall field of a therapist.

Some Conclusions

In the past, many conventional doctors accepted or at least tolerated Therapeutic Touch because it seemed harmless but doubted that the method had any real value. Medical research is changing this picture. We now know that the various energy therapies, including both complementary methods and those approved for medical practice (PEMF devices), have many similarities in terms of their effectiveness in stimulating tissue healing, and in terms of the mechanisms by which they influence tissues. A common denominator is the production of low intensity pulsating magnetic fields that induce tiny currents to flow within tissues. Infrared energy (heat) and other forms of energy are probably involved as well (Figure 15.10). As similar cellular and molecular mechanisms appear to be involved, the extensive research on the effectiveness and safety of PEMF devices, non-contact Therapeutic Touch, acupuncture (see Eskinazi, 1996) and a variety of other energy methods tend to support each other.

It is fascinating that practitioners of Therapeutic Touch and related methods seem to produce measurable biomagnetic fields that are not steady in frequency. The emitted field appears to sweep or scan through a variety of frequencies in the ELF range (see Figure 15.8). This is the same range of frequencies that biomedical researchers are finding effective for jump-starting healing in a variety of soft and hard tissues.

References

Adrian, E.D., Bronk, D.W., 1929. Motor nerve fibers. Part II. The frequency of discharge in reflex and voluntary contractions. J. Physiol. 67, 19–51.

Andersen, P., Andersson, S.A., 1968. Physiological Basis of the Alpha Rhythm. Appleton-Century Crofts, New York, NY.

Babbitt, E.D., 1896. The Principles of Light and Color. College of Fine Forces, East Orange, NJ.

Baldwin, A.L., Rand, W.L., Schwartz, G.E., 2013. Practicing Reiki does not appear to routinely produce high-intensity electromagnetic fields from the heart or hands of Reiki practitioners. J. Altern. Complement. Med. 19 (6), 518–526.

Balser, M., Wagner, C.A., 1960. Observation of earth: ionosphere cavity resonances. Nature 188, 4751.

Bassett, C.A.L., 1995. Bioelectromagnetics in the service of medicine. In: Blank, M. (Ed.), Electromagnetic Fields: Biological Interactions and Mechanisms. Advances in Chemistry Series, vol. 250. American Chemical Society, Washington, DC, pp. 261–275.

Bassett, C.A.L., Mitchell, S.N., Gaston, S.R., 1982. Pulsing electromagnetic field treatment in ununited fractures and failed arthrodeses. J. Am. Med. Assoc. 247, 623–628.

Becker, R.O., 1961. Search for evidence of axial current flow in the peripheral nerves of the salamander. Science 134, 101–102.

Becker, R.O., 1963. Relationship of geomagnetic environment to human biology. N. Y. State J. Med. 1, 2215–2219.

Becker, R.O., 1990a. Cross Currents: The Perils of Electropollution, The Promise of Electromedicine. Jeremy P. Tarcher, Los Angeles, CA, p. 80 (Figs 3-4).

Becker, R.O., 1990b. The machine brain and properties of the mind. Subtle Energies 1, 79–87.

Becker, R.O., 1991. Evidence for a primitive DC electrical analog system controlling brain function. Subtle Energies 2, 71–88.

Bentov, I., 1976. Micromotion of the body as a factor in the development of the nervous system. In: Sannella, L. (Ed.), Kundalini: Psychosis or Transcendence? Integral Publishing, Lower Lake, CA (appendix A).

Berger, H., 1929. Uber das Elektrenkephalogramm des Menschen. Archiv fur Psykchiatrica 87, 527–570.

Brighton, C.T., Black, J., Friedenberg, Z.B., Esterhai, J.L., Connolly, J.F., 1981. A multicenter study of the treatment of non-union with constant direct current. J. Bone Joint Surg. Am. 63A, 1–13.

Chaitow, L., 1987. Soft-Tissue Manipulation. Thorsons, Wellingborough, UK.

Chien, C.-H., Tsuei, J.J., Lee, S.C., Huang, Y.-C., Wei, Y.-H., 1991. Effect of emitted bioenergy on biochemical functions of cells. Am. J. Chin. Med. 19, 285–292.

Cram, J.R., Steger, J.C., 1983. EMG scanning in the diagnosis of chronic pain. Biofeedback Self Regul. 8 (2), 229–241.

Cremer-Bartels, G., Krause, K., Mitoskas, G., 1984. Magnetic field of the earth as additional zeitgeber for endogenous rhythms? Naturwissenschaften 71, 567–574.

Davson, H., 1970. A Textbook of General Physiology, fourth ed. Williams and Wilkins, Baltimore, MD, p. 559.

Destexhe, A., Babloyantz, A., Sejnowski, T.J., 1993. Ionic mechanisms for intrinsic slow oscillations in thalamic relay neurons. Biophys. J. 65, 1538–1552.

Direnfeld, L.K., 1983. The genesis of the EEG and its relation to electromagnetic radiation. J. Bioelec. 2, 111–121.

Dubrov, A.P., 1978. The Geomagnetic Field and Life: Geomagnetobiology. Plenum Press, New York, NY.

Einthoven, W., 1906. Le télécardiogramme. Arch. Int. physiol. 4, 132–174.

Enander, B., Larson, G., 1977. Microwave radiometric measurements of the temperature inside a body. Electron. Lett. 10, 317.

Eskinazi, D.P. (Ed.), 1996. NIH Technology Assessment Workshop on Alternative Medicine: Acupuncture. J. Altern. Complement. Med., vol. 2. pp. 1–256.

Eyster, J.A.E., Maresch, F., Krasno, M.R., 1933. The nature of the electric field around the heart. Am. J. Physiol. 106, 574–588.

Fregly, M.J., Fregly, M.S., 1982. Edward F. Adolph. Physiologist 25 (1), 1.

Friedman, H., Becker, R.O., Bachman, C., 1963. Geomagnetic parameters and psychiatric hospital admissions. Nature 200, 626–628.

Friedman, H., Becker, R.O., Bachman, C., 1965. Psychiatric ward behaviour and geophysical parameters. Nature 205, 1050–1052.

Friedman, H., Becker, R.O., Bachman, C., 1967. Effect of magnetic fields on reaction time performance. Nature 213, 949–956.

Galejs, J., 1972. Terrestrial Propagation of Long Electromagnetic Waves. Pergamon Press, Oxford, UK, New York, NY.

Gauguelin, M., 1974. The Cosmic Clocks. Avon Books, New York, NY.

Goodwin, T.J., 2003. Physiological and Molecular Genetic Effects of Time-Varying Electromagnetic Fields on Human Neuronal Cells. NASA/TP-2003-212054.

Gotch, F., 1903. The time relations of the photoelectric changes on the eyeball of the frog. J. Physiol. 29, 388–416.

Gould, J.L., 1984. Magnetic field sensitivity in animals. Annu. Rev. Physiol. 46, 585–598.

Guyton, A.C., 1991. Textbook of Medical Biology, eighth ed. W.B. Saunders, Philadelphia, PA, fig 59.1, p. 662.

Hamer, J.R., 1968. Effects of low level, low frequency electric fields on human time. Comm. Behav. Biol. 2 (Part A), 217–222.

Hamer, J.R., 1969. Effects of low level, low frequency electric fields on human time judgment. In: Fifth International Biometeorological Congress, Montreux, Switzerland.

Holmgren, F., 1865. Method att objectivera effecten af ljusintryck på retina. Uppsala Läk. För. Förh. 1, 184–198.

Kandel, E.R., Schwartz, J.H., Jessell, T.M., Siegelbaum, S.A., Hudspeth, A.J. (Eds.), 2012. Principles of Neural Science, fifth ed. McGraw-Hill Professional, New York, NY.

Khalil, A.M., Qassem, W., 1991. Cytogenetic effects of pulsing electromagnetic field on human lymphocytes in vitro: chromosome aberrations, sister-chromatid exchanges and cell kinetics. Mutat. Res. 247 (1), 141–146.

Kobayashi, A.J., Kirschvink, L., 1995. Magnetoreception and EMF effects: sensory perception of the geomagnetic field in Animals & Humans. In: Blank, M. (Ed.), Electromagnetic Fields: Biological Interactions and Mechanisms. American Chemical Society Books, Washington, DC, pp. 367–394.

Konig, H.L., 1974. ELF and VLF signal properties: physical characteristics. In: Persinger, M.A. (Ed.), ELF and VLF Electromagnetic Field Effects. Plenum Press, New York, NY, pp. 9–34.

Krieger, D., 1975. Therapeutic touch: the imprimatur of nursing. Am. J. Nurs. 5, 784–787.

Lee, R.H. (Ed.), 1999. Scientific Investigations into Chinese Qigong. China Healthways Institute, San Clemente, CA.

Leonard, G., 1978. The Silent Pulse: A Search for the Perfect Rhythm that Exists in Each of Us. Dutton, New York, NY.

Lerchl, A., Zachmann, A., Ali, M.A., Reiter, R.J., 1998. The effects of pulsing magnetic fields on pineal melatonin synthesis in a teleost fish (brook trout, Salvelinus fontinalis). Neurosci. Lett. 256 (3), 171–173.

Liboff, A.R., MeLeod, B.R., Smith, S.D., 1993. Method and Apparatus for the Treatment of Cancer. Patent No. 5,211,622.

Lin, Y., Nishimura, R., Nozaki, K., Sasaki, N., Kadosawa, T., Goto, N., Date, M., Takeuchi, A., 1992. Effects of pulsing electromagnetic fields on the ligament healing in rabbits. J. Vet. Med. Sci. 54 (5), 1017–1022.

Lin, Y., Nishimura, R., Nozaki, K., Sasaki, N., Kadosawa, T., Goto, N., Date, M., Takeuchi, A., 1993. Collagen production and maturation at the experimental ligament defect stimulated by pulsing electromagnetic fields in rabbits. J. Vet. Med. Sci. 55 (4), 527–531.

Mackean, D.G., 1973. Introduction to Biology. John Murray, London.

Marinelli, R., van der Furst, B., Zee, H., McGinn, A., Marinelli, W., 1995. The heart is not a pump: a refutation of the pressure propulsion premise of heart function. Frontier Perspectives 5, 15–24.

Matsunaga, S., Sakou, T., Ijiri, K., 1996. Osteogenesis by pulsing electromagnetic fields (PEMFs): optimum stimulation setting. In Vivo 10 (3), 351–356.

McCraty, R., Atkinson, M., Tomasino, D., Tiller, W.A., 1998. The electricity of touch: detection and measurement of cardiac energy exchange between people. In: Pribram, K.H. (Ed.), Brain and Values: Is a Biological Science of Values Possible. Lawrence Erlbaum Associates, Publishers, Mahwah, NJ, pp. 359–379.

Mesmer, A., 1948. Mesmerism: With an Introduction by Gilbert Frankau. Macdonald, London (This is Mesmer's Memoir of 1779.).

Miyagi, N., Sato, K., Rong, Y., Yamamura, S., Katagiri, H., Kobayashi, K., Iwata, H., 2000. Effects of PEMF on a murine osteosarcoma cell line: drug-resistant (P-glycoprotein-positive) and non-resistant cells. Bioelectromagnetics 21 (2), 112–121.

Muehsam, D.J., Markov, M.S., Muehsam, P.A., Pilla, A.A., Shen, R., Wu, Y., 1994. Effects of Qigong on cell-free myosin phosphorylation: preliminary experiments. Subtle Energies 5, 93–108.

Niu, X., Liu, G., Yu, Z., 1992. Secondary acoustic biological response. In: Lee, R.H. (Ed.), Scientific Investigations into Chinese QiGong. China Healthways Institute, San Clemente, CA.

Oschman, J.L., 1993. A biophysical basis for acupuncture. In: Proceedings of the First Symposium of the Society for Acupuncture Research, Rockville, MD, 23-24 January.

Oschman, J.L., Oschman, N.H., 1994. Physiological and emotional effects of acupuncture needle insertion. In: Proceedings of the Second Symposium of the Society for Acupuncture Research, Washington, DC, 17-18 September.

Perry, F.S., Reichmanis, M., Marino, A., Becker, R.O., 1981. Environmental power-frequency magnetic fields and suicide. Health Phys. 41, 267–277.

Popp, F.A., Li, K.H., Gu, Q. (Eds.), 1992. Recent Advances in Biophoton Research and Its Applications. World Scientific, Singapore.

Pressman, A.S., 1970. Electromagnetic Fields and Life. Plenum Press, New York, NY.

QiGong Institute, 1995. The QiGong database is available for Macintosh and IBM or DOS compatible computers from the QiGong Institute. East West Academy of Healing Arts, San Francisco, CA.

Quinn, J.F., 1984. Therapeutic touch as energy exchange: testing the theory. Adv. Nurs. Sci. 6, 42–49.

Quinn, J.F., 1992. The Senior's Therapeutic Touch Education Program. Holistic Nurse Practitioner 7, 32–37.

Quinn, J.F., 1993. Psychoimmunologic effects of therapeutic touch on practitioners and recently bereaved recipients: a pilot study. Adv. Nurs. Sci. 15, 13–26.

Rajaram, M., Mitra, S., 1981. Correlation between convulsive seizure and geomagnetic activity. Neurosci. Lett. 24, 187–191.

Ratner, S., 1979. The dynamic state of body proteins. Ann. N. Y. Acad. Sci. 325, 189–209.

Rattemeyer, M., Popp, F.A., Nagl, W., 1981. Evidence of photon emission from DNA in living systems. Naturwissenschaften 68, 572–573.

Reilly, W., Reeve, V.E., Quinn, C., McMakin, C. Anti-inflammatory Effects of Interferential Frequency-Specific Applied Microcurrent. Abstract ID: ABSLN-3TVEH-RYZ99-A78C8.

Reite, M., Zimmerman, J., 1978. Magnetic phenomena of the central nervous system. Annu. Rev. Biophys. Bioeng. 7, 167–188.

Reiter, R., 1953. Neuere Untersuchungen zum Problem der Wetterabhangigkeit des Menschen. Archie fair Meterologie. Geophysik and Bioclimatologie B4, 327 (For a review of Reiter's work in English, see Konig, 1974b.).

Russek, L.G., Schwartz, G.E., 1996. Energy cardiology: a dynamical energy systems approach for integrating conventional and alternative medicine. Adv.: J. Mind-Body Health 12, 4–24.

Sakai, A., Suzuki, K., Nakamura, T., Norimura, T., Tsuchiya, T., 1991. Effects of pulsing electromagnetic fields on cultured cartilage cells. Int. Orthop. 15 (4), 341–346.

Sandyk, R., 1995. Treatment of Neurological and Mental Disorders. Patent No. 5,470,846.

Schienle, A., Stark, R., Vaitl, D., 1998. Biological effects of very low frequency (VLF) atmospherics in humans: a review. J. Sci. Explor. 12 (3), 455–468.

Schoenheimer, R., 1942. The Dynamic State of Body Constituents. Harvard University Press, Cambridge, MA.

Schumann, W.O., 1952. On the characteristic oscillations of a conducting sphere which is surrounded by an air layer and an ionospheric shell. Zeitschrift fur Naturforschung 7a, 149–154 (In German. For a summary of Schumann's research in English, see Konig, 1974a.).

Schumann, W.O., Konig, H., 1954. Ober die Beobachtung von Atmospheics bei geringstein Frequenzen. Naturwissenschaften 41, 183.

Schwartz, S.A., DeMattei, R.J., Brame, K.G., Spottiswoode, S.J.P., 1990. Infrared spectra alteration in water proximate to the palms of therapeutic practitioners. Subtle Energies 1, 43–72.

Sentman, D.D., 1995. Schumann resonances. In: Volland, H. (Ed.), Handbook of Atmospheric Electrodynamics, vol. 1. CRC Press, Boca Raton, FL, pp. 267–295.

Seto, A., Kusaka, C., Nakazato, S., et al., 1992. Detection of extraordinary large biomagnetic field strength from human hand. Acupunct. Electrother. Res. 17, 75–94.

Sisken, B.F., Walker, J., 1995. Therapeutic aspects of electromagnetic fields for soft-tissue healing. In: Blank, M. (Ed.), Electromagnetic Fields: Biological Interactions and Mechanisms. Advances in Chemistry Series, vol. 250. American Chemical Society, Washington, DC, pp. 277–285.

Strogatz, S., 2004. Sync: How Order Emerges from Chaos in the Universe, Nature and Daily Life, reprint ed. Hyperion, Santa Clara, CA, 352 pp.

Takahashi, K., Kaneko, I., Date, M., Fukada, E., 1986. Effect of pulsing electromagnetic fields on DNA synthesis in mammalian cells in culture. Experientia 42 (2), 185–186.

Takano-Yamamoto, T., Kawakami, M., Sakuda, M., 1992. Effect of a pulsing electromagnetic field on demineralized bone-matrix-induced bone formation in a bony defect in the premaxilla of rats. J. Dent. Res. 71 (12), 1920–1925.

Takayama, K., Nomura, H., Tanaka, J., Zborowski, M., Harasaki, H., Jacobs, G.B., Malchesky, P.S., Licata, A.A., Nosé, Y., 1990. Effect of a pulsing electromagnetic field on metabolically derived osteoporosis in rats: a pilot study. ASAIO Trans. 36 (3), M426–M428.

Venkatraman, K., 1976. Epilepsy and solar activity: an hypothesis. Neurol. India 24, 1–5.

Verzeano, M., 1970. Evoked responses and network dynamics. In: Whalen, R.E., et al. (Eds.), Neuronal Control of Behavior. Academic Press, New York, NY, pp. 27–54.

Vogt, P.M., Thompson, S., Andree, C., et al., 1994. Genetically modified keratinocytes transplanted to wounds reconstitute the epidermis. Proc. Natl. Acad. Sci. U. S. A. 91, 9307–9311.

Walker, M., 1994. The healing powers of QiGong, Part 3. Townsend Letter for Doctors (April) 296–303.

Wallenstein, G.V., 1994. A model of the electrophysiological properties of nucleus reticularis thalami neurons. Biophys. J. 66, 978–988.

Wever, R., 1968. Einfluss schwacher elektro-magnetischer Felder auf die circadiane Periodik des Menschen. Naturwissenschaften 55. , 29–32. (In German. For a summary of Wever's work in English, see Wever, 1974).

Wever, R., 1974. ELF-effects on human circadian rhythms. In: Persinger, M.A. (Ed.), ELF and VLF Electromagnetic Field Effects. Plenum Press, New York, NY, pp. 101–144.

Zimmerman, J., 1990. Laying-on-of-hands healing and therapeutic touch: a testable theory. BEMI Currents. J. Bio-Electro-Magnetics Inst. 24, 8–17 (Available from Dr. John Zimmerman. See also an article published in 1985: New technologies detect effects of healing hands. Brain/Mind Bulletin 10 (September 30):3).

CHAPTER 16

The Electromagnetic Environment

Introduction

This chapter discusses what may well be the most important health issue of our times, an issue that is intimately involved with energetics and energy medicine. A close look at energetic processes taking place in the human body reveals a great variety of electrical, magnetic, and photonic processes. Every cell and every molecule is 'listening' to its environment and receiving information that enables it to function in concert with the whole body. For example, electrical processes are intimately involved in virtually all cellular processes:

> *Cells undergo a variety of physiological processes, including division, migration and differentiation, under the influence of endogenous electrical cues, which are generated physiologically and pathologically in the extracellular and sometimes intracellular spaces. These signals are transduced to regulate cell behaviours profoundly, both in vitro and in vivo. Bioelectricity influences cellular processes as fundamental as control of the cell cycle, cell proliferation, cancer–cell migration, electrical signaling in the adult brain, embryonic neuronal cell migration, axon outgrowth, spinal-cord repair, epithelial wound repair, tissue regeneration and establishment of left–right body asymmetry. In addition to direct effects on cells, electrical gradients interact with coexisting extracellular chemical gradients. Indeed, cells can integrate and respond to electrical and chemical cues in combination. This Commentary details how electrical signals control multiple cell behaviours and argues that study of the interplay between combined electrical and chemical gradients is underdeveloped yet necessary.*
>
> MCCAIG ET AL. (2009)

Knowledgeable biologists, physicians, and scientists from many fields are recognizing that our technology has been far outpacing our understanding of the effects our favourite devices, such as cellular telephones, are having on our biology. In *Cross Currents: The Perils of Electropollution and the Promise of Electromedicine*, Becker (1990), points out the paradox we find ourselves in with the emergence of electromagnetic medicine, which promises to unlock the secrets of healing, and the growth of electromagnetic pollution, which poses a clear environmental danger. He explains the effectiveness of alternative healing methods that use parts of the body's innate electrical healing systems and warns that these same systems are being adversely affected by power lines, computers, microwaves, and satellite dishes. He predicted that electromagnetic pollution could become more significant than air and water pollution in terms of health effects.

In this chapter, we look first at the natural electromagnetic environment and then at the possible biological effects of electromagnetic pollution. We begin with geophysical and meteorological phenomena that are not widely known to the public. To what extent do these energies complement or interfere with the delicate and intricate electrical and electronic signaling systems that regulate vital biological processes? Can these energies enhance or compromise the nurturing environment of the therapeutic setting? What do patients need to know about this subject to get the most benefit from their therapies? Historical detail is included to help the reader understand that there is an extensive literature on these subjects. Some of this literature is very reliable; some is completely outdated.

Biology and Physics at Odds

Biologists have repeatedly documented the great sensitivity organisms have to exceedingly tiny signals in their environment. A host of sensory systems are employed for a variety of survival purposes. Organisms use energetic cues to locate and orient themselves geographically; to set their biological rhythms; to detect prey, predators, and mates; and to anticipate meteorological and Earth changes, including seasonal variations, weather fronts, hurricanes, tornadoes, and earthquakes (Dubrov, 1978; Ho et al., 1994; Presman, 1970).

Extreme examples of energy sensitivity have been discovered for virtually all living systems at all levels of organization: bacteria, algae, higher plants, protozoa, flatworms, insects such as honeybees, snails, fish, birds such as carrier pigeons, green turtles, sharks, whales, and humans (summarized by Adey and Bawin, 1977; Kalmijn, 1971; Warnke, 1994).

For several decades, physics seemed to be at odds with these discoveries. Physicists treat living systems like other forms of matter. Known or measurable properties of cells and tissues and the established laws of electricity and magnetism are employed to calculate the currents induced in tissues by environmental fields of various sorts. The calculations are based on the degree that fields of different frequencies penetrate into the body, tissue conductivity, viscosity and dielectric properties, interactions of induced currents with larger currents from other sources, the 'noise' from random thermal agitation at body temperature, and so on. A consistent but entirely incorrect conclusion is that environmental fields can have no biological effects on living matter unless the energy intensity is sufficient to ionize or heat tissues (e.g., Foster and Guy, 1986; Foster and Pickard, 1987; Wachtel, 1995). Weaker fields may induce microcurrents in living tissues, but these are millions of times smaller than the noise from thermal agitation and normal physiological signaling processes and should therefore have no biological effects. The biology must be wrong.

The Dilemma Resolved

This physics/biology dilemma was resolved when careful research revealed that biological systems completely defy a simple and obvious logic: Larger stimuli should produce larger responses. In living systems, extremely weak fields may have potent effects, while there may be little or no response to strong fields. A turning point in the controversy came about when scientists from the prestigious Massachusetts Institute of Technology (MIT) Neurosciences Research Program examined the evidence and concluded that:

> ... a striking range of biological interactions has been described in experiments where control procedures appear to have been adequately considered ... The existence of biological effects of very weak electromagnetic fields suggests an extraordinarily efficient mechanism for detecting these fields and discriminating them from much higher levels of noise. The underlying mechanisms must necessarily involve ever increasing numbers of elements in the sensing system, ordered in particular ways to form a cooperative organization and manifesting similar forms and levels of energy over long distances.
>
> ADEY AND BAWIN (1977)

This statement signalled the emergence of a new paradigm in biology that has led to extensive research and clinical investigation into the beneficial and harmful effects of electromagnetic fields. We now know that cells and tissues are highly nonlinear, non-equilibrium, cooperative, and coherent systems, capable of responding to very specific 'windows' (Figure 16.1) in terms of frequency and intensity (Adey, 1990).

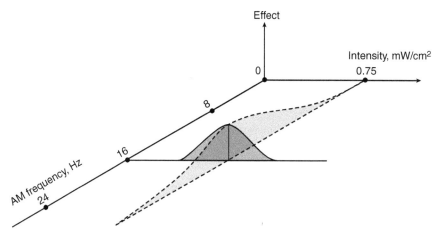

Figure 16.1   A frequency–power window, the frequency–power–density 'window' or 'response surface' for the brain. The measured response was calcium ion efflux from chick forebrain tissue. The fundamental signal frequency was 147 MHz (million cycles per second). This signal was amplitude modulated sinusoidally at selected frequencies and power densities. This study, published by Blackman and colleagues (1979) confirmed earlier work by Bawin et al. (1975) who reported that brain tissue has a maximum frequency sensitivity in the extremely low frequency (ELF) range between 6 and 20 Hz and intensity of 10^{-7} V/cm. This is the level associated with navigation and prey detection in marine vertebrates and with control of human biological rhythms. The amplitude modulated microwave signal has an intensity window around 10^{-1} V/cm. This is at the level of the electroencephalogram (EEG) in brain tissue (see also Adey, 1980). *(Blackman, C.F., Elder, J.A., Weil, C.M., Benane, S.G., Eichinger, D.C., House, D.E., 1979. Induction of calcium-ion efflux from brain tissue by radio-frequency radiation: effects of modulation frequency and field strength. Radio Sci. 14 (6S), 93–98.)*

Clinical Applications

Biomedical researchers have been testing the use of pulsing magnetic fields originating outside the organism to induce microcurrents within tissues to stimulate healing (see Chapter 6). A consistent observation is that triggering a cellular response requires the application of energy in a very narrow range of frequencies and intensities (Bassett, 1978, 1995). Extensive research on fracture nonunions led to the statement that 'jump starting a car with a dead battery creates an operational machine; exposure of a nonunion to PEMFs can convert a stalled healing process to active repair, even in patients unhealed for as long as 40 years!' (Bassett, 1995).

Microampere currents induced from outside the body restart the healing process by recruiting bone-forming cells in a manner similar to a natural repair response. Field effects are highly specific and confined to a narrow power frequency window. Too high an induced current stimulates tissue necrosis rather than repair. And the characteristics of a 'bone healing pulse' are different from those of an 'osteonecrosis pulse'.

In Chapter 15 it was also shown that there is a similarity between the frequencies and intensities of low energy emissions from the hands of therapists and the signals from pulsed electromagnetic field (PEMF) devices used in clinical medicine. Medical researchers have documented a cascade of signal transduction processes from the cell membrane to the nucleus and on to the genetic material that are facilitated by PEMF therapies (Bassett, 1995). Polarity, Reiki, Therapeutic Touch, acupuncture, and many hands-on therapies probably affect the same signal pathways. Evidence presented later will describe how electromagnetic pollution at somewhat higher frequencies (50 or 60 Hz) appears to have negative effects on the same pathways.

Mechanisms

Much is being learned about the biophysical mechanisms involved in the amplification of tiny signals to produce significant physiological and behavioural effects (e.g., Ho et al., 1994; Oschman, 2000). All of this information has relevance to energy therapists who wish to validate and explain their experiences.

Biologists accept that living molecules exist in the context of a myriad of violent and random thermal fluctuations. Yet cells and tissues and organs must maintain their precise and intricate actions and reactions, responses and adjustments, unperturbed by the thermal noise. In order to survive, living systems have developed a variety of tricks to get around the more obvious physical limits to sensitivity.

Of particular importance in understanding the physical mechanisms involved was the realization that molecular 'sensors' in living systems are actually highly ordered arrays of molecules. These are the 'ever increasing numbers of elements in the sensing system, ordered in particular ways to form a cooperative organization and manifesting similar forms and levels of energy over long distances' mentioned in the Adey and Bawin (1977) quotation above.

Frohlich and others have described the physics and sensitivity of molecular arrays in great detail (Fröhlich, 1968a,b, 1970, 1974, 1975, 1988; Ho, 1998). Fröhlich focused on the arrays of phospholipid molecules in cell membranes, but there are many other arrays in living tissues (Figure 16.2). All of these are electrically polarized and are probable components of the sensing apparatus:

- Arrays of phospholipid molecules in cell membranes
- Collagen arrays in connective tissues
- Arrays of chlorophyll molecules in the leaf
- Myelin sheaths of nerves
- Contractile arrays in muscles
- Arrays of sensory endings in the retina
- Arrays of microtubules, microfilaments, and other fibrous components of the cytoskeleton in nerves and other kinds of cells, including the cilia of sensory organs such as those responsible for detecting odours, sounds, and gravity (the vestibular apparatus)

In general, organisms are poised to respond to minute 'whispers' in the electromagnetic environment. Bassett (1995) suggested a fascinating analogy between the arrays of bone cells in the osteon and the phased arrays of radio-telescope antennas, such as those at Jodrell Bank in Cheshire, England (Figure 16.3). Radio-telescope arrays enable astrophysicists to detect extremely weak electromagnetic signals from nebulae thousands of millions of light years away. Bassett suggested that tissues extract information from fields originating outside the body by a physical process akin to that involved in radio astronomy (Figure 16.3). This author (Oschman, 2000) hypothesized that the collagen and mineral arrays of the bone probably serve as the antenna array, while the cellular osteon contains the electronic solid state circuitry that detects and interprets the information contained in electromagnetic fields. This hypothetical concept could apply to all of the cellular and tissue arrays listed above and shown in Figure 16.2. Note that these arrays make up much of the structural features of the living organism.

The physical mechanisms suggested by Fröhlich and Bassett are not the only models that have been proposed. Other concepts are described by Bridges and Preache (1981), Lednev (1991), and Liboff (1985).

Biosensors

We now examine some of the specific sensory systems found in nature.

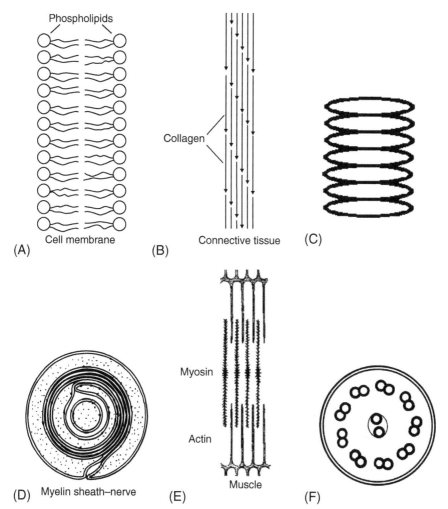

Phospholipids

Cell membrane
(A)

Collagen

Connective tissue
(B)

(C)

Myosin

Actin

Muscle

(D) Myelin sheath–nerve

(E)

(F)

Figure 16.2 Crystalline arrays in living systems. Crystalline arrangements are the rule and not the exception in living systems. (A) Arrays of phospholipid molecules form cell membranes. (B) Collagen arrays form connective tissue. (C) Arrays of chlorophyll molecules in the leaf. (D) The myelin sheath of nerves. (E) The contractile array in muscle is composed of actin and myosin molecules organized around each other. (F) Arrays of microtubules, microfilaments, and other fibrous components of cytoskeleton occur in nerves and other kinds of cells. The example shown here is the cilium of sensory organs such as those responsible for detecting odours and sounds. *(Illustration (D) is reproduced with permission of Arnold.)*

THE RETINA

The most remarkable and thoroughly studied sensor in the human body is the eye. The retina contains a protein, rhodopsin, which absorbs light. Careful research, which is still in progress, is showing how the rhodopsin molecule is designed for its task. Energy is stored within its structure in such a way that a single photon can activate a large shift in molecular structure. This shift triggers a cascade of chemical reactions, the flow of millions of sodium ions across the rod cell membrane, and an electrical signal that is transmitted by the optic nerves to the brain. In essence, the absorption of each photon is amplified many times to produce a nerve impulse (Stryer, 1985, 1987, 1988).

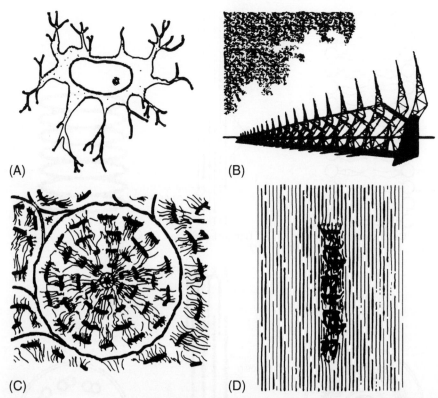

Figure 16.3 Bone compared to a radio-telescope array. Bassett (1995) made the analogy between the array of osteocytes in the osteon and the phased radio-telescope array. (A) A single osteocyte. There is a central nucleus and a large number of slender processes or extensions of the cell surface. (B) A phased array of radio-telescope antennas such as those at Jodrell Bank in England. (C) An osteon, the cylindrical unit of compact bone. Each osteon has a blood vessel running through its center, and this is surrounded by an array of electrically interconnected osteocytes. (D) The osteon is embedded in another array composed of collagen molecules. These are precisely offset, like the elements of a radio-telescope array. *(Panel B: Redrawn from Hoyle (1962), p. 202, and used with kind permission from Sir Fred Hoyle. Panel C: Adapted with permission from Bassett (1995), Copyright © 1995, American Chemical Society.)*

OTHER SENSES

The retina is just one of the sensory systems that enable the organism to build up an accurate image and awareness of itself in relation to its surroundings. The traditional five senses are sight, hearing, smell, taste, and touch. However, it is obvious that there are other senses besides the traditional five. Murchie (1978) lists 32. As an example, some people can 'hear' radar, an electromagnetic signal in the microwave region of the electromagnetic spectrum (Guy et al., 1975). An ability to detect cosmic rays with the eye has been documented (D'Arcy and Porter, 1962; Wick, 1972). There is discussion of whether these sensory systems are also able to respond to a single quantum of energy, as the retina appears to be able to do (Bialek, 1987).

The Natural Electromagnetic Energy Spectrum

GEOMAGNETISM

Geomagnetism is far more widely researched than most people realize. Chapman and Bartels (1940) wrote a 1000-page book that collected and reviewed some 100,000 pages of printed matter on the subject. In 1967, 27 years later, Matsushita and Campbell (1967) edited a two-volume work that attempted to cover the enormous amount of new literature that followed the earlier review. By 1987, four volumes, written by more than 25 authors, were required to treat the phenomenally growing area of research (Jacobs, 1987). A bimonthly journal, *Geomagnetism and Aeronomy*, was begun in 1961 and continues to publish research articles on the ionosphere, geomagnetism, and atmospheric radio noise.

GEOMAGNETIC VARIATIONS

The magnetic field of the Earth, called the geomagnetic field, causes the compass needle to point towards the North Pole. However, if you look carefully at a compass needle with a microscope, you will see that the needle is rarely still – it dances back and forth in a variety of rhythms.

Oscillations of the compass needle were first observed by the great London clockmaker George Graham. In 1722 and 1723, Graham made over 1000 observations of the compass declination at his house on Fleet Street (Graham, 1724). He observed the declination at different times during the day, using three 12-inch compasses that had delicate pivots and fine graduations so that the slightest movements could be detected. He noted that 'all of the needles … would not only vary in their direction on different days but at different times on the same day, and this difference would sometimes amount to upwards of 30 minutes or 1/degree in 1 day, sometimes in a few hours'.

- These results were confirmed by Celsius and Hiorter in Uppsala, Sweden, during the period 1740–1747. On the clear night of March 1, 1741, Hiorter noticed a large oscillation of the needle, through several degrees, in sympathy with the northern lights or aurora borealis (quoted by Hansteen, 1819). In the same year (1741), Celsius and Graham collaborated to determine if the compass variations occurred simultaneously in different places. On April 5, 1741, the magnetic needle at London had an unusual motion at the same time that a disturbance of nearly 2° was recorded in Uppsala. Alexander von Humboldt termed these disturbances 'magnetic storms' (see Malin, 1987).
- On quiet, undisturbed days there are still variations in the direction of north. Geomagnetic rhythms range in frequency from moment-to-moment to millions of years. The rhythmic variations over the past 4 million years have been documented by studying magnetic minerals in deep-sea sediments collected by drilling core samples (Valet and Meynadier, 1993).
- In the late 1830s, von Humboldt, in collaboration with Gauss, formed the Gottingen Magnetic Union to organize the data from observatories that maintained records of the magnetic variations. Intensive observations were made on certain days each year. The results were published in six Annual Reports of the Magnetic Union (1836–1841).
- By 1987, there were some 150 magnetic observatories around the world. Here the direction of the magnetic field is monitored continuously using a variometer and recorded on a magnetogram. A light beam is reflected from a mirror attached to the compass and focused onto a sheet of photographic paper on a drum rotating once per day. The recorded data are tabulated, sent to World Data centers, and published in yearbooks that are distributed to libraries around the world (see Wienert, 1970).

Some of the geomagnetic rhythms are diurnal (24 h), some are much slower, and others are quite fast, in the extremely low frequency (ELF) range in the electromagnetic spectrum. The latter are now called geomagnetic micropulsations. They are caused by a unique geophysical mechanism known as the Schumann resonance.

Other Extraterrestrial Sources

In addition to the Schumann resonance and VLF-atmospherics or sferics (see Chapter 15), the surface of the Earth is exposed to a variety of other extraterrestrial electromagnetic signals, including X-rays and cosmic rays. Volland (1984) is a good source of information on this subject.

We have described the Schumann resonance and VLF-sferics because they are the phenomena most widely studied for their possible biological effects.

Geopathic Stress

Many investigators have identified 'earth radiations' occurring at particular 'pathogenic sites' that can be detected with sensitive magnetometers, dowsing, or by observing animals. European traditions describe observing a herd of sheep before building a house. The spot where sheep bed down for the night is free of geopathic stress and is thus the best area for the master bedroom. Dowsers recognize that sheep, like most mammals (except cats) instinctively know how to avoid geopathic zones.

Some scientists are highly skeptical about both geopathic stress and dowsing. However, some European and American physicians take them extremely seriously. The author was convinced about dowsing after watching the head of the local water department using dowsing rods to successfully locate underground water pipes.

Underground fluid flows, as in springs or pipes, are thought to distort natural magnetic fields and other radiations from the Earth or atmosphere. Where water and/or electric currents flow at different depths and cross each other, beneficial or harmful interference patterns can be set up.

Modern investigation began in 1922 with a study of unusually high cancer deaths in Vilsbiburg, Germany. Health records were compared with geopathic lines mapped by a dowser. There was a 100% correlation between geopathic stress zones and cancer deaths (von Pohl, 1985). The study was repeated in larger and smaller German and Austrian towns, with always the same results - 100% correlation. Hence geopathic stress is widely recognized in Germany, where efforts are made to keep health records on individual homes (Best, 1988a,b; Smith and Best, 1989a; and Miller, 1998).

Some clinicians can identify signs of geopathic stress in cancer patients and find the information essential to their treatments. It is important that one's bed not be located above a geopathic zone (Figure 16.4). Sleeping in such a region can affect the body's energetic communication

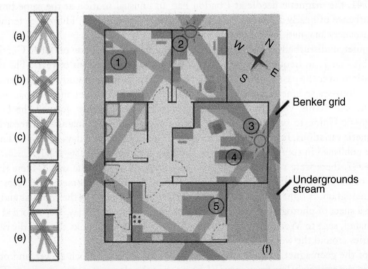

Figure 16.4 Geopathic stress zones can be detected with a sensitive recording magnetometer that profiles the magnetic variations in an area such as a bed place (Wooster 1988). Dowsing can also map these zones. The grids are referred to as Ley lines, Curry lines, the Hartmann grid, or the Benker grid. Sometimes moving a bed or chair a short distance reduces the geopathic stress on the occupant and enables them to recover from a seemingly incurable condition. Rolf Gordon and Dulwich Health, UK (2013) reported that in all cancer cases studied, the tumors first developed where two or more geopathic stress lines crossed: (a) brain tumor, (b) cervical cancer, (c) tumor in right lung, (d) prostate cancer, (e) cancer in right breast. A floor plan (f) shows sources of geopathic stress, including a Benker grid and an underground water stream. The evaluation: Position 1: master bed touches the grid only slightly, mostly o.k. Position 2: child's bed is badly affected and should be moved. Positions 3&4: living room, chair (3) and sofa (4) should be moved. Position 5: kitchen is ok, as the time spent there is limited, but avoid the seat on the right bench, if possible. *(a-e from Gordon, 2013; (f) is from http://geopathology.com/geopathic-stress.html.)*

systems, compromise the immune system, and make one vulnerable to serious disease (Aschoff and Aschoff, 1986). In Britain, the Dulwich Health Society has documented many case histories and published methods for assessing and preventing geopathic stress (Gordon, 2013). Moving a bed or chair a few feet can certainly do no harm, and sometimes seems to have great health benefits.

The Energy Spectrum of Technology

It is only within the last 100 years that electricity has become abundantly available throughout much of the world. This has led to the evolution of the enormous range of devices, appliances, and technologies that we take for granted, seldom appreciating that none of this existed but a short time ago. The 'filling in' of the electromagnetic spectrum over the last century is dramatically illustrated by Figure 16.5. In a very short time, in a few generations, we have gone from a relatively quiet natural electromagnetic environment to one that is literally packed with signals of every sort.

Our technologies expose us to far more than a mixture of frequencies emitted by a host of devices. We enjoy a variety of appliances, such as electric blankets, hair dryers, food mixers, coffee mills, refrigerators, stoves, microwave ovens, sewing machines, coffee pots, heating pads, computers, televisions, radios, cell phones, water beds, and others. Each device produces a variety of signals while it is being used. Some of these energies are radiated directly into the tissues of nearby organisms, while some energy goes back into the power grid and travels a certain distance through it. Moreover, each device has controls that we use to turn it on and off, or to adjust its operations. Using each of these adjustments can set up transients, or pulses, or spikes with complex harmonics. These signals too are radiated into nearby tissues and also enter the power distribution system and travel a certain distance. The pulses can interact with other fields and transients to produce complex interference patterns. These intricate and unpredictable signals can be conducted from

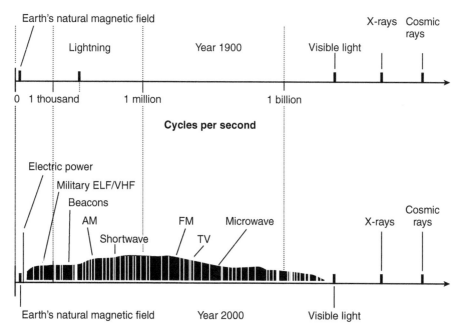

Figure 16.5 The filling-in of the electromagnetic spectrum. During the last 100 years, our electromagnetic environment has gone from a naturally quiet place to one that is literally packed with signals of every sort. *(After Becker (1990), pp. 79, 188, 189, with kind permission from Robert O. Becker, MD.)*

one appliance to another, where they interact with another set of electrical or electronic components and the fields they are generating. Signals from radio, TV, cell phones, wireless pagers, satellite uplinks and downlinks, and natural geomagnetic and geoelectric phenomena can also be collected by the power distribution grid, which acts as a huge antenna. All of these signals can interact to produce intense but unpredictable energetic 'hot spots' in particular regions of space.

'We have never encountered poor engineering in nature' (Albrecht-Buehler, 1985). The electrical and electronic signals within the living system are honed to perfection. Each molecule has its electromagnetic signature (Benveniste, 1998; Oschman, 1997b). Each molecular interaction and each physiological process generates fields as well. All of these fields are compatible. In normal tissues, interferences and incompatibilities do not occur. Within the body, thousands of physiological and biochemical and electronic processes take place each second. Each heartbeat, each breath, each emotion generates characteristic electromagnetic fields that travel through the body to cells and tissues a distance away. The result is coordination, integration, interdigitation of processes. When problems arise in this marvellous and intricate web, bodywork and movement therapies can restore order. In contrast to our organized and smoothly operating internal environment, the external electromagnetic background is chaotic and unpredictable.

Conclusions About Our Natural Environment

Our present understanding of the natural and artificial energy fields in our environment is based on much careful research. This chapter provides a taste of the enormous amount of information that is available. The details are relevant to hands-on therapists of all schools who wish to educate themselves and their clients about both energy therapies and the invisible energies in their environment.

Three areas of investigation are particularly significant for developing a theoretical basis for energetic therapies of all kinds:

- Studies of the mechanisms by which sensory systems extract information from the environment
- Studies of the ways PEMF therapies trigger beneficial effects at the same frequencies and strengths as the signals emitted from the hands of therapists
- Studies of the tissue and cell effects of 50 and 60 cycle power signals, as well as microwaves and other radio frequencies

The last of these will be discussed in the next part of this chapter, which will also consider the potential hazards present in our electromagnetic environment and what can be done about them.

The Electromagnetic Environment: Biological Effects

The question of all questions for humanity, the problem which lies behind all others and is more interesting than any of them, is that of the determination of [our] place in nature and [our] relation to the cosmos.

T.H. HUXLEY QUOTED IN SEYMOUR (1988), P. 211

About 2500 years ago, Hippocrates recognized the significance of the weather and climate on living systems (Jones, 1948). In the twentieth century, the relations between natural electromagnetic rhythms and living systems were explored in the pioneering work of Harold Saxton Burr and his colleagues at Yale University School of Medicine (for references, see Burr, 1957). In the 1950s, a visitor to Burr's ancestral home, Mansewood, in Lyme, Connecticut, would discover various kinds of trees connected to recording voltmeters. Burr was studying how the electric fields of trees change in advance of weather patterns and other atmospheric phenomena. His research had convinced him that life on Earth is not isolated from the rest of the universe but is susceptible to forces extending across vast distances of space. The fields within the human body are inevitably affected by the larger fields of the planet and other celestial bodies. The mechanisms involved are not mystical or obscure – they involve well-documented pathways of interaction. For example, sunspots and the cycles of the moon cause changes in ionospheric currents and geophysical fields that in turn influence the fields within us.

To Burr it was obvious that the energies so thoroughly studied by physicists surround, penetrate, and are produced by every organism. He was convinced that all living things, from mice to men, from seeds to trees, are formed and controlled by fields that can be measured with standard detectors. The fields reflect physical and mental conditions and can therefore be useful for diagnosis. Burr obtained evidence that abnormal fields show up before serious pathology sets in and that balancing or restoring the field can reverse disease processes.

These concepts are also part of the core theory of acupuncture and related methods and are being validated by modern biomedical research on cancer and acquired immunodeficiency syndrome (AIDS) (Brewitt, 1996, 1999).

Burr's discoveries paralleled those of another controversial scientist, Frank A. Brown, Jr., who documented the abilities of plants and animals to synchronize their biological clocks with the large-scale rhythms of nature (Brown, 1973). In addition to a lifetime of research on biological clocks, Brown was responsible for the translations into English of two valuable books, *Electromagnetic Fields and Life* (Presman, 1970) and *The Geomagnetic Field and Life* (Dubrov, 1978).

Another important investigator in this area was Gauquelin (1966, 1974). The conclusions of all of these scientists regarding the externally driven biological clocks were confirmed by Wever (1968), who showed that shielding humans from natural electromagnetic fields desynchronized their biological rhythms. Further confirmation came from studies of the relations between reaction time and ELF micropulsations from approaching thunderstorms (Moore-Ede et al., 1992; Reiter, 1953) as detailed in Chapter 15.

All of the scientists mentioned above were following in the footsteps of one of the world's foremost chemists, Svante Arrhenius, who developed the theory for the way salts dissolve in water and then went on to study the relationships between environmental fields and health (see Ward, 1971). Arrhenius' profound insight came in a flash on the night of May 17, 1883. After a sleepless night working through the concept, Arrhenius raced to his thesis advisor to present his theory. His professor looked at him through skeptical eyes and said, 'You have a new theory? That is very interesting. Goodbye'.

Arrhenius's doctoral thesis was graded 'fourth class' by the then-conservative faculty at the University of Uppsala. His ideas challenged concepts of the establishment and were strongly opposed. It was years before his theory came to be accepted by chemists everywhere, leading to great progress. In 1903, Arrhenius received the Nobel Prize, and in 1909, King Oscar II installed him as director of the Nobel Institute for Physical Chemistry at Stockholm. Here Arrhenius was given the situation every scientist dreams of: ideal conditions to study whatever interested him.

Soon Arrhenius turned his attention to cosmic influences on the behaviour of plants, animals, and humans. He found data on the periodic occurrence of bronchitis, epilepsy, birth and death rates, and the human ovulation cycle. He concluded that biological rhythms correlate with rhythms and tides in the cosmic forces that surround the Earth. He suggested that the electrical tension in the air influences biochemical reactions and thereby affects all living things. His work laid the groundwork for one of the stormiest controversies of modern biology.

Weather Sensitivity

A large percentage of the population is weather sensitive (reviewed by Schienle et al., 1998). Those who are unaware of this phenomenon are puzzled by the sudden onset of headaches, sleepiness, indigestion, phantom limb pain, asthma, sleep disorders, fatigue, confusion, or other symptoms, often prior to weather changes. Part of the problem is that a lightning storm can precipitate physiological changes, and then swerve off in a different direction, leaving the weather-sensitive individual unaware of the cause of discomfort. Emotional and behavioural changes and their consequences have also been observed: increases in crime rates, suicides, memory loss, lack of concentration, prolonged reaction times, and automobile and industrial accidents.

Allergies

Information about environmental electromagnetic fields is of increasing importance as more and more people are developing electromagnetic sensitivities (Best, 1984, 1988a,b; Choy et al., 1987; Smith and Best, 1989). The father of electrical engineering, Nikolai Tesla, was probably the first well-documented but nondiagnosed case of electromagnetic hypersensitivity (Smith and Best, 1989). Some individuals are, in essence, allergic to 50 or 60 Hz electromagnetic fields. These are people who immediately react when they are near transformers, fluorescent lights, microwave ovens, refrigerators, and other appliances. Often these are multiple allergy patients.

Multiple sensitivity begins when a person is exposed to a chemical agent, such as a pesticide, drug, solvent, perfume, smoke, exhaust, or chemicals in food or in carpets. The agent (or its electromagnetic signature; see below) triggers a reaction in one or more of the body's regulatory systems. The result of the initial encounter can be fatigue, respiratory problems, or difficulty concentrating. After one is sensitized, future exposures to even minute amounts of the allergen can trigger an immediate reaction. The problem is compounded when the sensitized person is exposed to a second agent or to an electromagnetic field while reacting to the first allergen. In this way, people can develop allergies to hundreds of substances and their electromagnetic signatures. Few physicians understand electromagnetic sensitivities, and therefore treat the symptoms without recognizing the source of the problem.

To treat electromagnetic allergies, Smith and colleagues use a clinical confrontation–neutralization protocol. The principle is the same as that used in the classical skin tests for chemical allergies. A signal generator a distance from the patient is used to find the frequency that will trigger the allergic reaction. Then other frequencies are tested to find the neutralizing frequencies that stop the reaction. Signals at these frequencies can 'potentize' vials of water that can be carried by the patient and used to stop the reaction. The allergic response is inhibited by holding the vial of water in the hand. In a given patient, the symptoms provoked electrically are similar to those provoked chemically and those provoked by the patient's environment. Electrical and chemical stimuli and neutralization appear to be interchangeable (Choy et al., 1987; Smith and Best, 1989).

'Billiard-Ball' Regulations Versus Electromagnetic Signaling

The research of Smith (1987) and Benveniste (1998) and others cited below provides dramatic documentation of an important phenomenon that underlies a number of energetic therapies as well as environmental electromagnetic effects.

In the conventional picture of biological regulations (left side of Figure 16.6), structurally matching molecules exchange energy and information by billiard ball-type direct impacts. Signal molecules diffuse, wiggle, and bump about randomly until they chance to approach a receptor site, at which time electrostatic, short-range (two to three times the molecule size) forces draw them together so that 'the key can fit into the lock'. It is not generally appreciated that this kind of random encounter, taking place in a sea of other molecules, gives these molecular meetings a statistically low probability. The simplest biological event or regulatory process should require a very long time to happen (also discussed in Chapter 9).

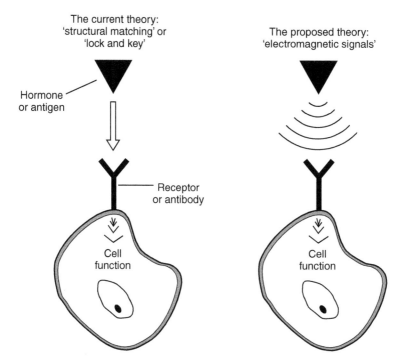

The current theory:
'structural matching' or
'lock and key'

The proposed theory:
'electromagnetic signals'

Hormone
or antigen

Receptor
or antibody

Cell
function

Cell
function

Figure 16.6 Theories of molecular signaling. Left, the conventional structural matching or 'lock and key' model of biological regulations. The three-dimensional structure of a ligand molecule, such as a hormone, antigen, or other signal molecule matches the three-dimensional structure of the receptor or antibody. This physical contact activates a particular cell function. Right, the proposed electromagnetic model. The signal molecule emits an electromagnetic signal (signature) that coresonates with the receptor molecule, thereby activating it and triggering the cell function. *(After Benveniste (1998), with kind permission from Dr. J. Benveniste.)*

In the energetic model of biological regulations (shown to the right in Figure 16.6), communication occurs between signal and receptor molecules that are not touching (Benveniste, 1998). The term 'molecular signal' acquires an electromagnetic meaning. In essence, the molecules can interact by coresonance, like radio transmitters and receivers. If you tune a receiver to 92.6 MHz, you tune in Station A, because electrons in the antennas of the receiver and the transmitter are oscillating at the same frequency. If you tune the receiver to a different frequency, say 91.6 MHz, you receive Station B instead. In living systems, long-range electromagnetic fields transmit messages between distant molecules, as long as their emission and absorption spectra match. Non-resonating, unwanted random signals are excluded. From basic electronics, we know that particularly good reception – meaning good separation of signal from noise – takes place if the transmitting and receiving antennas have the same shape, length and orientation.

Molecular electromagnetic communications can account for the rapid and subtle and integrated functioning of living systems. Millions of molecules can communicate with each other in this way. The upper limit on the signal velocity is the speed of light.

Dramatic evidence for this electromagnetic resonance model comes from studies of molecular signals recorded and digitized with a multimedia computer sound card (Benveniste, 1998). A molecular signal is represented by a spectrum of frequencies in the range 20–20,000 Hz, similar to the range of human hearing and music. In thousands of experiments, repeated over many years, Benveniste showed that playing recordings of the electromagnetic signatures of signal molecules can trigger various kinds of receptors to respond, just as though they were in the presence of the molecules that normally trigger them.

The mechanisms behind molecular coresonance are well understood. We have known for over a century that atoms and molecules vibrate when they absorb or emit electromagnetic waves. The resulting electromagnetic 'signatures' are used by spectroscopists to determine molecular structure and to identify unknown molecules. Most of what we know about the molecular structure of drugs and antibiotics comes from spectroscopic data. And, radio-telescopes detect characteristic molecular signals at distances of billions of light years.

From the research of Smith (1987) and Benveniste (1998) and their colleagues, there is every reason to think that signal molecules can activate their corresponding receptor sites without physical contact. The signal molecule vibrates and emits frequencies that resonate with the receptor and cause it to vibrate as well. For example, when you are in a dangerous situation, adrenalin 'tells' its various receptors, and those receptors alone, to make your heart beat faster, to dilate pupils and superficial blood vessels, and to trigger the other reactions of the 'fight-or-flight' response. Benveniste has suggested that the specific actions of biomolecules (e.g., histamine, caffeine, nicotine, adrenaline, insulin), as well as the antigens of viruses and bacteria, are due more to electromagnetic interactions than to direct contact.

These findings, while controversial, have enormous therapeutic implications and provide new insights into the energetic interactions taking place between and within organisms. They also provide clues about how environmental fields can influence physiological processes.

The Legacy of Lucretian Biochemistry

Smith (1987) and Benveniste (1998) are among the minority of scientists who have considered the possibility that electromagnetic signaling can play a direct communication role in living matter (see also Chapter 10). Albert Szent-Györgyi was another. In the following quotation he refers to the biochemistry based on the ancient concepts of Lucretius and Epicurus, who pioneered the idea that matter is composed of hard, indivisible 'billiard-ball' units, atoms:

> *Lucretian biochemistry involves the assumption that no interaction can take place between molecules without their touching one another. Support is given in this book (Szent-Györgyi, 1957) to the idea that manifold interactions can take place without such bodily contact, either through energy bands or through the electromagnetic field, which thus appears with water and its structures as the matrix of biological reactions. Water does not merely fill the space between molecules. Water is more than this; it is part and parcel of the living matter itself. One of the main functions of the protoplasmic structures (cytoskeleton and nuclear matrix) may be to generate in water those specific structures which make forms of electronic excitations and energy transmissions possible which would be improbable outside these structures.*
> SZENT-GYÖRGYI (1957) [STATEMENTS IN PARENTHESES ADDED].

The importance of water cannot be overemphasized. In terms of electronics, the essential role of water structure Szent-Györgyi referred to is impedance matching between the oscillating molecule and the surrounding medium. Impedance matching is essential for efficient transmission of energy and information from one medium to another, while minimizing reflections. Stated another way, water both conditions and is conditioned by the molecular framework in cells and tissues, the living matrix.

In spite of all of the documentation and its conceptual simplicity, electromagnetic interactions have been difficult for many scientists to grasp. This is remarkable, considering that action at a distance is an accepted part of Newtonian mechanics and accounts for the motions of the celestial bodies. Newtonian mechanics justifies movements other than those produced by impulsion.

None of the work on electromagnetic interactions between molecules violates any of the known laws of chemistry, physics, or biology. The passage from a biology of rigid structures randomly bumping into each other to one of information travelling at the speed of light can be accomplished without a 'scientific revolution'. All of the pieces of the puzzle are well accepted.

Acute Pathology

Geomagnetic storms often begin with turmoil on the sun. The sun spews very fast and energetic blobs of matter and magnetic energy that are carried earthward by the solar wind. When this energy crashes into the Earth's magnetosphere, enormous electrical currents are set up. These currents, in turn, influence the huge electric currents flowing in the ionosphere. Geomagnetic storms can be so intense that they damage satellites, power lines, telephone cables, and pipelines, and disrupt radio communications. It is not surprising that these events, which can be intense enough to prevent your automobile from starting, can affect physiology and behaviour. Geomagnetic disturbances have been correlated with the onset of a variety of disorders and death. The following list includes a sample of the enormous literature on this subject:

- Cardiovascular problems (Bellossi et al., 1985; Knox et al., 1979; Stoupel, 1993; Stoupel et al., 1993, 1994, 1995; Watanabe et al., 1994)
- Seizures, epilepsy, convulsions (Mikulecky et al., 1996; Persinger and Psych, 1995; Stoupel et al., 1991)
- Hypothermia (Bureau et al., 1996)
- Headache (De Matteis et al., 1994)
- Vestibular problems (Persinger and Richards, 1995)
- Bacterial growth (Polikarpov, 1996)
- Intraocular pressure (Stoupel et al., 1993)
- Sleep (Conesa, 1995; Kotleba et al., 1973)
- Death (Lipa et al., 1976; Stocks, 1925)

In addition, a variety of behavioural changes have been noted:

- Crime (Chibrikin et al., 1995)
- Aggression (St Pierre and Persinger, 1998)
- Anxiety (Usenko and Panin, 1993)
- Depression (Kay, 1994)
- Loss of attention and memory (Tambiev et al., 1995)
- Accidents (Grigor'ev, 1995)

Efforts to replicate these studies have yielded conflicting results. The reasons such studies are difficult to reproduce have been discussed in detail by Hainsworth (1983). The main problem is that living systems are exquisitely sensitive to low-energy signals, and individuals vary widely in their responses. Some individuals are affected negatively, some are neutral, and others seem to benefit from geomagnetic storms and related meteorological phenomena. Because of this, massive amounts of data are needed to establish valid relationships. (See section 'Scalar Waves' below for a perspective on individual variation that relates to structural bodywork.)

To complement the correlation studies, some researchers have simulated geomagnetic variations to induce seizures (e.g., Michon and Persinger, 1997; Michon et al., 1996; Persinger, 1996; Schienle et al., 1998), changes in reaction time (Reiter, 1953), and other effects.

Reviews of earlier literature have been published by Rajaram and Mitra (1981) and Venkataraman (1976). The latter author suggests that the effects of pulsing magnetic fields are similar to the well-known photoflash phenomenon that induces seizures. This is a reasonable hypothesis, given that virtually any form of pulsating energy can entrain brain waves (see Alexander and Gray, 1972; Di Perri, 1972; Foster, 1975; Oschman, 1997a,b).

Electromagnetic Pollution and Other Diseases

While there is heated debate, many serious health problems, including cancer, are being correlated with exposure to the invisible electromagnetic radiation produced by 50- and 60-cycle appliances, microwaves, radio transmitters, computers, etc. Serious problems have also been correlated with 'geopathic stress' (Figure 16.4).

Chapter 11 described the great sensitivity organisms have to exceedingly tiny signals in their environment and the reasons many physicists reached the conclusion that the biology was simply wrong. This physics/biology dilemma was resolved in the late 1970s when it became clear that living systems completely defy the logic that larger stimuli should produce larger responses. Living tissues are nonlinear, cooperative, and coherent, and are capable of responding to very specific 'windows' in terms of frequency and intensity (see Chapter 9 and Figure 16.1). Thus information on the health effects of natural and artificial electromagnetic fields is understandable on the basis of what has been learned about the sensitivities of all living systems to minute environmental signals. Interference with the molecular electromagnetic regulatory systems depicted in Figure 3.11 undoubtedly also plays a role.

Previous chapters (11 and 15) have described the Fröhlich model, in which the sensitivity of living systems is accounted for on the basis of the large numbers of molecules that form regular arrays, similar to those found in radio-telescope antennas (Figure 16.3). Teneforde and Kaune (1987) list a number of other models that are under consideration. In any case, electromagnetic fields in the ELF range (which includes the 50- and 60-Hz power distribution system) now have well-documented effects on a wide range of cellular systems.

R.P. Liburdy and colleagues have studied the effects of electromagnetic fields on cultured cells. Under well-controlled conditions, they established unequivocal field effects and identified the sites of action in the cellular regulatory process. However, a Federal Ethics Inquiry has found Liburdy guilty of 'scientific misconduct'. Supposedly he falsified and fabricated data published in two papers published in 1992.

After discussions with experts in the field, many researchers suspect Liburdy was treated unfairly by the engineering of absurd and irrelevant statements prominently reported in the media. On page 1 of the *New York Times* (July 24, 1999) we find: 'The disclosure [of Liburdy's 'misconduct'] appears to strengthen the case that electric power is safe'. In the *Wall Street Journal* (July 27, 1999, p. A22): 'A government-funded scientist systematically distorted data to support the hypothesis that electromagnetic fields near power lines cause cancer'. And, in *Science* (July 2, 1999): 'EMF researcher made up data'. These preposterous headlines have virtually nothing to do with Liburdy and his research. Liburdy never stated that 'electromagnetic fields near power lines cause cancer'. Actually, his data and interpretations were not challenged in the ethics review, just how the data were graphed. Moreover, Liburdy is widely respected, and his key conclusions have been confirmed in other laboratories. Here are some of the findings:

- Radiofrequency radiation affects the immune system by altering human immunoglobulin on T- and B-lymphocytes. The effect takes place at power levels below the current U.S. recommended safety limit of $0.4\,W\,kg^{-1}$ (Liburdy and Wyant, 1984).
- Microwaves at 2450 MHz increase the sodium permeability of rabbit erythrocytes (Liburdy and Vanek, 1985) and cause the shedding of at least 11 proteins from the cell surface (Liburdy et al., 1988).
- The calcium channel is the site of field interactions (Liburdy, 1992, confirmed by Pall, 2013).
- The findings on calcium metabolism are consistent with a proposed parametric resonance theory of the interaction of low-intensity magnetic fields with biological systems (Lednev, 1991; Yost and Liburdy, 1992).
- 60-Hz magnetic fields enhance breast cancer cell proliferation by blocking melatonin's natural oncostatic action. The effect is 'windowed' between 2 and 12 mG (milli Gauss) (Liburdy et al., 1993a).
- Magnetic fields, mitogens, and carcinogens influence the cascade of regulatory signal transduction processes. An early effect is on calcium influx into the cell, followed by an effect on the expression of a specific gene. A very weak dose of a mitogen, insufficient to trigger cell proliferation by itself, will stimulate cell division if it is combined with 60-Hz field treatment (Liburdy et al., 1993b).

- Both melatonin and tamoxifen inhibit the growth of cultured human breast cancer cells. 60-Hz fields block these inhibitions (Harland and Liburdy, 1997).

Statements by physicists such as Bennett (1994) that the fields from appliances cannot possibly affect living systems are simply outdated. Much more up-to-date information can be found in a wide variety of scientific journals, in a biannual series entitled 'Advances in Electromagnetic Fields in Living Systems' (Lin, 1994, 1997) and has been the subject of at least two Congressional hearings.

The relevance to the energy therapist is that the studies are showing that electromagnetic fields, at the frequencies and intensities emitted from the hands of a therapist, are capable of producing biological effects. It appears that the low frequencies emitted from the hands of therapists and from pulsing electromagnetic field therapy devices (in the range of 2–30 Hz) are beneficial, whereas somewhat higher frequencies of the power distribution system (50 and 60 Hz) can be harmful.

Scalar Waves

Physics has a little-known framework for a deeper understanding of electric and magnetic fields and their biological effects. Research in this area has considerable therapeutic significance. The concepts involved go to the heart of the quantum mechanical interpretation of reality and consciousness.

Briefly, we learn in classical physics that waves can interfere with each other. When two waves are of the same frequency and are in phase (the timing of their variations is identical), their amplitudes add together to create larger waves. This is termed *constructive interference*. When the waves are exactly out of phase, their amplitudes subtract, and they can partially or completely cancel or destroy each other. This is termed *destructive interference* (Figure 16.7A). In nature, interacting waves usually have a mix of frequencies and phases, and therefore add and subtract in a complex manner.

The field concept originated with Michael Faraday in 1846. However, the introduction of relativity and quantum mechanics shortly after the beginning of the twentieth century required

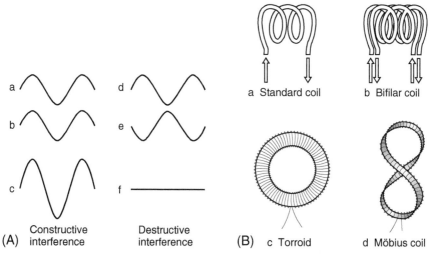

Figure 16.7 (A) Interference: In constructive interference (a, b, c), waves that are in phase (a and b) add together to produce a larger wave (c). In destructive interference (d, e, f), waves that are out of phase with each other can cancel or destroy each other (f). (B) Coils used to emit fields and potentials. (a) Is a standard coil that emits electric and magnetic fields into the surrounding space. (b) Is a bifilar coil, in which the electric and magnetic fields are cancelled, and electric scalar and magnetic vector waves are produced. (c) Is a torroidal coil that has the same effect as the bifilar coil. (d) Is a Möbius coil that produces only scalar waves. *(The information of coil properties is from Abraham, personal communication (1998).)*

that fields be expressed in terms of more fundamental entities, called potentials. Whittaker (1903, 1904) recognized this; Tesla (1904) generated potential waves and called them 'non-Hertzian waves'. When we say that a magnetic field induces a current flow in a conductor, such as a wire or a living tissue, it is actually the potential component of the field, and not the field itself, that underlies the effect. The potentials are of two kinds, called *electric scalar potentials* and *magnetic vector potentials*. The way these concepts were phased-out of physics is summarized in a book on Oliver Heaviside (Nahin 1988). Also see a book on Scalar Waves by Konstantin Meyl (2003).

For a long time, it was thought that these potentials had no real existence or significance. They were thought of as abstractions that were needed to simplify and balance quantum equations. That there was far more to the story was revealed in a classic paper by Aharonov and Bohm (1959). These authors showed that the potentials must have a physical reality and suggested some experiments to demonstrate them. For more recent work, see Batelaan & Tonomura, 2009.

The first demonstration of a magnetic vector potential was done with a coil designed so that the electric and magnetic fields remained entirely within its core, and absolutely no field existed on the outside. A beam of electrons passing through the 'force-free' region around the coil nonetheless underwent a phase change, indicating that some non-electric, non-magnetic physical 'entity' must be acting on it. This entity is the magnetic vector potential or magnetic A field.

Subsequent work documented the existence of an electric scalar potential in a region where no electric field exists. Both of these phenomena are referred to as the Aharonov–Bohm effect, a cornerstone of quantum mechanics. Technical details were published by Olariu and Popescu (1985). (For a less technical but still challenging account, see Imry and Webb, 1989.)

Hence, in destructive interference, where the classical fields cancel each other, there nonetheless remain electrostatic scalar potentials and magnetic vector potentials. In essence, the energy and information contained in the original waves is not destroyed by interference. In fact, the classical electromagnetic field is actually derived from two potential waves interfering with each other.

The Aharonov–Bohm effect began as an abstraction needed to balance quantum equations, but gradually found its way into down-to-earth applications in electronics. Scalar waves have been utilized for a communication system (Gelinas, 1984), for a device for locating humans and other animals during search and rescue operations (Afilani, 1998) and for wireless power transmission (Meyl 2003).

Various kinds of coil designs enable the vectors (the directions and magnitudes) of the electric and magnetic fields to destructively interfere or cancel each other (Figure 16.7). The figure caption describes the kinds of waves and fields they produce.

Scalar waves appear to interact with atomic nuclei, rather than with electrons. Such interactions are described by quantum chromodynamics (Yndurain, 1983). The waves are not blocked by Faraday cages or other kinds of shielding; they are probably emitted by living systems, and they appear to be intimately involved in healing (see, e.g., Jacobs, 1997; Rein, 1998).

The scalar potential has a peculiarity: It propagates instantaneously everywhere in space, undiminished by distance. In contrast, the vector potential has a finite velocity (Jackson, 1975). In the real world, scalar waves encounter environmental fields, and complex interactions take place that prevent them from extending indefinitely into space. Mathematical physics justifies the instantaneous propagation of scalar waves, but this is often dismissed as 'obviously unphysical behaviour' (e.g., Jackson, 1975).

The present situation parallels what happened over a century ago with regard to electromagnetic fields. When Maxwell combined the understandings that had been reached by Faraday, Ampère, and Gauss, he declared that there must exist an 'electromagnetic wave' capable of transmitting energy at a speed of 300 million m/s. At the time, the suggestion was considered to be completely outrageous. Subsequently, Hertz showed that Maxwell was correct, and Marconi applied the phenomenon when he developed practical radio transmission. Many times in our history, the mathematics requires a phenomenon to exist, but it takes years to demonstrate it.

Much more is known about electric and magnetic fields than about scalar waves and vector potentials simply because fields are easy to measure. Experimental demonstration of scalar waves and vector potentials and their biological effects is extremely difficult. At present, the best way to document their presence is by testing on electromagnetically sensitive individuals. It is widely assumed that it is the electric and magnetic fields that interact with organisms, but some researchers suspect that scalar and potential waves actually underlie these effects.

Scalar Waves and Bodywork

For the evolution of energetic bodywork and energy medicine, a number of important consequences are emerging from research on scalar waves. Each bioelectric and biomagnetic field produced by the human body – whether emitted by the brain, the heart, the eye, the muscles, an organ, or by the hand of a therapist or a QiGong practitioner – will also be associated with scalar waves and vector potentials.

It is important to look at the ways in which the energetic anatomy of the body might give rise to self-cancelling fields that result in biological scalar waves. Moreover, the energy fields in the environment, whether natural or created by technology, also have scalar and vector components. For example, the Schumann resonance (see Chapter 15) is described by five quantities: velocity of propagation, electric field, magnetic field, electric scalar potential, and magnetic vector potential (Abraham, personal communication, 1998). Further research is needed to determine the extent to which the biological effects of the Schumann resonance, VLF-sferics, and geopathic stress, as well as the phenomenon of dowsing, may be related to the Aharonov–Bohm effect.

Near-field interactions occur when the interacting elements, such as a therapist and patient, are close enough that their energy fields, which abruptly drop off in strength with distance, can interact. What about other healing modalities that seem independent of distance? A large and growing body of reliable evidence shows that distant healing and intercessory prayer are effective, even when the individuals involved are separated by great distances (Dossey, 1993).

The idea of subtle interactions at a distance is embodied in the 'synchronicity' concept of Jung (Peat, 1987) and is also part of radionics and related methods (e.g., Fellows, 1997). While these and kindred phenomena, such as telepathy and clairvoyance, are too far-fetched for some scientists, there is now too much evidence to ignore them (see a thorough discussion in Woodhouse, 1996 and Radin, 1997).

Some scholars look to the well-documented peculiarities of quantum mechanics for explanations, such as quantum non-locality (Rohrlich, 1983). It is often stated that non-local phenomena are mediated by unknown forms of energy, sometimes vaguely referred to as 'subtle energies'. Some look to these phenomena for clues about the nature of consciousness and the structure of the physical universe. Others suggest the word 'energy' is inadequate, and its use in relation to healing should be discontinued. The philosophical and metaphysical implications are the subject of ongoing discussions (e.g., exchanges between Dossey and Woodhouse in Network 64, 1997).

Key studies of non-local interactions have been published by Grinberg-Zylberbaum and colleagues (1992, 1994). Pairs of subjects who achieve a feeling of emotional connection (empathy) can develop correlated electroencephalographic patterns that are not attenuated by spatial separation or by electromagnetic shielding (Faraday cages). When one of the subjects was stimulated, as with a flash of light, the evoked brainwave was 'transferred' to a non-stimulated subject in another electromagnetically shielded room. The researchers assert that these findings represent a genuinely non-local, macroscopic manifestation of consciousness that is physiologically relevant.

Studies like this, using shielded rooms, seem to rule out energetic interactions. But do they? What about the scalar and vector potentials described above? Could the Aharonov–Bohm effect account for non-local interactions?

One possibility is that long-range biological interactions may be due to modulation of the scalar component of the Schumann resonance (Oschman, 2000). While this may seem far-fetched, it is fascinating that well-documented 'telepathic experiences' are reliably and systematically correlated with calm periods of global geomagnetic activity (Persinger and Krippner, 1993).

Implications for Structural Bodywork

Ida Rolf emphasized the importance of the relationship between fields of the living body and the larger fields of the planet (Rolf, 1962). As deep tissue alignment methods (e.g., Rolfing®, Structural Integration) and related techniques bring the body into anatomical and energetic balance with the field of gravity, it is possible that conditions may also develop such that the bioelectric and/or biomagnetic fields partly cancel each other. In such circumstances, the measured biomagnetic field would be converted into scalar and/or vector potentials. How this would affect an individual can only be a fascinating speculation at the present time. One possibility is that an individual capable of generating significant scalar waves would be relatively protected from negative effects of environmental energies. Perhaps this can explain the phenomenon mentioned above – that there is a wide range in responses in weather-sensitive people. While some individuals suffer, others seem to enjoy the stimulatory effects of geomagnetic storms and related meteorological events.

Prudent Avoidance

In the 1980s, several personal electromagnetic shielding devices were developed – based on the use of coils of the Möbius design that emit scalar waves – that were said to be safe for living systems. One of these devices was a watch containing a microchip that produced a Schumann-type signal at about 8.0 Hz. This device purportedly stabilized a person's brain waves at a frequency that was considered safe and beneficial. Many of these devices were sold, and there were reports of benefits from wearing them, including reduction of jet lag, more energy, lower blood pressure, and feelings of well-being. These qualitative effects have been difficult to document.

Rein (1998) has summarized more recent work on the biological effects of scalar waves. Scalar waves can inhibit neurotransmitter uptake into nerve cells and stimulate the growth of human lymphocytes. There are indications that the effects are in part mediated by effects on the properties of cell and tissue water.

More powerful emitters of scalar waves, in the range 6–60 mW power consumption, have been developed (Abraham, personal communication, 1998). The devices emit scalar waves at the average Schumann frequency, 7.83 Hz. Preliminary tests indicate that scalar waves at this frequency are safe and protect those who suffer from electromagnetic field sensitivity. Moreover, preliminary clinical trials indicated a variety of health benefits, including improvement of symptoms of chronic fatigue syndrome, fibromyalgia, cognitive impairments, and sleep disorders (Abraham, personal communication, 1998).

The development of a reliable and powerful source of potential waves opens up many possibilities for studies of the clinical effects of this form of energy, and, possibly, for resolving some of the mysteries and variability of both local and non-local biological effects.

There is widespread confusion and misinformation about our electromagnetic environment. Key information widely available in technical circles is virtually unknown to the general public. This is due to several factors that reinforce each other. One is the strong bias many biologists have against geophysical pacemakers for biological rhythms. This bias arises in part because evidence of this sort might be taken as support for astrology, a subject that is widely considered to be scientifically unfounded (see, however, Seymour, 1988). Another is the threat to the ego posed by the possibility that our lives might be influenced by events very far away from us. The idea that the human body both radiates and is sensitive to invisible energy fields may be menacing to some.

Finally, a documentation of health effects from fields generated by power distribution systems and technological devices have enormous economic and legal consequences.

Therapists are careful to make their treatment spaces as pleasant and comfortable as possible. But what about the ubiquitous invisible energies present in the treatment environment? No matter how well you treat individuals with electromagnetic or geopathic sensitivities and related disorders, they will continue to have problems when they go back to their homes and/or workplaces where they are immersed in disturbing energy fields. Treating the whole person involves education about the possible health effects of the invisible electromagnetic environment so that suitable precautions can be taken.

These considerations are of increasing importance for a variety of reasons that have been discussed here. Moreover, the likely physiological effects of environmental fields have been more widely researched than many people realize. Virtually every disease and disorder has been linked by one investigator or another to electromagnetic pollution. As one example, Sobel and colleagues have noted an elevated risk of Alzheimer's disease among those who work in areas where they are exposed to high electromagnetic fields (Sobel and Davanipour, 1996; Sobel et al., 1995a,b).

Preliminary clinical trials with devices that shield against electromagnetic pollution show relief from a wide range of symptoms, suggesting that those problems may actually be caused or aggravated by electromagnetic pollution. Whether these correlations will stand up to long-term research is unknown, but enough information is available on electromagnetic bioeffects to have led the U.S. government to warn that prudent avoidance is a good policy until more is learned. At present we do not know what constitutes a 'safe limit' for electromagnetic field exposure. It is interesting that the Russian standard for maximum safe microwave exposure to avoid changes in brain activity is 1000 times less than the U.S. legal maximum.

Low-cost detectors of magnetic fields are available, and these devices are invaluable for those who wish to get a better appreciation of the fields present in their homes and workplaces. One of these devices (TriField from AlphaLab) is reasonably inexpensive and combines magnetic, electric, and radio/microwave detectors. The magnetic section has three detecting coils oriented in the three directions of space, which is important. With such devices, one can locate the 'hot spots' in the home and work environment, such as near electric blankets and heaters, fluorescent lights, light dimmers, microwave ovens with bad seals, cellular phones, computers, televisions, transformers, and motors in devices such as refrigerators and clocks. Sometimes moving furniture, cribs, or beds a short distance can significantly reduce long-term exposure.

Some people have taken steps to rewire their homes and workplaces to reduce the levels of 50- or 60-Hz magnetic fields. Simple changes in wiring configuration can make an enormous difference in the levels of magnetic fields in the home (Maxey, 1991). However, Abraham, personal communication (1998) has cautioned that any method of field cancellation, such as twisting conductors together, can lead to the generation of undetectable 50- or 60-Hz scalar waves that could also have serious health effects. Obviously, we have much to learn about our electromagnetic environment and its relations to therapeutics.

Avoidance of geopathic stress is also important. Hall (1997) presents some techniques, and dowsers are also a good source of suggestions.

Therapists are being introduced to a variety of devices that are promoted as shields against electromagnetic pollution. The consumer must be cautioned, however, that it is easy to be deceived in a situation where the effects are invisible and unmeasurable and benefits are subjective. At present, the best way to assess such devices is by testing on a person who has electromagnetic sensitivity. This may seem unscientific, but there is a good precedent for it. Many of the important discoveries in biology began with sensitive biological assays in which the strength of an unknown compound or other factor is estimated by testing it on a living system. This is called a bioassay (e.g., Glass, 1973). The 'confrontation–neutralization technique' used by Choy and colleagues (1987) to study electrical sensitivities in allergy patients is a form of bioassay. The construction of an effective shield against electromagnetic effects is technically challenging and will be greatly facilitated when reliable detectors of scalar waves have been developed. Some researchers are developing devices that absorb environmental signals and convert them to beneficial frequencies. And Earthing or grounding has been shown to reduce induced electrical fields (discussed in Chapter 17).

Some Conclusions

To the biologist, the advent of the electronic age represents a major evolutionary event, a dramatic step into the unknown. Developments in electricity and electronics have greatly expanded the limits of what humans can achieve. But advances often have unanticipated costs. Some of the scientists who did the early research on radioactivity, X-rays, and microwaves lost their lives because of the cumulative effects of exposure to the energies they had discovered.

We have introduced a wide spectrum of invisible and potentially dangerous factors into our environment. Physicists continue to calculate how these energies may or may not influence living systems, but the biological concepts upon which they base their calculations are often rudimentary and inaccurate. Living tissue is far more sophisticated than any material physicists work with in the laboratory. Living tissue has remarkable properties that continue to astonish us. The truth is that we simply will not know the long-term biological effects of electromagnetic technologies for several generations. We are participants in a long-term study, with an unknown outcome. At this stage, however, there is more than enough evidence to be concerned and to take precautions and to revise safety standards (Johannson 2013, Pall 2014, Sage and Carpenter 2012).

There is reliable evidence that electromagnetic fields are a double-edged sword. Some frequencies are not good for you, others can stimulate healing. Some of the negative effects are uncomfortable, others are life-threatening. The research on cells in culture is particularly valuable in documenting the biological effects of electromagnetic fields at the cellular level. At the same time, this research has important implications for energetic bodyworkers by revealing the sensitive regulatory pathways in living tissues. It now appears that a minute field oscillating at 50 or 60 Hz can be harmful, while a field of similar strength but lower in frequency (e.g., 2, 7, 10, and 15 Hz) can stimulate healing of tissues such as nerve, bone, ligament, and capillaries, respectively (see Chapter 15).

References

Abraham, G., 1998. Potential shields against electromagnetic pollution: Synchroton Scalar Synchronizer. Optimox Corporation, PO Box 3378, Torrance, CA 90510–3378. Tel: 800-223-1601.

Adey, W.R., 1980. Frequency and power windowing in tissue interactions with weak electromagnetic fields. Proc. IEEE 68 (1), 119–125.

Adey, W.R., 1990. Electromagnetic Fields and the Essence of Living Systems: Modern Radio Science. Oxford University Press, Oxford, pp. 1–36.

Adey, W.R., Bawin, S.M., 1977. Brain interactions with weak electric and magnetic fields. Neurosci. Res. Program Bull. 15 (1), 1–129.

Afilani, T.L., 1998. Device and method using dielectrokinesis to locate entities. US Patent 5,748,088.

Aharonov, Y., Bohm, E., 1959. Significance of electromagnetic potentials in the quantum theory. Phys. Rev. 115 (3), 485–491.

Albrecht-Buehler, G., 1985. Is the cytoplasm intelligent too? Cell Muscle Motil. 6, 1–21.

Alexander, G.J., Gray, R., 1972. Induction of convulsive seizures in sound sensitive albino mice: response to various signal frequencies: 1. Proc. Soc. Exp. Biol. Med. 140 (4), 1284–1288.

Aschoff, D., Aschoff, J., 1986. Neue Grundlegende Erkeninisse. Verlag Mehr Wissen, Diisseldorf.

Bassett, C.A.L., 1978. Pulsing electromagnetic fields: a new approach to surgical problems. In: Buchwald, H., Varco, R.L. (Eds.), Metabolic Surgery. Grune and Stratton, New York, NY, pp. 255–306.

Bassett, C.A.L., 1995. Bioelectromagnetics in the service of medicine. In: Blank, M. (Ed.), Electromagnetic Fields: Biological Interactions and Mechanisms. Advances in Chemistry Series, vol. 250. American Chemical Society, Washington, DC, pp. 261–275 (Chapter 14).

Batelaan, H., Tonomura, A., 2009. The Aharonov–Bohm effects: variations on a subtle theme. Phys. Today 62 (9), 38–43.

Bawin, S.M., Kaczmarek, L.K., Adey, W.R., 1975. Effects of modulated very high frequency fields on specific brain rhythms in cats. Brain Res. 58, 365–384.

Becker, R.O., 1990. Cross Currents: The Perils of Electropollution, the Promise of Electromedicine. Jeremy P. Tarcher, Los Angeles, CA.

Bellossi, A., DeCertaines, J., Bernard, A.M., 1985. Is there an association between myocardial infarction and geomagnetic activity? Int. J. Biometeorol. 29 (1), 1–6.

Bennett, W.R., 1994. Health and Low-Frequency Electromagnetic Fields. Yale University Press, New Haven, CT.

Benveniste, J., 1998. From 'water memory effects' to 'digital biology'. On the web at: http://www.digibio.com/.

Best, S.T., 1984. Laying it on the power line. Guardian, October 24, 1984.

Best, S.T., 1988a. The electropollution effect. J. Alternat. Complement. Med. (May), 17, 18, 26, 30, 34, 43.

Best, S.T., 1988b. What we don't know about earth radiation. J. Altern. Complement. Med. (November), 17–18, 30.

Bialek, W., 1987. Physical limits to sensation and perception. Annu. Rev. Biophys. Biophys. Chem. 16, 455–478.

Blackman, C.F., Elder, J.A., Weil, C.M., Benane, S.G., Eichinger, D.C., House, D.E., 1979. Induction of calcium-ion efflux from brain tissue by radio-frequency radiation: effects of modulation frequency and field strength. Radio Sci. 14 (6S), 93–98.

Brewitt, B., 1996. Quantitative analysis of electrical skin conductance in diagnosis and current views of bio-electric medicine. J. Naturopathic Med. 6 (1), 66–75.

Brewitt, B., 1999. Electromagnetic medicine and HIV/AIDS treatment: clinical data and hypothesis for mechanism of action. In: Standish, L.J., Calabrese, C., Galatino, M.L. (Eds.), AIDS and Alternative Medicine: The Current State of the Science. Harcourt Brace, New York, NY.

Bridges, J.E., Preache, M., 1981. Biological influences of power frequency electric fields: a tutorial review from a physical and experimental viewpoint. Proc. IEEE 69 (9), 1092–1120.

Brown Jr., F.A., 1973. Biological rhythms. In: Prosser, C.L. (Ed.), Comparative Animal Physiology. third ed.. W B Saunders, Philadelphia, PA, pp. 429–456, Chapter 10.

Bureau, Y.R., Persinger, M.A., Parker, G.H., 1996. Effect of enhanced geomagnetic activity on hypothermia and mortality in rats. Int. J. Biometeorol. 39 (4), 197–200.

Burr, H.S., 1957. Harold Saxton Burr. Yale J. Biol. Med. 30 (3), 161–167.

Chapman, S., Bartels, J., 1940. Geomagnetism. Clarendon Press, Oxford, UK.

Chibrikin, V.M., Samovichev, E.G., Kashinskaya, I.V., et al., 1995. Dynamics of social processes and geomagnetic activity, 1: periodic components of variations in the number of recorded crimes in Moscow. Biofizika 40 (5), 1050–1053.

Choy, R.V.S., Monro, J.A., Smith, C.W., 1987. Electrical sensitivities in allergy patients. Clin. Ecol. 4 (3), 93–102.

Conesa, J., 1995. Relationship between isolated sleep paralysis and geomagnetic influences: a case study. Percept. Mot. Skills 80 (3/2), 1263–1273.

D'Arcy, F.J., Porter, N.A., 1962. Detection of cosmic ray p-mesons by the human eye. Nature 196 (4858), 1013–1014.

De Matteis, G., Vellante, M., Marrelli, A., Villante, U., Santalucia, P., Tuzi, P., Perncipe, M., 1994. Geomagnetic activity, humidity, temperature and headache: is there any correlation? Headache 34 (1), 41–43.

Di Perri, R., 1972. Photoprecipitable epilepsy: clinical observations and pathogenetic considerations. Acta Neurolgia (Napoli) 27 (5), 429–442.

Dossey, L., 1993. Healing Words: The Power of Prayer and the Practice of Medicine. Harper Collins, San Francisco, CA.

Dubrov, A.P., 1978. The Geomagnetic Field and Life: Geomagnetobiology. Plenum Press, New York, NY.

Fellows, L., 1997. Opening up the 'black box'. Int. J. Alternative Complementary Med. 15 (8), 9–13.

Foster, H., 1975. Letter. Photic fit near a helicopter. Lancet 2 (7926), 186.

Foster, K.R., Guy, A.W., 1986. The microwave problem. Sci. Am. 255 (3), 32–39.

Foster, K.R., Pickard, W.F., 1987. Microwaves: the risks of risk research. Nature 330, 531–532.

Fröhlich, H., 1968a. Bose condensation of strongly excited longitudinal electric modes. Phys. Lett. 26A, 402–403.

Fröhlich, H., 1968b. Long-range coherence and energy storage in biological systems. Int. J. Quantum Chem. 2, 641–649.

Fröhlich, H., 1970. Long-range coherence and the action of enzymes. Nature 228, 1093.

Fröhlich, H., 1974. Possibilities of long- and short-range electric interactions of biological systems. In: Adey, W.R., Bawin, S.M. (Eds.), Brain Interactions with Weak Electric and Magnetic Fields. Neurosciences Research Program Bulletin, MIT Press, Cambridge, MA; 15. pp. 1–129.

Fröhlich, H., 1975. Evidence for bose condensation-like excitation of coherent modes in biological systems. Phys. Lett. 51A, 21–22.

Fröhlich, H. (Ed.), 1988. Biological Coherence and Response to External Stimuli. Springer-Verlag, Berlin.

Gauquelin, M., 1966. Effets biologiques des champs magnetiques. Ann. Biol. 11–12, 595–611.

Gauquelin, M., 1974. The Cosmic Clocks. Avon Books, New York, NY.

Gelinas, R.C., 1984. Apparatus and method for transfer of information by means of a curl-free magnetic vector potential field. US Patent No 4,432,098.

Glass, G.E. (Ed.), 1973. Bioassay Techniques and Environmental Chemistry. Ann Arbor Science, Ann Arbor, MI.

Gordon, R., 2013. The Big Four. Health problems found affecting all people seriously ill with Cancer, Multiple Sclerosis, Lupus, Parkinson's, Alzheimer's disease etc., which very few doctors investigate. All four can easily be put right with very good results. This is common sense not alternative medicine. Dulwich Health Ltd., London.

Graham, G., 1724. An account of observations made of the variation of the horizontal needle at London, in the latter part of the year 1722. Philos. Trans. R. Soc. Lond. Ser. A 32, 96–107.

Grigor'ev, Iu.G., 1995. Mild geomagnetic field as a risk factor in work in screened buildings. Meditsina Truda Promyshlennaya Ekologiya (4),7–12.

Grinberg-Zylberbaum, J., Delaflor, M., Sanchez Arellano, M.E., Guevara, M.A., Perez, M., 1992. Human communication and the electrophysiological activity of the brain. Subtle Energies 3 (3), 25–43.

Grinberg-Zylberbaum, J., Delaflor, M., Attie, L., Goswami, A., 1994. The Einstein–Podolsky–Rosen paradox in the brain: the transferred potential. Phys. Essays 7 (4), 422–428.

Guy, A.W., Chou, C.K., Lin, J.C., Christensen, D., 1975. Microwave induced acoustic effects in mammalian auditory systems and physical materials. Ann. N. Y. Acad. Sci. 247, 194–218.

Hainsworth, L.B., 1983. The effect of geophysical phenomena on human health. Specul. Sci. Technol. 6 (5), 439–444.

Hall, A., 1997. Water, Electricity and Health: Protecting Yourself From Electrostress at Home and Work. Hawthorn Press, Stroud, UK.

Hansteen, C., 1819. Untersuchungen Ober den Magnetismus der Erde. Lehmann & GrOndahl, Christiania.

Harland, J.D., Liburdy, R.P., 1997. Environmental magnetic fields inhibit the antiproliferative action of tamoxifen and melatonin in a human breast cancer cell line. Bioelectromagnetics 18 (8), 555–562.

Ho, M.-W., 1998. The Rainbow and the Worm: The Physics of Organisms, second ed. World Scientific, River Edge, NJ.

Ho, M.-W., Popp, F.-A., Warnke, U., 1994. Bioelectrodynamics and Biocommunication. World Scientific, Singapore.

Hoyle, F., 1962. Astronomy. Crescent Books Inc. Wingdale, NY.

Imry, Y., Webb, R.A., 1989. Quantum interference and the Aharonov–Bohm effect: these counterintuitive effects play important roles in the theory of electromagnetic interactions, in solid-state physics and possibly in the development of new microelectronic devices. Sci. Am. 260 (4), 56–62.

Jackson, J.D., 1975. Classical Electrodynamics, second ed. John Wiley, New York.

Jacobs, J.A. (Ed.), 1987. Geomagnetism, 4 vols. Academic Press, London.

Jacobs, R., 1997. 21st century medicine. Kindred Spirit 3 (10), 37–40.

Johannson, O., 2013. Health effects of electromagnetic fields. A neuroscientist's view. Presentation at an international medical conference on electrosensitivity held in Barcelona, Spain on November 23. http://http//www.youtube.com/watch?v=I5udG8OCZWY.

Jones, W.H.S., 1948. Hippocrates. vol. 1. Harvard University Press, Cambridge, MA, pp. 73, 115.

Kalmijn, A.J., 1971. The electric sense of sharks and rays. J. Exp. Biol. 55 (2), 371–383.

Kay, R.W., 1994. Geomagnetic storms: association with incidence of depression as measured by hospital admission. Br. J. Psychiatry 164 (3), 403–409.

Knox, E.G., Armstrong, E., Lancashire, R., Wall, M., Haynes, R., 1979. Heart attacks and geomagnetic activity. Nature 281 (5732), 564–565.

Kotleba, J., Bielek, J., Glos, J., et al., 1973. Possible effect of the geomagnetic field on human sleep. Cesk. Fysiol. 22 (5), 459–460.

Lednev, V.V., 1991. Possible mechanism for the influence of weak magnetic fields on biological systems. Bioelectromagnetics 12, 71–75.

Liboff, A.R., 1985. Cyclotron resonance in membrane transport. In: Chiabrera, A., Nicolini, C., Schwan, H.P. (Eds.), Interactions Between Electromagnetic Fields and Cells. Plenum Press, New York, NY, pp. 281–296.

Liburdy, R.P., 1992. Calcium signaling in lymphocytes and ELF fields: evidence for an electric field metric and a site of interaction involving the calcium ion channel. FEBS Lett. 301 (1), 53–59.

Liburdy, R.P., Vanek Jr., P.F., 1985. Microwaves and the cell membrane, II: temperature, plasma, and oxygen mediate microwave-induced membrane permeability in the erythrocyte. Radiat. Res. 102 (2), 190–205.

Liburdy, R.P., Wyant, A., 1984. Radiofrequency radiation and the immune system, part 3: in vitro effects on human immunoglobin and on murine T- and B-lymphocytes. Int. J. Radiat. Biol. Relat. Stud. Phys. Chem. Med. 46 (1), 67–81.

Liburdy, R.P., Rowe, A.W., Vanek Jr., P.F., 1988. Microwaves and the cell membrane, IV: protein shedding in the human erythrocyte: quantitative analysis by high-performance liquid chromatography. Radiat. Res. 114 (3), 500–514.

Liburdy, R.P., Callahan, D.E., Harland, J., Dunham, E., Sloma, T.R., Yaswen, P., 1993a. Experimental evidence for 60 Hz magnetic fields operating through the signal transduction cascade: effects on calcium influx and c-MYC mRNA induction. FEBS Lett. 334 (3), 301–308.

Liburdy, R.P., Sloma, T.R., Sokolic, R., Yaswen, P., 1993b. ELF magnetic fields, breast cancer, and melatonin: 60 Hz fields block melatonin's oncostatic action on ER+ breast cancer cell proliferation. J. Pineal Res. 14 (2), 89–97.

Lin, J.C., 1994. In: Advances in Electromagnetic Fields in Living Systems, vol. 1. Plenum Press, New York, NY.

Lin, J.C., 1997. In: Advances in Electromagnetic Fields in Living Systems, vol. 2. Plenum Press, New York, NY.

Lipa, B.J., Sturrock, P.A., Rogot, E., 1976. Search for correlation between geomagnetic disturbances and mortality. Nature 259 (5541), 302–304.

Malin, S., 1987. Historical introduction to geomagnetism. In: Jacobs, J.A. (Ed.), Geomagnetism, vol. 1. Academic Press, London, pp. 1–49 (Chapter 1).

Matsushita, S., Campbell, W.H. (Eds.), 1967. Physics of Geomagnetic Phenomena. Academic Press, New York.

Maxey, E.S., 1991. A lethal subtle energy. Subtle Energies 2 (2), 55–70.

McCaig, C.D., Song, B., Rajnicek, M., 2009. Electrical dimesntions in cell science. Commentary. J. Cell Sci. 122 (23), 4267–4276.

Meyl, K., 2003. Scalar Waves. INDEL GmbH, Verlagsbteilung.

Michon, A.L., Persinger, M.A., 1997. Experimental simulation of the effects of increased geomagnetic activity upon nocturnal seizures in epileptic rats. Neurosci. Lett. 224 (1), 53–56.

Michon, A., Koren, S.A., Persinger, M.A., 1996. Attempts to simulate the association between geomagnetic activity and spontaneous seizures in rats using experimentally generated magnetic fields. Percept. Mot. Skills 82 (2), 619–626.

Mikulecky, M., Moravclova, G., Czanner, S., 1996. Lunisolar tidal waves, geomagnetic activity and epilepsy in the light of multivariate coherence. Braz. J. Med. Biol. Res. 29 (8), 1069–1072.

Miller, A., 1998. Dowsing: a review. Network 66, 3–8.

Moore-Ede, M.C., Campbell, S.S., Reiter, R.J., 1992. Electromagnetic Fields and Circadian Rhythmicity. Birkhauser, Boston, MA.

Murchie, G., 1978. The Seven Mysteries of Life. Houghton Mifflin, Boston, MA.

Nahin, P.J., 1988. Oliver Heaviside. Johns Hopkins University Press, Baltimore, MD.

Olariu, S., Popescu, I.I., 1985. The quantum effects of electromagnetic fluxes. Rev. Modem Phys. 57, 339–436.

Oschman, J.L., 1997a. Healing energy, part 3: silent pulses. J. Bodyw. Mov. Ther. 1 (3), 179–194.

Oschman, J.L., 1997b. Healing energy, part 4: vibrational medicines. J. Bodyw. Mov. Ther. 1 (4), 239–250.

Oschman, J.L., 2000. Energy medicine: the new paradigm. In: Charman, R. (Ed.), Complementary Therapies for Physical Therapists: A Theoretical and Clinical Exploration. Butterworth Heinemann, Oxford, introductory chapter.

Pall, M.L., 2013. Electromagnetic fields act via activation of voltage-gated calcium channels to produce beneficial or adverse effects. J. Cell. Mol. Med. 17 (8), 958–965.

Pall, M.L., 2014. Presentation in Oslo, Norway, at the Litteraturhuset, October 18, 2014, https://www.youtube.com/watch?v=_Up8bqiJN2k.

Peat, F.D., 1987. Synchronicity: The Bridge Between Matter and Mind. Bantam Books, Toronto.

Persinger, M.A., 1996. Enhancement of limbic seizures by nocturnal application of experimental magnetic fields that simulate the magnitude and morphology of increases in geomagnetic activity. Int. J. Neurosci. 86 (3–4), 271–280.

Persinger, M.A., Krippner, S., 1993. Dream ESP experiments and geomagnetic activity. In: Kane, B., Millay, J., Brown, D. (Eds.), Silver Threads: 25 years of Parapsychology Research. Praeger, Westport, Connecticut, pp. 39–53 (Chapter 3).

Persinger, M.A., Psych, C., 1995. Sudden unexpected death in epileptics following sudden, intense, increases in geomagnetic activity: prevalence of effect and potential mechanisms. Int. J. Biometeorol. 38 (4), 180–187.

Persinger, M.A., Richards, M., 1995. Vestibular experiences of humans during brief periods of partial sensory deprivation are enhanced when daily geomagnetic activity exceeds 15-20 nT. Neurosci. Lett. 194 (1–2), 69–72.

Polikarpov, N.A., 1996. The relationship of the indices of solar-geomagnetic activity and the autofluctuations in the biological properties of Staphylococcus aureus 209 subcultures in vitro. Zh Mikrobiol Epidemiol Immunobiol. 1, 27–30.

Presman, A.S., 1970. Electromagnetic Fields and Life. Plenum Press, New York, NY.

Radin, D.I., 1997. The Conscious Universe. The Scientific Truth of Psychic Phenomena. Harper Collins, New York, NY.

Rajaram, M., Mitra, S., 1981. Correlation between convulsive seizure and geomagnetic activity. Neurosci. Lett. 24, 187–191.

Rein, G., 1998. Biological effects of quantum fields and their role in the natural healing process. Front. Perspect. 7 (1), 16–23.

Reiter, R., 1953. Neuere Untersuchungen zum Problem der Wetterabhangigkeit des Menschen. Archie für Meterologie. Geophys. Bioclimatol. B4, 327 (For a review of Reiter's work in English, see Konig, H.L., 1974. Behavioral changes in human subjects associated with ELF electric fields. In: Persinger, M.A. (Ed.), ELF and VLF Electromagnetic Field Effects. Plenum Press, New York, NY, pp. 81-99. Also, see Moore-Ede, et al., 1992).

Rohrlich, F., 1983. Facing quantum mechanical reality. Science 221 (4617), 1251–1255.

Rolf, I.P., 1962. Structural integration: gravity: an unexplored factor in a more human use of human beings. J. Inst. Comp. Stud. Hist. Philos. Sci. 1, 3–20 (Available from the Rolf Institute, Boulder, CO, 800-530-8875).

Sage, C., Carpenter, D.O., 2012. The Bioinitiative Report. A Rationale for a Biologically-Based Exposure Standards for Low Intensity Electromagnetic Radiation. http://www.bioinitiative.org/ (accessed 12.21.14).

Schienle, A., Stark, R., Vaitl, D., 1998. Biological effects of very low frequency (VLF) atmospherics in humans: a review. J. Sci. Exploration 12 (3), 455–468.

Seymour, P., 1988. Astrology: The Evidence of Science. Penguin, London.

Smith, C.W., 1987. Electromagnetic effects in humans. In: Fröhlich, H. (Ed.), Biological Coherence and Response to External Stimuli. Springer-Verlag, Berlin, pp. 205–232.

Smith, C.W., Best, S., 1989. Electromagnetic Man: Health and Hazard in the Electrical Environment. Dent, London.

Sobel, E., Davanipour, Z., 1996. Electromagnetic field exposure may cause increased production of amyloid beta and eventually lead to Alzheimer's disease. Neurology 47 (6), 1477–1481.

Sobel, E., Davanipour, Z., Sulkava, R., et al., 1995a. Occupational exposure to electromagnetic fields: a possible risk factor for Alzheimer's disease. In: Iqbal, K., Mortimer, J.A., Winblad, B., Wisniewski, H.M. (Eds.), Research Advances in Alzheimer's Disease and Related Disorders. John Wiley, Chichester.

Sobel, E., Dunn, M., Davanipour, Z., Qian, Z., Chui, H.C., 1995b. Elevated risk of Alzheimer's disease among workers with likely electromagnetic field exposure. Am. J. Epidemiol. 142 (5), 515–524.

St Pierre, L., Persinger, M.A., 1998. Geophysical variables and behavior, LXXXIV: quantitative increases in group aggression in male epileptic rats during increases in geomagnetic activity. Percept. Mot. Skills 86 (3/2), 1392–1394.

Stocks, P., 1925. High barometer and sudden deaths. Br. Med. J. 2, 1188.

Stoupel, E., 1993. Sudden cardiac deaths and ventricular extrasystoles on days with four levels of geomagnetic activity. J. Basic Clin. Physiol. Pharmacol. 4 (4), 357–366.

Stoupel, E., Martfel, J., Rotenberg, Z., 1991. Admissions of patients with epileptic seizures (E) and dizziness (D) related to geomagnetic and solar activity levels: differences in female and male patients. Med. Hypotheses 36 (4), 384–388.

Stoupel, E., Goldenfeld, M., Shimshoni, M., Siegel, R., 1993. Intraocular pressure (TOP) in relation to four levels of daily geomagnetic and extreme yearly solar activity. Int. J. Biometeorol. 37 (1), 42–45.

Stoupel, E., Martfel, J., Rotenberg, Z., 1994. Paroxysmal atrial fibrillation and stroke (cerebrovascular accidents) in males and females above and below age 65 on days of different geomagnetic activity levels. J. Basic Clin. Physiol. Pharmacol. 5 (3–4), 315–329.

Stoupel, E., Wittenberg, C., Zabludowski, J., Boner, G., 1995. Ambulatory blood pressure monitoring in patients with hypertension on days of high and low geomagnetic activity. J. Hum. Hypertens. 9 (4), 293–294.

Stryer, L., 1985. Molecular design of an amplification cascade in vision. Biopolymers 24 (1), 29–47.

Stryer, L., 1987. The molecules of visual excitation. Sci. Am. 257 (1), 42–50.

Stryer, L., 1988. Molecular basis of visual excitation. Cold Spring Harb. Symp. Quant. Biol. 52, 283–294.

Szent-Györgyi, A., 1957. Bioenergetics. Academic Press, New York, NY.

Tambiev, A.E., Medvedev, S.D., Egorova, E.V., 1995. The effect of geomagnetic disturbances on the functions of attention and memory. Aviakosm Ekolog Med 29 (3), 43–45.

Teneforde, T.S., Kaune, W.T., 1987. Interaction of extremely low frequency electric and magnetic fields with humans. Health Phys. 53 (6), 585–606.

Tesla, N., 1904. Transmission of energy without wires. Sci. Am. Suppl. 57, 237.

Usenko, G.A., Panin, L.E., 1993. Blood system reactions in flight operators with high and low levels of anxiousness during geomagnetic disturbances. Aviakosm Ekolog Med 27 (2), 39–44.

Valet, J.-P., Meynadier, L., 1993. Geomagnetic field intensity and reversals during the past four million years. Nature 366 (6452), 234–238.

Venkataraman, K., 1976. Epilepsy and solar activity: an hypothesis. Neurol. India 24, 148–152.

Volland, H., 1984. Handbook of Atmospheric Electrodynamics. CRC Press, Boca Raton, FL.

von Pohl, G.F., 1985. Earth Currents: Causative Factor of Cancer and Other Diseases. Translation of 1932 original by I Lang Frech-Verlag, Stuttgart.

Wachtel, H., 1995. Comparison of endogenous currents in and around cells with those induced by exogenous extremely low frequency magnetic fields. In: Blank, M. (Ed.), Electromagnetic Fields: Biological Interactions and Mechanisms. Advances in Chemistry Series, vol. 250. American Chemical Society, Washington, DC, pp. 99–107 (Chapter 6).

Ward, R.R., 1971. The Living Clocks. In: Alfred A Knopf, New York, NY, p 64 et seq.

Warnke, U., 1994. Electromagnetic sensitivity of animals and humans: biological and clinical implications. In: Ho, M.-W., Popp, F.-A., Warnke, U. (Eds.), Bioelectrodynamics and Biocommunication. World Scientific, Singapore, pp. 365–386 (Chapter 15).

Watanabe, Y., Hillman, D.C., Otsuka, K., Bingham, C., Breus, T.K., Cornelissen, G., Halberg, F., 1994. Cross-spectral coherence between geomagnetic disturbance and human cardiovascular variables at non-societal frequencies. Chronobiologia 21 (3–4), 265–272.

Wever, R., 1968. Einfluss Schwacher Elektromagnetischer Felder auf die Circadiane Periodik des Menschen. Naturwissenschaften 55, 29–32, [For a summary of Wever's work in English, see Wever, R., 1974. ELF-effects on human circadian rhythms. In: Persinger, M.A. (Ed.), ELF and VLF Electromagnetic Field Effects. Plenum Press, New York, NY, pp. 101–144.

Whittaker, E.T., 1903. On the partial differential equations of mathematical physics. Mathematische Annalen 57, 333–355.

Whittaker, E.T., 1904. On an expression of the electromagnetic field due to electrons by means of two scalar potential functions. Proc. Lond. Math. Soc. 1, 367–372.

Wick, G.L., 1972. Cosmic rays: detection with the eye. Science 175, 615–616.

Wienert, K.A., 1970. Notes on Geomagnetic Observatory and Survey Practice. UNESCO, Paris.

Woodhouse, M.B., 1996. Paradigm Wars: Worldviews for a New Age. Frog, Berkeley, CA.

Wooster, S.M., 1988. Geopathogenic stress and cancer. Townsend Lett. Doctors Patients 64, 482–483.

Yndurain, F.J., 1983. Quantum Chromodynamics: An Introduction to the Theory of Quarks and Gluons. Springer-Verlag, New York, NY.

Yost, M.G., Liburdy, R.P., 1992. Time-varying and static magnetic fields act in combination to alter calcium signal transduction in the lymphocyte. FEBS Lett. 296 (2), 117–122.

CHAPTER 17

Energy Medicine in Daily Life

The study of energy medicine will give you a clearer picture of the world around and within you. The information can make a huge difference for your personal health and happiness and your comprehension of nature and of exciting new clinical tools should you need them.

From the Preface to the Second Edition, page xiv

… life springs and proliferates under the influence of a balanced environment.

Dittman (2007)

Introduction

The Preface asserts that the information presented in this book can make a huge difference in the reader's personal health. To help the reader experience such benefits, this chapter introduces examples of the role energy medicine can play in health, happiness and longevity. We mention some of the most costly and debilitating diseases and disorders of our times, and we offer insights into how these conditions can be avoided or minimized by following the lessons learned from the art and science of energy medicine. Some approaches are very easy to apply, but they are simply not known in mainstream medicine or discussed in the mainstream media. Nonetheless, many energy medicine practices have the potential to clear away the blind spots in conventional medical science that are preventing us from addressing the most serious global health crises.

As with other chapters in this book, this chapter mentions certain diseases, as well as methods that patients have reported to be therapeutic. Again, the reader is advised to look at the note at the beginning of the book. Nothing in this chapter is intended to be medical advice regarding diagnosis or recommendations for treatment. When experiencing a health challenge, the reader should consult a licensed healthcare provider. The information presented here is intended to give the reader some ideas about available approaches and to provide a basis for thoughtful conversations between the reader and a physician or other healthcare providers.

To this end, this chapter shows how various energy medicine techniques can be used to successfully prevent or ease some of the most costly, debilitating, and painful disorders. These methods are gradually being incorporated into conventional American and international medical facilities. For example, an American hospital survey conducted in 2005 found that 30% of 1400 responding hospitals offered Therapeutic Touch (Anath 2006). A closely related method called Healing Touch is offered in many hospices, doctors' offices and long-term care facilities, as well as home health care throughout the United States and the world. Elite centers, such as the Mayo Clinic, Duke University Medical Center, and the University of California – San Francisco, now offer acupuncture, massage, and other energetic approaches. All 18 hospitals on *U.S. News*'s most recent 'America's Best Hospitals' superselective 'Honor Roll' provide some form of complementary and alternative medicine.

At hospitals and clinics across America, Reiki is beginning to gain acceptance as a meaningful and cost-effective way to improve patient care. Personal interviews conducted with medical professionals corroborate this view. "Reiki sessions cause patients to heal faster with less pain," says Marilyn Vega, RN, a private-duty nurse at the Manhattan Eye, Ear and Throat Hospital in New York. [Reiki] accelerates recovery from surgery, improves mental attitude and reduces the negative effects of medication and other medical procedures.

RAND (1997)

This chapter considers some additional methods that could contribute greatly to reducing the physical, emotional and financial strains that many people experience as a result of disease, injury or aging. The methods described here are only the tip of the iceberg in terms of what energy medicine has to offer, however. We must remember that medicine is often referred to as the 'medical arts'. According to a classic medical treatise, *Cecil's Textbook of Medicine* (Goldman and Ausiello, 2004),

The art of caring and comfort, guided by millennia of common sense as well as a more recent systematic approach to medical ethics, remains the cornerstone of medicine – without these humanistic qualities the application of modern science of "medicine" is suboptimal, useless, even detrimental.

Tilden (2010) also explains,

Medicine is supposed to be a scientific study and its practice an art. The study of disease requires the aid of science. Consummate art is required to affect a cure when nature is no longer able to help herself.

TILDEN (2010)

Any scientist who ventures into unknown territory, such as the study of a presently incurable disease, has to be an explorer. The path to discovery is often not obvious and linear. In a classic article, Albert Szent-Györgyi (1972) described the process of scientific discovery and progress as follows:

Wilhelm Ostwald (1909) divided scientists into the classical and the romantic. One could call them also systematic and intuitive. John R. Platt calls them Apollonian and Dionysian. These classifications reflect extremes of two different attitudes of the mind that can be found equally in art, painting, sculpture, music, or dance. One could probably discover them in other alleys of life. In science the Apollonian tends to develop established lines to perfection, while the Dionysian rather relies on intuition and is more likely to open new, unexpected directions for research. Nobody knows what "intuition" really is. My guess is that it is a sort of subconscious reasoning, only the end result of which becomes conscious.

These are not merely academic problems. They have most important corollaries and consequences. The future of mankind depends on the progress of science, and the progress of science depends on the support it can find. Support mostly takes the form of grants, and the present methods of distributing grants unduly favor the Apollonian. Applying for a grant begins with writing a project. The Apollonian clearly sees the future lines of his research and has no difficulty writing a clear project. Not so the Dionysian, who knows only the direction in which he wants to go out into the unknown; he has no idea what he is going to find there and how he is going to find it.

ALBERT SZENT-GYÖRGYI (1972)

Practitioners of complementary and alternative medicine often describe themselves as being more artistic than scientific. They would not be doing what they are doing without the influence of their teachers, who are usually careful, creative, and sensitive observers willing to rely on intuitions and flashes of insight when creating new and successful clinical protocols.

Many experienced physicians confess that they are often able to 'read' a new patient at a glance, only to later have lab tests and medical imaging confirm their original flashes of insight. The value of such intuitive leaps is described in *Blink: The Power of Thinking Without Thinking* by Gladwell (2007).

Sometimes the logical treatment paradigm fails, and the patient gets worse rather than better. When this happens, the intuitive physician may step away from the conventional path and apply a new and creative method. These creative moments allow biomedicine to take a big step forward. By combining the work of these insightful and artful physicians, medical researchers, and alternative therapists, a growing proportion of modern medicine relies at least as much on intuition and art as it does on science.

Inflammation

We now know that many of the most common and debilitating health disorders and diseases are partly or entirely energetic in nature and are therefore difficult to prevent, treat, or even comprehend without embracing the role of energy in the patient's health. Moreover, cures for the most serious health problems will remain elusive until medical researchers take energetics into consideration. This does not mean we need to look more closely at biochemical or molecular energetics. Rather, we need to explore the energetics described by physics, biophysics, and quantum physics. This need to focus on the energetics related to physics is demonstrated by one of the most significant biomedical advances to occur since the publication of this book's first edition. Specifically, the study of inflammation has become a major area of biomedical research, with over 450,000 peer-reviewed studies completed during the period from 1967 to 2014 (see Figure p-1 in the Preface to the Second Edition), and inflammation is incomprehensible without an energetic perspective.

Chronic disease is the primary cause of death and disability worldwide. Treating patients with chronic diseases accounts for 75% of US healthcare spending, which surpassed $2.3 trillion in 2008, the most recent period for which we have accurate data. The most common and costly chronic diseases are heart disease, cancer, stroke, chronic obstructive pulmonary disease, osteoporosis, and diabetes (Swartz, 2011). Diabetes alone accounts for 10% of all healthcare dollars spent, and age-related osteoporosis affects about 28 million Americans (Partnership to Fight Chronic Disease, 2011).

> *The world is losing the battle against diabetes as the number of people estimated to be living with the disease soars to a new record of 382 million this year, medical experts said on Thursday. The vast majority have type 2 diabetes – the kind linked to obesity and lack of exercise – and the epidemic is spreading as more people in the developing world adopt Western, urban lifestyles. The latest estimate from the International Diabetes Federation is equivalent to a global prevalence rate of 8.4 percent of the adult population and compares to 371 million cases in 2012.*
>
> REUTERS, LONDON, NOVEMBER 14, 2013

Other significant conditions include Alzheimer's disease, asthma, bowel disorders, cirrhosis of the liver, cystic fibrosis, lupus, meningitis, multiple sclerosis, psoriasis, and arthritis. Many patients suffer from several of these problems simultaneously, and modern research has shown that all of these conditions are related to inflammation.

Major news sources have been informing the public about the connection between inflammation and health (e.g., *Time Magazine* cover story, February 23, 2004, 'Inflammation: The Secret Killer'; *Business Week* cover story, January 24, 2004, 'I can't Sleep'; and *Newsweek* cover story, April 25, 2006, 'Why women can't sleep', Kantrowitz 2006). While abundant research has documented a relationship between chronic inflammation and almost all chronic diseases, including all the diseases of aging, profoundly important questions remain unanswered. In fact, for some reason, these questions are rarely discussed:

- What causes chronic inflammation?
- Precisely why is inflammation associated with so many different chronic diseases?
- Why have these chronic diseases reached epidemic proportions?
- What can an individual do about it?
- What does successful energy therapy tell us about human biology and ways to stay healthy or recover from problems as quickly as possible?

The examples given in this chapter relate to health considerations that are 'of the Earth' and that have been recognized since ancient times. We begin by considering the benefits of direct physical contact with the surface of the Earth, as with bare feet or hands. This type of contact is termed 'grounding' or 'Earthing'. In the process of studying why Earthing is so beneficial, a group of scientists has uncovered some of the missing pieces of the inflammatory response, adding to our understanding of how the immune system works. Other examples of ancient and modern 'Earth remedies' include aromatherapy or essential oils, herbal medicines, and marine plasma.

Grounding or Earthing

People who work barefoot in the garden or walk barefoot along the beach often experience a special sense of wellbeing from being in direct physical contact with the Earth. Some teachers of ancient practices such as yoga and QiGong recommend that all such practices be done barefoot on the Earth. There is no comparison between practising any form of movement therapy or martial arts indoors and practising while in direct contact with the Earth. Since ancient times, Native American elders have also discussed the value of direct Earth contact in their traditional storytelling:

> *It was good for the skin to touch the bare earth, and the old people liked to remove their moccasins and walk with their bare feet on the sacred Earth ... they sat on the ground with the feeling of being close to a mothering power ... the soil was soothing, strengthening, cleansing and healing.*
>
> LUTHER STANDING BEAR (1868–1939), SIOUX TRIBAL LEADER

In the late nineteenth century, a back-to-nature movement in Germany claimed that being barefoot outdoors produced many health benefits, even in cold weather (Just, 1903). In the 1920s, George Starr White, a medical doctor, investigated the practice of sleeping grounded after being informed by some individuals that they could not sleep properly 'unless they were on the ground or connected to the ground in some way', as with copper wires attached to grounded-to-Earth water, gas, or radiator pipes. White (1929) reported improved sleeping using these techniques. However, these ideas never caught on in mainstream society.

Modern research, to be described next, has documented the following effects of grounding or Earthing, in the order in which they were discovered:

- improved sleep
- reduced pain
- reduced inflammation
- relaxation (autonomic nervous system)
- accelerated healing of injuries
- increased heart rate variability
- less clumping of red blood cells
- reduced blood viscosity

Throughout history, humans most often walked barefoot or with footwear made of an-imal skins. They slept directly on the ground or on animal hides. Recent research shows the advantages provided by this lifestyle. Through direct contact with the Earth, or through contact via perspiration-dampened animal skins used as footwear or sleeping mats, the abundant free electrons in the ground were able to enter the body, which is electrically conductive. Through this mechanism, every part of the body could equilibrate with the electrical potential of the Earth, thereby stabilizing the electrical environment of all organs, tissues, cells and molecules.

Modern lifestyle has increasingly separated humans from the primordial flow of Earth's electrons. For example, since the 1960s, we have increasingly worn insulating rubber- or plastic-soled shoes, instead of shoes with traditional leather soles fashioned from hides. Some have lamented that the use of insulating materials in the soles of post-World War II shoes has separated us from the Earth's energy field (e.g., Rossi, 1989). Obviously, we no longer sleep and walk directly on the ground as we did in times past.

During recent decades, chronic illness, immune disorders, and inflammatory diseases have become much more prevalent, and some researchers have cited environmental factors as the cause. However, modern biomedicine has not considered the possibility that the increasing incidence of disease might result from a modern disconnection with the Earth's surface. The research summarized in this section points in that direction. We are experiencing a global epidemic of diabetes, and it is tempting to consider the possibility that this epidemic may, in part, be caused by the kinds of shoes we wear. Figure 17.1 shows a correlation between the incidence of diabetes and the growth in sales of athletic shoes, virtually all of which have insulating rubber or plastic soles. This apparent connection between increases in diabetes prevalence and shoe sales ties-in with the discovery by Sokal and Sokal (2011), who found that continually Earthing during rest and physical activity over a 72-h period decreased fasting glucose among patients with non-insulin-dependent diabetes mellitus.

A modern understanding of the value of Earth-to-skin contact began with Clint Ober's discovery that a simple grounding system placed on a mattress enabled a person to sleep better (Ober, 2003, 2004; Ober and Coghill, 2003). In Poland, the Sokals made similar discoveries in the early 1990's, but they were only recently able to publish their work (Sokal and Sokal, 2011).

The grounding or Earthing story is summarized by the cartoon in Figure 17.2. There is a continuous flow of electrons from the sun to the ionosphere, and thence to the Earth via lightning

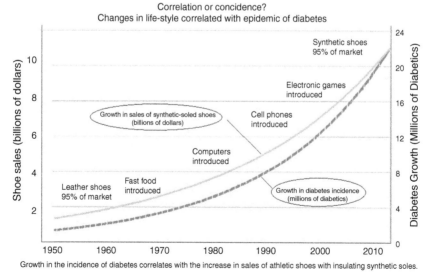

Growth in the incidence of diabetes correlates with the increase in sales of athletic shoes with insulating synthetic soles.

Figure 17.1 Sixty years of growth in synthetic-soled shoe sales compared with the growing incidence of diabetes during the same period. Diabetes incidence from Centers for Disease Control and Prevention (CDC 2014). Athletic shoe sales data from SGMA and Shoe Industry leading brand sales.

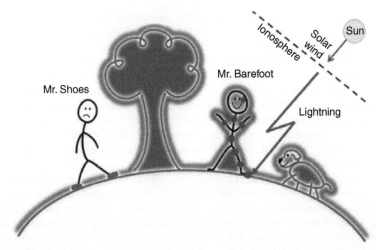

Figure 17.2 Electrons continuously flow from the sun to the ionosphere and then from the ionosphere to the Earth via lightning strikes. Lightning keeps the surface of the Earth electrically charged. The field of electrostatics teaches that when two conductive objects with different electrical potentials touch each other, a virtually instantaneous transfer of charge occurs, so that the two objects equilibrate to the same electrical potential. The human body is a conductor of electricity, as is the Earth. The terms 'grounded' and 'Earthed' refer to a state in which our bodies are connected to the surface of the Earth and its abundant supply of electrons. This is a natural condition in which Earth's electrons spread over and into our bodies, stabilizing our internal electrical environment.

strikes. Lightning keeps the conductive surface of the Earth electrically charged (Williams and Heckman, 1993). Electrostatics is the branch of physics teaching that, when two conductive objects with different electrical potentials touch each other, there is a virtually instantaneous transfer of charge so that the two objects equilibrate to the same electrical potential (e.g., Bertrand, 2013). The human body is a conductor of electricity and so is the Earth. When 'grounded' or 'Earthed', our bodies are conductively coupled or connected to the surface of the Earth and its abundant supply of electrons. This is a natural condition in which Earth's electrons spread over and into our bodies, stabilizing our internal electrical environment. As we shall see below, this stabilizing effect impacts all physiological systems, enhancing their functioning.

Ober's grounded sleep systems have included variations of bed sheets, pads, mats, and pillowcases utilizing conductive carbon particles or silver-plated threads woven into them. The conductive elements connect, via wire, to the ground port of a grounded wall outlet inside the residence or to a metal rod inserted into the soil outside. Sleeping on these systems connects the body to the Earth (Figure 17.3).

People using this system repeatedly reported that sleeping while grounded to the Earth improves the quality of sleep. Insomnia is a serious problem for approximately 30 percent of the people in the United States. Poor sleep is thought to lead to many automobile and other types of accidents, and lack of sleep costs U.S. businesses nearly $150 billion annually in absenteeism and lost productivity (National Institutes for Health State-of-the-Science Conference on Manifestations and Management of Chronic Insomnia in Adults, 2005). Therefore, further investigation of grounded sleep is worthwhile. A pilot study (Ghaly and Teplitz, 2004) showed that improved sleep was associated with the normalization of the day–night rhythm of the 'stress hormone' cortisol (Figure 17.4).

Many who had improved sleep also reported the reduction or elimination of pain from new or old injuries or from conditions such as arthritis. Increasing feedback over the years indicates that many other uncomfortable or debilitating conditions are partly or completely mitigated by grounding the body during sleep.

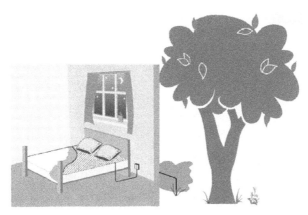

Figure 17.3 The grounded sleep system consists of a cotton sheet with conductive carbon or silver-plated threads woven into it. The threads connect to a wire that goes out the bedroom window or through the wall to a metal rod inserted into the earth. Sleeping on this system connects the body to the Earth. People using these systems have repeatedly reported that sleeping while grounded to the Earth improves the quality of sleep.

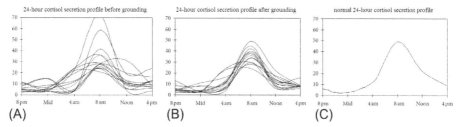

Figure 17.4 A pilot study (Ghaly and Teplitz, 2004) showed that improved sleep was associated with normalization of the day–night rhythm of the 'stress hormone' cortisol. (A) 24 hour cortisol secretion profile before grounding. (B) 24 hour cortisol secretion profile after grounding. (C) is the normal 24-h cortisol profile. *(Courtesy Earth FX, Inc.)*

When any method has a broad spectrum of benefits, as often happens with sleeping grounded, one can look for a common underlying mechanism. One mechanism is obvious: extensive scientific research from around the world has already shown that the lack of sleep stresses the body and has many detrimental health consequences. A procedure that improves sleep quality and duration could therefore provide relief from a host of disorders related to exhaustion, stress, and the resulting anxiety.

Looking further, we know that lack of sleep is often the result of pain, because people simply cannot sleep well when they are experiencing discomfort. Hence, the reduction of pain might lead to improved sleep, stress reduction, and relief from a wide variety of unpleasant and debilitating conditions. Pain reduction resulting from sleeping grounded has been documented in a controlled study of delayed onset muscle soreness (DOMS). This is a well-known result of excessive, unfamiliar, or intensive exercise. We all feel DOMS when we engage in new or infrequent forms of exertion, such as mowing a large lawn for the first time in the spring. Muscle cell breakdown occurs along the muscle Z-lines, which are the regions where tension that has developed within the muscle cell is conducted to the myofascial system and thence to bones. During breakdown, muscle cell membranes become leaky, and muscle soreness begins 24–48 h after the exercise, possibly lasting well over 96 h. DOMS is an excellent model for the study of acute inflammation. The excessive exercise can be standardized and does not produce any permanent injury to research subjects. Sleeping grounded is the first intervention ever discovered that speeds recovery from the pain of DOMS (Brown et al., 2010). See Figure 17.5.

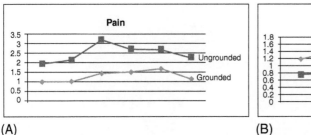
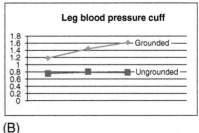

(A)   (B)

Figure 17.5   Delayed onset muscular soreness (DOMS) study. (A) During each measurement, the ungrounded subjects consistently expressed the perception of greater pain than the grounded subjects did. The differences in reported pain ranged from 61% to 126%. (B) Subjects were tested with a blood pressure cuff on the calf of the injured leg. At each measurement taken, subjects that had slept grounded could consistently withstand more pressure.

One of the documented causes of sleep disturbance is the environmental electric field generated by home wiring and appliances. The wires to a lamp or clock radio on a table next to the bed induce measurable voltages on the body, as do wires concealed within the walls, and the electric field created by the wires is present even when the appliances are turned off. An electrical engineer experienced in the design of electrostatic discharge systems for electronics, Applewhite (2005) measured home electric fields in relation to sleep. Measurements were taken while a subject was ungrounded and then while the subject was grounded using a conductive patch or conductive bed pad. Applewhite measured the induced fields at three positions: left breast, abdomen, and left thigh. Each method (patch and sheet) immediately reduced the alternating current (AC) 60-Hz ambient voltage induced on the body by a highly significant factor of about 70 on average. Figure 17.6 shows this effect.

The Applewhite (2005) study showed that, when the body is grounded, its electrical potential becomes equalized with the Earth's electrical potential through a transfer of electrons from the Earth to the body. This, in turn, prevents the 60-Hz fields in the environment from producing an alternating electric potential at the surface of the body and, thus, from agitating charged ions and molecules inside the body. The study thereby confirms the 'umbrella' effect of Earthing the body explained by Nobel Prize winner Richard Feynman in his famous *Lectures on Physics* (Feynman et al., 1964). Feynman said that when the body potential is the same as the Earth's electric

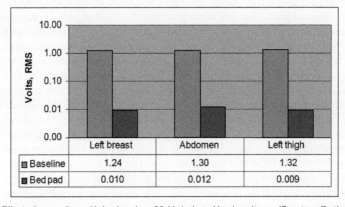

Figure 17.6   Effect of grounding with bed pad on 60-Hz induced body voltage. *(Courtesy Earth FX, Inc.)*

potential (and thus grounded), it becomes an extension of the Earth's gigantic electric system. The Earth's potential (ground) thus becomes the working agent that cancels, reduces, or pushes away electric fields from the body. This is the key to the effects of Earthing in reducing voltages induced on the body.

Nobel Prize winning physicist, Richard Feynman, said that, "When the body potential is the same as the Earth's electric potential (grounded), it becomes an extension of the Earth's gigantic electric system." Our planet's vast reservoir of electrons provides great stability for all of the many electrical processes taking place within us. These electrical processes are involved in every aspect of physiology and biochemistry.

As pointed out above, the surface of the Earth has an abundance of electrons that give it a negative electrical charge. If you are standing outside on a clear day, wearing shoes or standing on an insulating surface (e.g., wood or vinyl), there is an electrical charge of some 200 V between the Earth and the top of your head (Figure 17.7A).

Applewhite (2005) documented changes in the voltage induced on the body by monitoring the voltage drop across a resistor. The results showed the above-described 'umbrella effect'. The electrons in the body of a grounded person are not agitated by environmental electrical systems.

You might ask, 'If there really is a voltage difference of 200 V from head to toe, why don't I get a shock when I go outside?' The answer is that air is a relatively poor conductor and therefore allows almost no electrical current flow. If you are standing outside in your bare feet (Figure 17.7B), you are Earthed: your whole body is in electrical contact with the Earth's surface. Your body is a relatively good conductor, and, as a result, your skin and the Earth's surface make a continuous charged surface with the same electrical potential. Given that your skin is continuous with the mucous membranes of your digestive and respiratory systems, and because the respiratory system is associated with the blood capillaries in the alveoli of your lungs, the grounding effects reach your circulatory system and then every part of your body. This electrical balancing explains the rapid effect grounding has on red blood cells, as will be described below (see Figure 17.10A).

Figure 17.7B also shows that the charged area is pushed up and away from your head if you are grounded. Any object in direct contact with the Earth – a person, a dog, a tree – creates this shielding effect (also shown in Figure 17.2). Grounded objects essentially reside within the

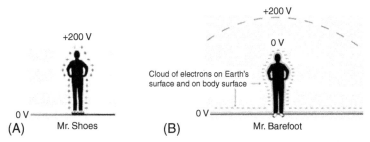

Figure 17.7 The surface of the Earth has an abundance of electrons that give it a negative electrical charge. (A) If you are standing outside on a clear day, wearing shoes or standing on an insulating surface, such as a wood or vinyl floor or asphalt, there is an electrical charge of around 200 V between the Earth and the top of your head. (B) If you are standing outside barefoot, your whole body is in electrical contact with the Earth's surface. Your body is a relatively good conductor. Your skin and the Earth's surface make a continuous charged surface with the same electrical potential. Also notice in (B) that the charged area is pushed up and away from your head if you are grounded. Any object in direct contact with the Earth (a person, a dog, a tree) creates this shielding effect. The object is essentially residing within the protective umbrella of Earth's natural electric field. This protective phenomenon also occurs inside your house or office if you are connected to the Earth with an Earthing device such as a grounding wrist pad or a foot pad.

protective umbrella of Earth's natural electric field. This protective phenomenon also occurs inside your home or office, if you are connected to the Earth with an Earthing device such as a grounded bed sheet or a grounded foot pad.

Jamieson et al. (2007) asked whether the failure to appropriately ground humans contributes to the potential consequences of electropollution in offices. Considerable debate exists on whether electromagnetic fields in our environment cause a risk to health (e.g., Genuis, 2008), but there is no question that the body reacts to the presence of environmental electric fields. Applewhite's study demonstrated that grounding essentially eliminates the ambient voltage induced on the body from common household electric power sources.

Evidence suggests that painful conditions are often the result of various kinds of acute or chronic inflammation, which are caused, in part, by highly reactive molecules known as reactive oxygen species or free radicals. These molecules are generated by normal metabolism and also by the immune system, as part of the body's response to injury or trauma. These reactive molecules are thought to be the immediate cause of the characteristic features of inflammation that have been recognized since ancient times: pain, redness, heat, swelling, and loss of function. Inflammation produces heat that can be measured with infrared medical imaging. A study using this approach (Amalu, 2004) revealed rapid reductions in inflammation at the same time as pain was reduced (Figure 17.8).

The apparatus shown in Figure 17.9 was assembled to track physiological changes produced by Earthing. A ground wire was connected to a switch box so that the grounding could be turned on or off during experiments without the subject knowing about whether or not grounding was taking place. The grounded patch was connected to the subject at the acupoints known as Kidney 1 (inset Figure 17.9). Acupuncturists refer to this point as the primary entry point for Qi, known in Hawaii as 'mana' and in Sanskrit as 'prana'. While the term is not

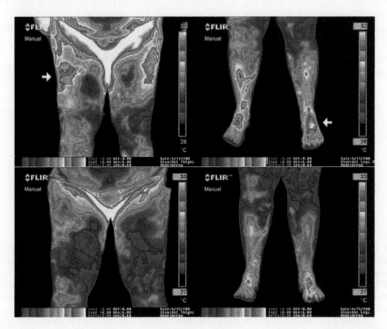

Figure 17.8 Reduction in inflammation and pain after sleeping grounded for four nights. Medical infrared imaging shows warm and painful areas (arrows). Sleeping grounded for four nights resolved the pain, and the hot areas cooled. *(Courtesy Earth FX, Inc., Thermal Image Photo.)*

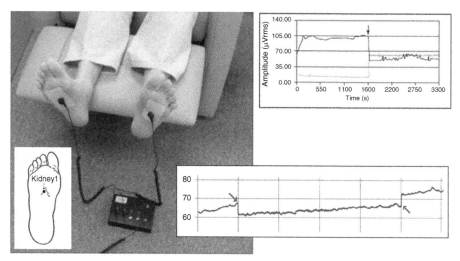

Figure 17.9 Technique for studying the flow of electrons from the Earth to the human body. Conductive patches are placed on the balls of the feet. Wires connect these patches to an Earthing rod inserted into the soil near a healthy outdoor plant to assure a good connection with the supply of free electrons on the Earth's surface. The inset shows the proximity of the conductive patch to the acupuncture meridian point known as Kidney 1. The photograph is from Chevalier and Mori (2008). The inset is from http://www.acupuncture.com/education/points/kidney/kid1.htm. The upper graphic shows virtually instantaneous normalization of muscle tension at the moment of grounding (arrow), as measured with electromyography of the trapezius muscle. The lower graphic shows a drop in skin conductance at the moment of grounding (left arrow) and a rebound in skin conductance at the moment of ungrounding (right arrow). *(The author thanks Drs. Chevalier and Mori for permission to reproduce these illustrations.)*

used in Western medicine, more than 65 cultures from around the world have words for Qi energy and incorporate the concept in their sciences, philosophy, culture, and healing arts. The Kidney 1 point is located near the ball of the foot. Chevalier & Mori (2008) performed a series of studies using the arrangement shown in Figure 17.9. They were able to establish a precisely timed Earth connection, and they recorded changes in various physiological parameters before, during, and after grounding.

How does grounding the body reduce inflammation? One logical explanation is that grounding the body allows antioxidant electrons from the Earth to enter the body and neutralize highly charged reactive oxygen species at sites of inflammation. If this theory is correct, one would expect changes in the well-researched profiles in blood chemistry and white blood cell counts associated with inflammation. Such changes have been documented (Brown et al., 2010).

Finally, stress reduction has been confirmed using various measures that show virtually instantaneous shifts from sympathetic to parasympathetic dominance of the autonomic nervous system, as well as the normalization of muscle tension. The upper-right graphic in Figure 17.9 shows virtually instantaneous normalization of muscle tension at the moment of grounding (arrow), as measured through electromyography of the trapezius muscle. The lower-right graphic in Figure 17.9 shows a drop in skin conductance at the moment of grounding (left arrow) and a rebound in skin conductance at the moment of ungrounding (right arrow). Thus, grounding the body produces a cascade of effects on sleep, inflammation, pain, and the debilitating consequences of stress. Now we look at important cardiovascular effects.

Earthing appears to have profound effects on the cardiovascular system. A barefoot connection with the Earth reduces blood viscosity and the clumping of red blood cells (Figure 17.10A). Blood

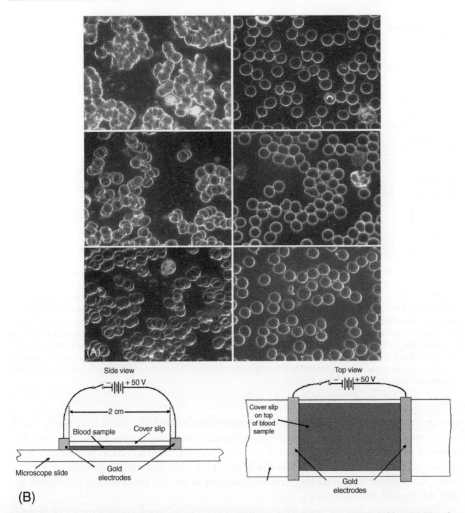

Figure 17.10 (A) The effect of Earthing on red blood cell (RBC) aggregation was measured by counting the numbers of clustered cells in each sample. (B) Side and top views of the experimental setup for zeta (ζ) potential measurement. Standard microscope slides and cover slips were used. The electrode system consisted of two gold bars placed directly on the microscope slide at the sides of the cover slip. The gold bars were connected to two 9-volt batteries in series. A switch controlled the application of the electric field. The field between the electrodes ranged from 14.3 to 28.0 V/cm For each sample, a drop of solution containing minerals and trace elements in the same proportions as they occur in blood serum (Quinton's isotonic water) was added to the drop of blood to decrease RBC concentration and to prevent electroendosmosis from affecting the RBCs' mobility. The proportion was 20% blood to isotonic solution. A cover slip was then placed over the sample and the gold bars moved into position. A drop of isotonic solution was added on each side of the cover slip to insure conductive contact between the gold electrodes and the diluted blood sample. A video camera mounted on a dark field microscope (Richardson RTM-3.0; combined magnification factor of 1000) recorded the movement of the RBCs. Observations were made for a few minutes, which was enough time to record the RBCs' terminal velocities for a period of at least 10 s at three different locations. A micrometer stage allowed the repositioning of the sample to find areas with appropriate RBC density for zeta potential and aggregation measurement. When a suitable area was located, the power to the gold bars was switched on. Suitable areas had a low enough RBC density that most of the RBCs could move about freely without collision for at least 10 s. Three separate measurements were made at each of three different such areas, yielding a total of nine measurements on each sample. The video images were recorded on digital videodiscs for subsequent determination of the velocity of RBC migration. The zeta potential (ζ) of RBCs maintains the fluidity of blood by preventing RBC aggregation. The combination of zeta potential and aggregation are important determinants of blood viscosity. For further details, see Chevalier et al. (2013).

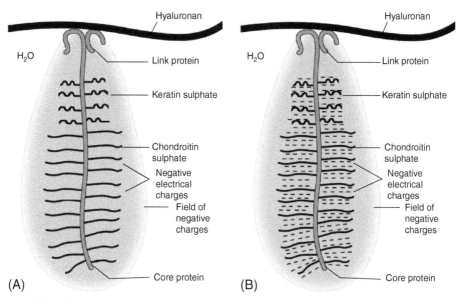

Figure 17.11 Charges on the ground substance (matrisome). In the ungrounded person (A) the ground substance is depleted of electrons. In the grounded person (B) the ground substance is saturated with electrons. The matrisome is a repeating proteoglycan unit consisting of the core protein linked to hyaluronan and glycosaminoglycan side chains. The glycosaminoglycans stand out straight from the proteoglycan backbones, and adjacent chains repel each other to form an arrangement like the bristles of a brush. The result of the charge density is a strong field or 'domain' of negative charge. *(Lee RP: Interface: Mechanisms of Spirit in Osteopathy, Stillness Press LLC, 2005)*

viscosity was measured with the apparatus shown in Figure 17.10B. Elevated blood viscosity has been implicated in virtually every aspect of cardiovascular disease, which is the number one cause of death worldwide. This is a most important finding in relation to global public health and the costs of healthcare, both in terms of personal suffering and the growing debts of many nations.

The mechanism by which Earthing affects inflammation has been postulated as follows:

- The polyelectrolyte ground substance (see Chapter 11 and Figure 11.4) extends throughout the body. The charged groups on the glycosaminoglycans have an enormous capacity to store electrons. In the ungrounded person, charge reservoirs in the connective tissue ground substance are depleted of electrons (Figure 17.11A). It is thought that the body continually uses electrons from the reservoirs to neutralize reactive oxygen species produced by metabolism, by responses to toxins and injuries, and by other oxidative processes. After disconnecting from the Earth, the whole body gradually becomes 'electron depleted'. In the grounded person, charge reservoirs in the connective tissue ground substance are rapidly saturated with electrons (Figure 17.11B). This is referred to as a state of 'inflammatory preparedness'.

- The reactions of ungrounded and grounded people to an injury are shown in Figure 17.12A and B, respectively. In the ungrounded person, the charge reservoirs in the connective tissue ground substance are depleted of electrons. As a result, an inflammatory barricade can form around the injury site. The barricade is formed from damaged cells and tissues (see Figures 17.12 and 17.13). In the grounded person, charge reservoirs in the connective tissue ground substance are saturated with electrons – inflammatory preparedness. The grounded person forms little or no inflammatory barricade around an injury because the living matrix and the electron-saturated ground substance provide electrons that can neutralize reactive oxygen species (free radicals) thereby avoiding damage to nearby healthy tissue (Oschman, 2008, 2009).

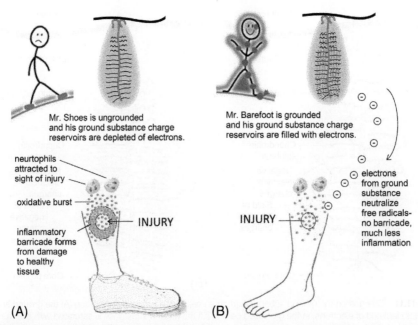

Figure 17.12 (A) Ungrounded person: charge reservoirs in the connective tissue ground substance are depleted of electrons. The whole body is 'electron depleted'. The ungrounded person will form an inflammatory barricade around the injury site. (B) Grounded person: charge reservoirs in the connective tissue ground substance are saturated with electrons. The electron saturation is referred to as a state of inflammatory preparedness. The grounded person will not form an inflammatory barricade because electrons from the living matrix and from the electron-saturated ground substance will immediately neutralize reactive oxygen species (free radicals) that could damage nearby healthy tissues.

These findings resonate with the work of Hans Selye, who developed the concept of stress and did pioneering studies of inflammation. Biomedical research from around the world is revealing that chronic or 'silent' inflammation is the culprit behind virtually every chronic disease (summarized by Oschman, 2007). Inflammation is defined as a localized response to trauma or infection that can wall off damaged tissues until the immune system removes foreign matter, damaged cells, and/or bacteria. Selye (1953, 1956) published micrographs and drawings of the way irritants can produce a walled-off area (Figure 17.13A–D). When the inflammatory response does not completely wind down, palpable 'inflammatory pockets' can form and can persist for many years, slowly releasing toxins that can damage organs anywhere in the body. Selye (1956) described the phenomenon of persistent localized inflammation in his classic book *The Stress of Life* and in an article he published in the *Journal of the American Medical Association* (Selye, 1953) and in other articles. A search of PubMed revealed more than 1600 references to the inflammatory or granuloma pouch, with some specifically referring to the use of the 'Selye Pouch' for the study of inflammatory reactions (e.g., Davis et al., 1981).

Selye's work connected inflammatory responses with stress, cortisol secretion, and adaptation. Selye and others have obtained evidence that the products of necrotic tissue breakdown can leak from inflammatory pockets into the blood and lymphatic circulation, producing slow but progressive atrophy in various organs, despite distance from the original site of trauma. For example, on page 161 of the first edition of *The Stress of Life*, Selye describes how he was able to inject irritants or microbes into inflammatory pouches under the skin of rats, producing inflammation of the heart valves (endocarditis) very similar to the inflammation that often occurs in

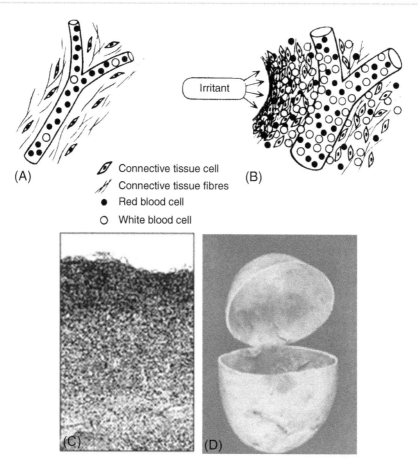

Figure 17.13 Formation of the inflammatory barricade and pouch, according to Selye (1956). (A) Normal connective tissue territory. (B) Same tissue exposed to irritant. The vessel dilates, blood cells migrate toward the irritant, and connective tissue cells and fibres form a thick impenetrable barricade that prevents the spread of the irritant into the blood, but that also prevents the entry of regenerative cells that could repair the tissue (Ben Harrison, Wake Forest Institute for Regenerative Medicine, personal communication). The result can be a long-lasting pocket of incompletely resolved inflammation that can eventually leak toxins into the system and disturb the functioning of an organ or tissue. (C) Histology of the inflammatory barricade. Electrons are the ultimate antioxidants. It is suggested that electrons can be semi-conducted into the inflammatory pouch where they can neutralize reactive oxygen species (free radicals). (D) The inflammatory pouch, a concept developed by Selye and widely used in studies of inflammation.

children suffering from rheumatic fever. Under some conditions, endocarditis was accompanied by inflammation of the kidney (nephritis) and excessive stimulation of the blood-forming organs. The inflammatory pouch concept explains how local pockets of inflammation can trigger a diversity of chronic diseases and disturbances, many of which frustrate the physician because it is difficult to locate the cause. 'Silent inflammation' refers to a condition in which the inflamed site is not painful and may go unnoticed, even though it is causing problems elsewhere in the body. The phenomenon was described long ago in dentistry, beginning with 25 years of important root canal research by Dr. Weston Price (see Meinig, 1994). Silent inflammation is now rarely recognized however, except by 'biological' dentists who are aware of the hazards of root canals and amalgam.

Reduction of Primary Indicators of Osteoporosis, Improvement of Glucose Regulation, and Immune Responses

Researchers in Poland have added another dimension to our understanding of Earthing, pointing out that grounding could have a protective effect against diabetes and osteoporosis. Karol Sokal and Pawel Sokal, a cardiologist father and neurosurgeon son in Poland, conducted a series of experiments to determine whether contact with the Earth via a copper conductor can affect physiological processes (Sokal and Sokal, 2011). Their pioneering investigations were prompted by questions regarding the possible relationship between the natural electric charge on the surface of the Earth and the regulation of human physiological processes. Double-blind experiments were conducted on groups ranging from 12 to 84 subjects who followed similar physical activity, diet, and fluid intake schedules during the trial periods. Grounding was achieved with a copper plate (30×80 mm) placed on the lower part of the leg and attached with a strip so that it would not come off during the night. A conductive wire connected the leg plate to a larger plate (60×250 mm) placed in contact with the Earth outside.

In one experiment with nonmedicated subjects, grounding during a single night of sleep resulted in statistically significant changes in concentrations of minerals and electrolytes in the blood serum, including iron, ionized calcium, inorganic phosphorus, sodium, potassium, and magnesium. Renal excretion of both calcium and phosphorus was significantly reduced as well, and the observed reductions in blood and urinary calcium and phosphorus directly relate to osteoporosis. Therefore, the results of the Sokals' experiments suggest that Earthing for only a single night reduces primary indicators of osteoporosis.

In addition, the Sokals showed that continuous Earthing during rest and physical activity over a 72-h period decreased fasting glucose among patients with non-insulin-dependent diabetes mellitus. Patients in the study had been well controlled with glibenclamide, an antidiabetic drug, for about 6 months, but at the time of study, the subjects had unsatisfactory glycemic control despite dietary and exercise advice and glibenclamide doses of 10 mg/day.

The Sokals also drew blood samples from six male and six female adults with no history of thyroid disease. A single night of grounding produced a significant decrease of free tri-iodothyronine and an increase of free thyroxin and thyroid-stimulating hormone. The significance of these results is unclear, but the logical explanation is that Earthing influences hepatic, hypothalamic, and pituitary relationships via adjusting thyroid function. Ober et al. (2014) have observed that many individuals on thyroid medication reported symptoms of hyperthyroid, such as heart palpitations, after starting grounding. Such symptoms typically vanish after medication is adjusted downward under medical supervision. Through a series of feedback regulations, thyroid hormones affect almost every physiological process in the body, including growth and development, metabolism, body temperature, and heart rate. Further study of Earthing effects on thyroid function will be valuable.

In another experiment done by the Sokals, the effect of grounding on the classic immune response following vaccination was examined. Earthing accelerated the immune response, as demonstrated by increases in gamma globulin concentration. This result confirms an association between Earthing and the immune response, as was suggested in the DOMS study (Brown et al., 2010).

Sokal and Sokal, 2011 concluded that grounding or Earthing the human body may be 'the primary factor regulating endocrine and nervous systems'. Grounding may therefore represent a 'universal regulating factor in Nature' that strongly influences bioelectrical, bioenergetic, and biochemical processes, and that can have a significant effect on the chronic diseases they encounter daily in their clinical practices.

The Earthing or grounding studies can be summarized in a single statement: connecting with the Earth is easy and can have many benefits. Anyone can practice Earthing at no cost by simply removing their shoes and socks and walking barefoot on the Earth. The research on Earthing has revealed a new picture of the nature of inflammation and the reasons it can lead to chronic and autoimmune diseases. We can see that grounding can lead to the reduction or elimination of inflammatory barricade formation, which Western medical science recognizes as a common response to injury. Formation of the inflammatory barricade is so common following injury because most people are not grounded. Therefore, prevention of chronic inflammation can be accomplished by saturating the ground substance in the connective tissues around an injury site with electrons, protecting against 'collateral damage' in healthy tissues, provided that the living matrix is functioning properly. Grounding immediately after an injury can be very valuable as 'first aid' until the doctor arrives.

The research on Earthing has revealed a new picture of the nature of inflammation and the reasons it can lead to chronic diseases.

Reports from people around the world have led to a new compilation of observations in the second edition of a book by Ober et al. (2014). In that edition, Clint Ober summarized:

Since 1998, I have been invited into the homes of probably several thousand people and reconnected them to the Earth. I have grounded newborns, kids, young adults, midlifers, seniors, and centenarians, and individuals deathly ill for whom the medical system had no more fixes to offer. Some understood what I was doing. Most didn't. They just understood that they felt better and had less pain.

For example, while Earthing is not a cure for autism, autistic children who use Earthing are often much more comfortable, sleep better, and are easier to care for. This can make a huge difference for families who are often engaged in a lifelong struggle. Many women also report relief from menstrual issues. Autoimmune diseases are not cured, but the pain associated with them becomes much more manageable; the pain after tattoos is greatly relieved; headaches often become less intense and less frequent, and sometimes go away altogether; for those who are bedridden, a grounded sheet reduces or eliminates bed sores; asthma, arthritis, respiratory and circulatory problems, constipation, eczema and psoriasis have been relieved; mobility has improved; inflammation of all kinds has been reduced; 'mystery disorders' that the best medicine is unable to treat are improved; the list goes on and on.

Implications for Aging

Finally, the leading theory of aging is the so-called free radical theory. Simply stated, it has been suggested that aging results from the cumulative damage done to cells and tissues by free radicals produced during normal biochemical processes such as oxidative metabolism and during the body's natural responses to injury and pollutants. Because the free radical is a molecule with one or more unpaired electrons, it has charge and magnetic properties that make it highly reactive, as well as attractive to free electrons. This is the physics that makes these molecules so destructive – they literally rip electrons from pathogens and damaged cells produced by an injury. Key work of Gershman et al. (1954) revealed that elevated oxygen atmospheres in incubators were causing retrolental fibroplasia (blindness) in premature babies. This was one of several clues that led Harman (1956) to propose his free radical theory of aging, the most widely studied model of the aging process. While some details require further study, the free radical model has stood the test of time.

Today, free radicals are being implicated in virtually all of the diseases of aging and in the aging process itself. Recognition of the free electron as the ideal antioxidant has led to an explanation of how Earthing and a number of microcurrent electrotherapy devices are so effective at reducing

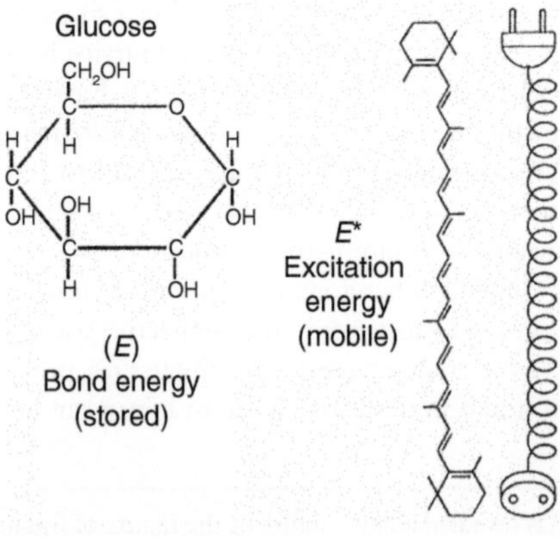

Figure 17.14 Albert Szent-Györgyi (1968) referred to the immobile electron energy stored in the bonds of the glucose molecule as E to distinguish them from mobile excited electrons E^*. The carotene molecule shown on the right contains a series of double bonds, each of which has one electron that is not confined to the bond but is free to move. In the diagram on the right he compares the carotene molecule with the power cord for a toaster.

inflammation and treating chronic diseases. The ability of charges to migrate through the living matrix is relevant to antiaging medicine because of the potential antioxidant nature of the mobile electrons. While a great deal of research is being done to correlate inflammation with disease states, there are few theories on the mechanisms involved. The research on Earthing has provided a logical and testable theory based on a variety of kinds of evidence (Oschman, Chevalier & Brown 2015). The antiinflammatory effects of connecting to the Earth arise because the Earth's surface is an abundant source of excited and mobile electrons.

Albert Szent-Györgyi (1957) made a distinction between E, energy stored in chemical bonds, and E^*, excited energy that is mobile (Figure 17.14). The basic hypothesis states that the living matrix is a semiconductor network extending throughout the body and is capable of rapidly delivering excited electrons, or E^*, to any point where a free radical appears. If the matrix is in a healthy state, it will be conductive to E^* at all points, and the mobile electrons will have an antiaging effect by neutralizing any reactive molecules as soon as they form. If the matrix conduction is blocked, or if electrons are not available (electron depletion, Figure 17.11A), the cumulative damage that leads to aging will take place. When the matrix is conductive, and when the ground substance is saturated with electrons, free radical damage will be minimized, and aging will be slower.

Following on Ober's original discovery (Ober, 2003), a number of technologies emerged for the purpose of simply and conveniently connecting the individual to the Earth without actually going barefoot. These technologies include conductive grounding sheets for the bed, as was shown in Figure 17.3; grounding pads for under the feet or wrists when working at a computer; bracelets that can be worn around the wrist or ankles or chest; and flip-flops and comfortable shoes that connect people with the Earth during the day as they are walking about (Figure 17.15). The shoes and flip-flops have conductive plugs positioned next to acupoint Kidney 1 to allow electrons to enter the body.

Aromatherapy and Essential Oils

Essential oils are the volatile liquids that are distilled or pressed from aromatic or fragrant parts of plants, such as seeds, bark, leaves, stems, roots, flowers, and fruit. These substances were among the earliest medicines, having been used by priests and physicians for thousands of years. Gradually, through millennia of experience, these substances were evaluated for their healing properties, and they came to be known as some of the most effective medicines in the world.

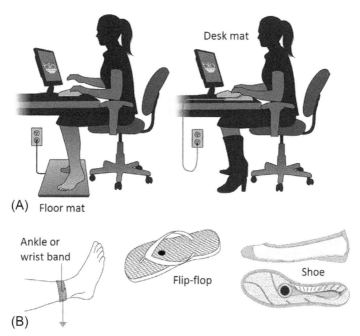

Figure 17.15 Grounding methods that do not require walking barefoot on the Earth. Earthing mats (A) can be used on or under the desk. (B) Earthing can also be achieved using ankle or wrist bands, flip-flops, and shoes. The flip-flops and shoes have conductive plugs located at Kidney 1. *(Courtesy Earth FX, Inc., Thermal Image Photo.)*

There are 188 references to essential oils in the Bible (frankincense, myrrh, rosemary, etc.).

In modern times, essential oils are prized for the speed with which they act on annoying discomforts, diseases, or skin problems. Because of their enormous popularity and widespread use, modern medical researchers are investigating the health effects of essential oils, with over 12,000 articles on essential oils and 850 on aromatherapy listed in the database of the US National Library of Medicine, PubMed. A valuable and extensive compilation of the literature can be found in *Modern Essentials* (Aroma Tools, 2013).

Antimicrobial resistance is one of our most serious health threats. Infections from resistant bacteria are now too common, and some pathogens have even become resistant to multiple types or classes of antibiotics (antimicrobials used to treat bacterial infections). The loss of effective antibiotics will undermine our ability to fight infectious diseases and manage the infectious complications common in vulnerable patients undergoing chemotherapy for cancer, dialysis for renal failure, and surgery, especially organ transplantation, for which the ability to treat secondary infections is crucial. When first-line and then second-line antibiotic treatment options are limited by resistance or are unavailable, healthcare providers are forced to use antibiotics that may be more toxic to the patient and frequently more expensive and less effective. Even when alternative treatments exist, research has shown that patients with resistant infections are often much more likely to die, and survivors have significantly longer hospital stays, delayed recuperation, and long-term disability. Efforts to prevent such threats build on the foundation of proven public health strategies: immunization, infection control, protecting the food supply, antibiotic stewardship, and reducing person-to-person spread through screening, treatment and education.

Frieden, 2013

One obvious mechanism for the behavioural and neurological effects of essential oils is the ability of volatile molecules to penetrate through the blood–brain barrier and thereby reach into parts of the brain that are inaccessible to many drugs. For example, nurses have used *Lavandula augustifolia* essential oil diffused nightly in a nursing home. The method was effective at reducing insomnia and anxiety in residents suffering from dementia, anxiety, and disturbed sleep patterns (Johannessen, 2013). The author can confirm that a few drops of lavender on the pillow at night is very relaxing. Aromatherapy also shows much promise for treating various neurological disorders.

Another recent study concerned a major issue in modern medicine, the treatment of methicillin-resistant *Staphylococus aureus* (MRSA). Conventional treatments cost billions of dollars worldwide each year; some $34 billion per year in the US alone. Many essential oils have demonstrated antimicrobial properties, but they are rarely used in hospitals, mainly because doctors are not aware that there is so much scientific evidence of their efficacy. Doctors also have concerns about the toxicity of essential oils and, therefore, they continue to rely on the conventional therapies with which they are familiar. Antimicrobial resistance is a very serious problem, however, as outlined by the US Centers for Disease Control in 2013 (see box above) and also by the World Health Organization (WHO) in 2014 (see box below).

New WHO Report Provides the most Comprehensive Picture of Antibiotic Resistance to Date, with Data from 114 Countries

30 April 2014|GENEVA – A new report by WHO – its first to look at antimicrobial resistance, including antibiotic resistance, globally – reveals that this serious threat is no longer a prediction for the future. It is happening right now in every region of the world and has the potential to affect anyone, of any age, in any country. Antibiotic resistance – when bacteria change so antibiotics no longer work in people who need them to treat infections – is now a major threat to public health.

Nelson (1997) tested a range of essential oils and extracts for their bacteriostatic and bactericidal properties. *Melaleuca alternifolia* (tea tree) was the most potent of the essential oils tested. In 2004, Edwards-Jones et al. placed wound dressings with essential oils over Petri dishes and demonstrated that the fumes of tea tree oil had antimicrobial effects. Chin and Cordell (2013) confirmed that tea tree oil works on patients with *Staph* infections as well. The results showed that treatment with tea tree oil speeded healing of the infections in all but one of the participants. The differences between tea tree and conventional treatment were striking.

Because of widespread optimism about the clinical use of these substances, research is under way to determine the safety and effectiveness of these substances in various medical situations. In this chapter we are not summarizing the growing data on this topic, as there is already an abundant literature. Instead, we focus on the possible mechanisms by which essential oils can have such rapid beneficial effects, even when given in minute quantities.

Martin L. Pall (2013) studied how very low energy electromagnetic fields (EMFs) produce beneficial or harmful biological effects. He was surprised to find that that the answer was "hiding in plain sight" in the scientific literature. Most investigators are too focused and highly specialized to take the time to read and organize the relevant literature. Pall found twenty-six reports showing that low energy EMF's act via voltage-gated calcium channels, and that blockers of these channels can prevent responses to such exposures.

In Chapter 9 we suggested that physiological regulations may in part be carried out by electromagnetic fields between resonant molecules. When turning a physiological process on or off, a mechanism of this kind can operate much faster (speed of light) than regulatory molecules randomly diffusing from place to place through the fluid compartments within the body. One can envision a network of electromagnetic informational or photonic signalling processes enabling every tissue, cell, or molecule to coordinate its activities with the organism as a whole – a process that has been termed *systemic cooperation* by Oschman (2003) and *gestaltbildung* by Popp and Beloussov (2003). It is also easy to see how specific frequencies produced by vibrations of the molecules in essential oils could interact with the key components of this signalling system to produce specific effects.

In one sense, these concepts place aromatherapy in the same category as other subtle interactions discussed earlier in this book. These interactions include the types of energy involved in the martial arts, external homeopathy, and noncontact energy treatments such as those used in Polarity Therapy, Therapeutic Touch, Healing Touch, Reiki, and so on, as well as the harmful or interfering effects of radiations used in technologies such as cellular telephones and Wi-Fi. The validity of these subtle interactions has been questioned because most scientists have been puzzled to the point of incredulity by claims that low-energy photons, which don't have enough energy to influence the chemistry or temperature of a cell, can still have weak electromagnetic field (EMF) effects on physiology. How can nonthermal effects of such tiny EMFs possibly do anything?

Satyendra Nath Bose was an Indian mathematician and physicist who wrote a paper in 1924 describing a statistical theory for light. Albert Einstein showed that the same rules apply to atoms, as in a gas. Bose and Einstein collaborated to develop a mathematics called Bose–Einstein statistics that describes the gas-like qualities of both electromagnetic radiation (light) and collections of coherent electrons or atoms. The theory describes the behaviour of a group of particles in the same energetic state and accounts for the cohesive streaming of laser light and other quantum phenomena. The Bose–Einstein condensate is a dense collection of bosons, which are elementary particles or atoms with integer spin, named after S.N. Bose.

In 2013, Pall summarized 23 studies demonstrating that voltage-gated calcium channels are responsible for the effects of weak EMFs (see box at the bottom of page 316). There is another mechanism that may be more general: weak fields may influence other parts of the cellular regulatory chains, including individual molecules in the signalling cascade.

This explanation is gaining strength because of recent discoveries about the quantum properties of water (Oschman, 2013). Specifically, the study of quantum coherence in living systems led Herbert Fröhlich to realize that liquid crystalline components of the living body can accomplish Bose–Einstein condensation of strongly excited longitudinal electric modes, long-range coherence, and energy storage (Fröhlich, 1968) (see box for an explanation of this phenomenon). Recent applications of quantum field theory reveal coherence domains of millions of molecules (Del Giudice et al., 2010). Finely tuned metastable energized states within arrays of spinning water molecules enable responses to exceedingly weak electromagnetic fields of appropriate frequency, releasing an amount of energy within the organism that is far in excess of that contained in the original EMF. This amplification enables coherence domains in physiological systems to function in a manner comparable to the oscillatory instabilities found in some sensory systems (Camalet et al., 2000).

Other processes make living systems sensitive to particular frequencies as well. In a mechanism known as Larmor precession, particular frequencies cause spinning electrons, protons, or water molecules to precess (see Figure 17.16 for a description of this process). Because of Larmor precession and quantum coherence, frequency becomes a more important parameter than intensity in terms of extremely weak field effects and the establishment of regulatory standards for limiting exposures.

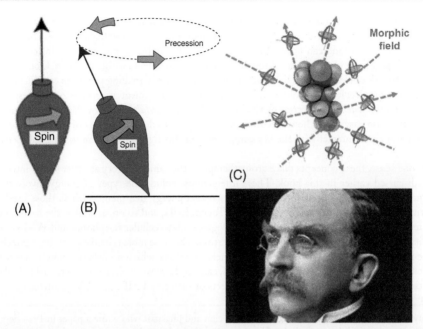

Figure 17.16 Protons and electrons have a property known as spin. The situation can be compared to the spinning top (A). In the absence of an external field, there will be a certain spin axis. If an external field is applied, the spin axis will tilt and the particle will precess, and the spin axis of the particle will sweep out a conical surface (B). The frequency causing the precession is known as the Larmor frequency, named after Sir Joseph Larmor, an Irish physicist and mathematician. (C) Hypothesis: spinning water molecules at the surface of larger molecules, such as this amino acid, lysine, act as the information exchange interface between the biomolecule and its surroundings.

In the case of aromatherapy, measurements of the frequencies of the oils are made during the manufacturing process to ensure their purity and content. These measurements can be used to determine the specific frequencies emitted or absorbed by the essential oils. This last statement should be noted because we can hypothesize that some therapeutic benefits may arise from the ability of an essential oil to absorb harmful frequencies caused by pathological processes taking place within the body. This is a good topic for future research (Figure 17.17).

Medicinal Herbs

Herbal medicine is distinct from aromatherapy in that its methods employ plants of all kinds, not just those that are aromatic or fragrant. Plants and parts of plants have been used for medicinal purposes through much of human history, and traditional herbal medicine is still widely practised today. Modern medicine and pharmacology makes use of many plant-derived compounds as the basis for evidence-tested pharmaceutical drugs. Phytotherapy applies modern standards of effectiveness testing to herbs and medicines that are derived from natural sources. The scope of herbal medicines sometimes includes fungal and bee products, as well as minerals, shells, and certain animal parts.

The WHO estimates that 80% of the populations of some Asian and African countries presently use herbal medicines as part of their primary healthcare. Pharmaceuticals are prohibitively expensive for most of the world's population, half of which live on less than US$2 per day. In comparison, anyone can grow herbal medicines from seed or gather them from nature for little or no cost.

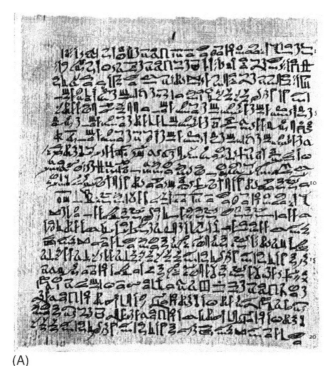

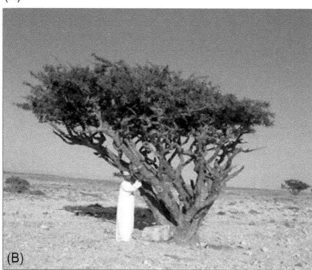

Figure 17.17 (A) The Egyptians may have been the first to use essential oils, as such substances are mentioned in the *Ebers Papyrus*, one of the oldest medical documents known, and possibly the oldest book in the world (Bryan 1930, Figure 17.21). This manuscript, dating from 1553 to 1550 BC, was compiled from other documents from five to twenty centuries earlier. Among its 811 treatments, the *Ebers Papyrus* describes the use of frankincense and other oils for treating various ailments. (B) The Omani frankincense tree, from http://www.mermadearts.com/article_info.php?articles_id=12.

We are interested in the extent to which energetic phenomena are involved in the action of herbal medicines. The same considerations that were applied to aromatherapy may apply equally to herbal medicines. Specifically, the usual model for the action of chemicals of any kind is a biochemical or molecular biology model along the lines of Lucretian biochemistry (see Chapter 16). In this book, we explore an alternative way of looking at these processes, however. Yes, molecules can enter into biochemical reaction pathways and alter them in various ways. This is the area that gets the most attention from biomedical researchers. But molecules are also dependent on the frequencies they exchange with the body's electromagnetic matrix and thereby with other molecules. This frequency-dependence provides a potential mechanism to explain the many subtle effects of herbs, aromas, and remedies of all kinds.

Herbal products are commonly used to treat clinical conditions. Scientific study of these medications is a fascinating topic, and many good reports have been published (PubMed has more than 22,000 entries as of the end of 2013). Anyone considering the use of botanicals or dietary supplements is advised to look into this growing scientific literature to research a substance's safety and effectiveness, possible adverse reactions, the risk–benefit profile, and potential herb–drug interactions. Herbs are often purchased online or at health food stores without the supervision of a healthcare provider. Herbal use is controversial in part because of widespread exaggerated claims of clinical efficacy and safety (Owens et al., 2014).

Case studies can be very valuable. A case study may involve only one or a few people, and, if properly done and accurately reported, this form of research can give a patient an idea of how others have responded to the same treatment. Potential users of herbal medicine must always remember that people are different, however, and what works for one person may have no effect or even a negative effect on another.

The box shows an example of a case study from the recent literature. Migraine is a common neurological condition characterized by the disabling effects it has on the patient. Despite efforts in drug development, better treatments for migraine are still needed. Takaku et al. (2013) provide a case study of treatment with an herbal medicine that had a strong pain-relieving effect for the type of migraine known as migraine without aura.

A 49-year-old woman had frequent episodes of migraine without aura (aura refers to strange feelings and symptoms noticed shortly before a headache). In spite of the use of antiepileptic drugs, she experienced severe migraines almost three times a week and had to take 100 mg of sumatriptan (Imitrex) orally for each attack. Because the pain relieving effect of the drug was inconsistent, the physicians decided to treat her with a traditional Japanese/Chinese herbal medicine, sanno-shashin-to (Xie Xin Tang) extract. Soon after she started taking this decoction the intensity of her headaches was markedly decreased. Therefore, she was told to continue with the herbal medicine once a day (two capsules before going to sleep at night) to prevent severe morning headaches. She was also allowed to continue taking the same antiepileptic drug. After 3 weeks of treatment, the frequency of her headaches had not changed. However, the intensity of her morning headaches had markedly decreased, even though she had stopped taking sumatriptan. Her residual headaches rapidly disappeared within about an hour when she started taking an additional capsule in the morning. The patient has now been undergoing the same treatment for almost 2 years without any exacerbation of her migraine attacks. She has not taken sumatriptan since she started taking this herbal medicine.

Takaku et al., 2013

Sanno-shashin-to was originally produced in ancient China and is described in early texts. It consists of *Rhei radix et rhizoma*, *Coptidis rhizoma*, and *Scutellariae radix*. The description of the clinical use of this decoction in traditional Japanese and Chinese medicine makes no sense to the Western-trained academic.

The formula is used to drain an excess of damp-heat, which is characterized by fever, irritability, restlessness, a flushed face, red eyes, dark urine, constipation, and a greasy and yellow tongue coating. More precisely, *Rhei radix et rhizoma* (rhubarb roots and rhizomes) is the chief herb that drains the heat, especially from the upper part of the body. The subcomponents, *Coptidis rhizoma* and *Scutellariae radix* (baikal skullcap), also drain heat from the upper and middle parts of the body.

Marine Plasma

Modern health science must focus on ensuring that our children and their children will live long, healthy, happy lives, despite the toxic world in which they now live. In these times, prospective parents seeking to birth and raise a healthy child are challenged by reduced sperm counts (Dindyal, 2004) and toxic chemicals in the air, water, food, and even in their blood (see box). By allowing the release of these toxins into our environment, we have compromised our health and even our future as a species.

Roy Dittmann, OMD, MH (Figure 17.18C) has taken on this issue with a passion. His popular book, *Brighton Baby: A Revolutionary Organic Approach to Having an Extraordinary Child* (Dittmann, 2012), has enabled countless parents to avoid the disastrous trends toward autism, attention-deficit disorder (ADD), birth defects, and infertility. Dr. Dittmann exposes the dangers of conceiving in our toxic world and focuses couples on how to prepare body, mind, and spirit for the moment of conception and afterwards. Dittmann describes *Brighton Baby* as a book 'about the art and science of gifting the best of who we are to our future children. It is about reducing human suffering by preventing birth defects before they occur.' (Dittmann, 2012).

One of Dittmann's most successful tools is 'marine plasma' obtained by the methods described by René Quinton (Figure 17.18A). In 1897, Quinton discovered, harvested, and purified seawater from special regions he found in the ocean. He referred to this as 'marine plasma' because it is isotonic with blood plasma. This fluid has extraordinary properties.

Dittmann & Brugioni (2006) describe Quinton Marine Plasma as a 'living fluid' produced by dense 'blooms' of zoo-plankton (microscopic animals) as they consume smaller phytoplankton (microscopic plants). 'Blooms' are large visible areas on the water surface containing huge numbers of microscopic plants that reproduce abundantly under ideal conditions of sunlight, nutrients, and warm water.

Quinton was fascinated with Darwin's concept that all life on earth evolved from a single-celled oceanic organism. Quinton asked where this actually took place. He eventually stumbled upon the properties of the ocean water from sites where large colonies of plankton form vast blooms. Huge numbers of these microscopic animals and plants instinctively swim in large circles. Together with oceanic tides, these organisms create oceanic vortices, hundreds of miles across, which are large enough to be seen in satellite photographs (Figure 17.19). The world's oceans sustain six or seven of these vortices at any one time. The vortices swirl deep down to the ocean floor and stir up rich mineral beds that would otherwise rarely mix with the upper layers of seawater. The walls of the vortices create natural barriers between the bloom and surrounding waters. Larger organisms congregate in the vortices to feed upon the plankton, creating a rich food chain and breeding ground for many species. The result is seawater that is rich in minerals, amino acids, RNA, antioxidants, polysaccharides, and fatty acids – an organic matrix that supports an explosion of life within the vortex. The world's largest living mammals, the great blue whales and their calves, travel thousands of miles to reach these blooms, where they feed on the plankton and krill (small crustaceans). The vegetation growing in these blooms has a larger biomass than all of the vegetation found on land put together.

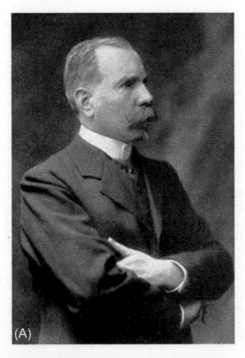

(A)

(B)

L'EAU DE MER

MILIEU ORGANIQUE

CONSTANCE DU MILIEU MARIN ORIGINEL,
COMME MILIEU VITAL DES CELLULES, A TRAVERS LA SÉRIE ANIMALE

PAR

RENÉ QUINTON

Assistant du Laboratoire de Physiologie pathologique des Hautes-Études,
au Collège de France

PARIS
MASSON ET Cⁱᵉ, ÉDITEURS
LIBRAIRES DE L'ACADÉMIE DE MÉDECINE
120, BOULEVARD SAINT-GERMAIN

1904

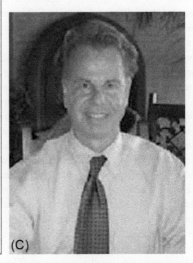

(C)

Figure 17.18 (A) René Quinton, MD. (B) René Quinton's 1912 publication on his clinical discoveries using the marine plasma he discovered. (C) Roy Dittmann, OMD, MH, author of a series of articles on Quinton's discoveries.

Pollutants Compromising Sperm Counts

Estrogen-like chemicals
Plastics
Drugs
Insecticides
Fungicides
Pesticides
Industrial chemicals
Heavy metals
Genetically modified foods
Artificial sweeteners
Rancid oils
Processed foods
Contaminated drinking water
Electrosmog
Preservatives in vaccines

The cells within us evolved from cells such as those forming the plankton blooms. Our cells continue to need a well-balanced ratio of trace elements. However, the soils we use to grow our food lack the full spectrum of essential trace minerals. This was recognized long ago when the United States Senate issued a report (Beach, 1936) warning that our crops were being grown on mineral-depleted soil and that human health was suffering as a result. From that report:

'*Sick soils mean sick plants, sick animals, and sick people. Physical, mental and moral fitness depends largely upon an ample supply and a proper proportion of minerals in our foods. Nerve function, nerve stability and nerve cell-building likewise depend upon trace minerals.*'

Essential trace minerals form about 3% of the electrolytes in the ocean and should be at the same levels in our internal environment.

In his landmark book, *L'eau de Mer Milieu Organique* (Figure 17.18B), René Quinton (1904) demonstrated that drying out or desiccating marine plasma irreversibly damaged the 'live' mineral and protein complexes:

'*The entirety of trace elements contained in marine plasma is to be found in the solution in their active states.*'

The quality of the minerals and water found within the extra-cellular fluid determines the quality of the communications that take place between cells (see Figures 3.1, 11.2, and 11.5). Alfred Pischinger (2004) asserted that:

'*Original seawater is the oldest system of communication between living cells.*'

After researching marine plasma, Passebecq & Soulier (1992) concluded that:

'*Upstream of most diseases there is an unbalanced terrain.*'

Healthcare practitioners throughout Europe have used marine plasma for over 100 years, but until recently, Quinton's discoveries and publications have remained untranslated and virtually unknown to the English-speaking world. However, Quinton repeatedly demonstrated that children with growth abnormalities could often be restored to normal development with injections of isotonic seawater obtained by his methods (Figure 17.19). Quinton suggested that trace minerals must

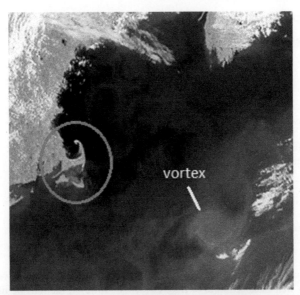

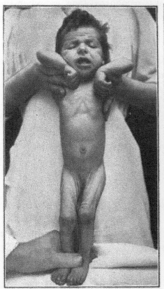 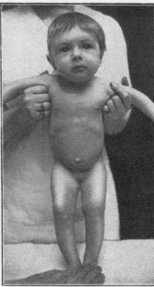 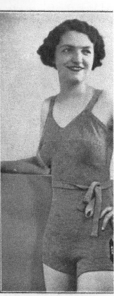

Figure 17.19 The vortices discovered by René Quinton are observable from satellite images. In this figure, a circle surrounds Cape Cod, Massachusetts, Martha's Vineyard, and Nantucket to orient the reader. Dr. Quinton repeatedly demonstrated that children with developmental disorders or growth abnormalities could be restored to normal development with injections of isotonic seawater obtained by his methods. The effects of isotonic seawater on individuals with such conditions suggests that abnormal development may be a consequence of a deficiency or lack of an essential minerals required for normal development. The series of three photos shows an example of a person who underwent the Quinton protocol. To the left, a baby girl at four months and 10 days of age, emaciated with weight 54% behind the weights of typically developing age peers. The image in the middle shows how the baby improved after 6 months of treatment. The image on the right shows her as a normal adult, at age 26. The photos document the individual's development from April 1911 to May 1937. René Quinton emphasized the importance of having all the elements of the periodic table available to the developing human body in a form that is 100% bioavailable. The elements in Quinton's ionic marine plasma are completely bioavailable to humans thanks to the action of the phytoplankton in the vortex. *(Images kindly provided by Dr. Francisco Coll of Laboratoires Quinton, Alicante, Spain.)*

undergo a transformation into a crystalloid state in order to be absorbed by the cells in our bodies. Microorganisms in vortical oceanic blooms accomplish this transformation. The microorganisms 'predigest' the organic minerals and other cofactors so that the human body does not need to actively digest the substances in order to absorb them across the intestinal walls. Our intestinal bacteria can also carry out this predigestion, but overuse of antibiotics has interfered with our intestinal flora.

In a series of three brilliant articles, Dittmann describes biological terrain theory and Quinton's unique clinical applications (Dittmann, 2006a,b, 2007). For example, during the 1918 flu pandemic, which killed many millions of people around the world, those who took Quinton's plasma did not become ill.

Quinton developed a method for harvesting, processing, and administering this fluid to produce remarkable clinical results. Using this fluid, Quinton helped hundreds of thousands of people around the world who were suffering from a vast array of health challenges related to a deficient bioterrain. Whatever the cause of a patient's imbalance, restoring the ailing person's 'inner ocean' or bioterrain was remarkably successful.

The works of PASTEUR bring us a thought conception of disease. Those of QUINTON bring us a conception of health. What is Pasteur's serum? It is a serum for and against a particular disease, a serum which attacks a given microbe and none other. What is sea water? It is a serum which attacks no microbe in particular, but provides the organic cell with the force to fight off all microbes.

L'INTRANSIGEANT PARIS 1907

This marine terrain is the microcosm of the sea itself. When you restore the quality of this internal sea aquarium to its original marine inheritance, every cell, organ, and tissue begins to respond and function as it was intended.

DITTMANN (2006A)

Marine plasma is still harvested from plankton blooms according to the original meticulous protocol developed by René Quinton in 1897. The water is cold-filtered to remove living plankton and microbes. It is never exposed to heat, radiation, or UV light during the course of packaging as René Quinton found that such exposures limit the biological activity. The pharmaceutical manufacturing facility is now located in Alicante, Spain.

Frequencies from Atoms

The reader may wonder about the relationship between trace minerals and energy medicine. One way to answer this question is to look at the work of therapists and musicians who have studied the frequencies of the elements in the periodic table (e.g., Boehm, 2007; Thut, 2013). A practical example is a phototherapy device developed by Robert James (2001). The technology differs from previous light devices because it employs the emission spectra of the elements that are most abundant in the human body: carbon, oxygen, hydrogen, and nitrogen. Together, these four elements comprise 96% of the body by weight. The spectral wavelengths of all these elements are known to the thousandth of an Angstrom (Å) (Haynes 2014, *Handbook of Chemistry and Physics*).

Number of emission lines listed in the Handbook:	
Oxygen	401
Carbon	222
Hydrogen	26
Nitrogen	450
Total	1099

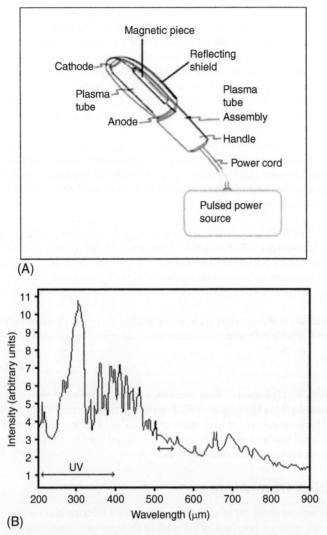

Figure 17.20 The device developed by Robert James and described in United States Patent 6,328,760, issued December 11, 2001. The device emits a soft purple-violet light that appears to benefit patients with dry macular degeneration and also patients with burn wounds of intermediate depth.

The device consists of a quartz tube (Figure 17.20A) that emits over 1000 different frequencies (Figure 17.20B). The soft purple-violet light created by the device has appeared to benefit patients with dry macular degeneration and burn wounds of intermediate depth. Unfortunately, clinical trials were suspended after the death of the inventor. However, he leaves behind a potentially valuable therapeutic technology.

Conclusions

This chapter demonstrates some practical applications of energy medicine in everyday life. All of the described methods are natural, because they relate to the properties of the Earth's surface

(Earthing), plant products grown on the Earth (aromatherapy and herbal medicines), minerals from the sea (Quinton's marine plasma), and light created by electrifying organic gases. These approaches are the discoveries of individuals who have been creative, intuitive, and sensitive observers of nature and natural phenomena. Some methods have been used in various cultures around the world for thousands of years, and in some countries they have been the most effective medicines available. Basic physics can help explain the effectiveness of these approaches. Energy medicine is largely concerned with frequencies, and, as a result, it concerns the ways specific vibrations are emitted and absorbed by therapists, patients, and natural products. Many of these approaches are so effective that they could play a central role in the medicine of the future. A shift toward energy medicine could also inexpensively solve some of the intractable disease conditions that are so costly when treated by our present healthcare system. For this dream to be realized, the public and the medical establishment must recognize those who are able to integrate scientific, artistic, intuitive, and natural phenomena into clinical medicine. Given the astronomical costs and the painful realities caused by chronic diseases, antibiotic resistance, autism, abnormal child growth, and the diseases of aging, there is an urgent need for medical researchers, hospitals and other clinical facilities to recognize the value of energy therapists and the treatments they provide. By developing the flexibility to incorporate safe and effective energetic approaches in clinical practice, medical institutions will lay the foundation for the healthcare system everyone desires.

References

Amalu, R. undated, Medical thermography case studies. Clinical Earthing Application in 20 Case Studies. http://www.earthinginstitute.net/wp-content/uploads/2013/06/Amalu_thermographic_case_studies_2004.pdf.

Ananth, S., 2006. Health Forum 2005 Complementary and Alternative Medicine Survey of Hospitals, July 19, 2006. News release, American Hospital Association.

Applewhite, R., 2005. The effectiveness of a conductive patch and a conductive bed pad in reducing induced human body voltage via the application of earth ground. Eur. Biol. Bioelectromagnet. 1, 23–40.

Aroma Tools, 2013. Modern Essentials: A Contemporary Guide to the Therapeutic Use of Essential Oils, fifth ed. Aroma Tools, Orem, UT.

Bertrand, C.L. (Ed.), 2013. Electrostatics: Theory and Applications. Nova Science Publishers, New York, NY, 332 pp.

Boehm, C.A., 2007. Methods for determining therapeutic resonant frequencies. United States Patent 7,280,874, issued October 9, 2007.

Brown, D., Chevalier, G., Hill, M., 2010. Pilot study on the effect of grounding on delayed-onset muscle soreness. J. Altern. Complement. Med. 16 (3), 265–273.

Bryan, C.P. (translator), 1930. The papyrus Ebers. Translated from the German. Geoffrey Bles, London, http://oilib.uchicago.edu/books/bryan_the_papyrus_ebers_1930.pdf (accessed 13.12.2013).

Camalet, S., et al., 2000. Auditory sensitivity provided by self-tuned critical oscillations of hair cells. Proc. Natl. Acad. Sci. U. S. A. 97 (7), 3183.

CDC, 2014. Centers for Disease Control and Prevention. http://www.cdc.gov/diabetes/statistics/prev/national/figpersons.htm (accessed 12.30.14).

Chevalier, G., Mori, K., 2008. The effects of earthing on human physiology part 2: electrodermal measurements. Subtle Energies & Energy Medicine 18 (3), 11–34.

Chevalier, G., Sinatra, S.T., Oschman, J.L., Delany, R.M., 2013. Earthing (grounding) the human body reduces blood viscosity—a major factor in cardiovascular disease. J. Altern. Complement. Med. 19 (2), 102–110.

Chin, K.B., Cordell, B., 2013. The effect of tea tree oil (*Melaleuca alternifolia*) on wound healing using a dressing model. J. Altern. Complement. Med. 19 (12), 942–945.

Davis, R.H., Pitkow, H.S., Shovlin, K.A., 1981. Anti-inflammatory effect of tryptophan in Selye pouch. J. Am. Podiatr. Med. Assoc. 71 (12), 690–691.

Del Giudice, E., et al., 2010. Water dynamics at the root of metamorphosis in living organisms. Water 2, 566–586.

Dindyal, S., 2004. The sperm count has been decreasing steadily for many years in Western industrialized countries: Is there an endocrine basis for this decrease? Internet J. Urol. 2 (1)Available at: http://archive.is/CEup7 (accessed 16.12.2013).

Dittmann, R., 2006. Evolutionary development of our internal ocean: restoring bio-terrain with Quinton Marine Plasma. Explore 15 (6), 1–5.

Dittmann, R., 2006a. Bio-terrain, evolutionary biology, and the practice of medicine in the early 1900s: an intro to René Quinton's marine plasma. Explore 15 (4), 1–4.

Dittmann, R., 2006b. René Quinton's integral approach to maintaining the internal/external terrain. Explore 16 (6): 1–5.

Dittmann, R., 2012. Brighton Baby: A Revolutionary Organic Approach to Having an Extraordinary Child. Balboa Press, Bloomington, IN, 1030 pp.

Edwards-Jones, V., Buck, R., Shawcross, S.G., Dawson, M.M., Dunn, K., 2004. The effect of essential oils on methicillin-resistant *Staphylococcus aureus* using a dressing model. Burns 30 (8), 772–777.

Feynman, R.P., Layton, R.B., Sands, M., 1964. In: The Feynman Lectures on Physics, vol. II. (Chapter 9, p. 1).

Frieden, T., 2013. Director, U.S. Centers for Disease Control and Prevention, Meeting the Challenges of Drug-Resistant Diseases in Developing Countries Committee on Foreign Affairs Subcommittee on Africa, Global Health, Human Rights, and International Organizations, United States House of Representatives, April 23, 2013.

Fröhlich, H., 1968. Long-range coherence and energy storage in biological systems. Int. J. Quant. Chem. 2, 641.

Genuis, S.J., 2008. Fielding a current idea: exploring the public health impact of electromagnetic radiation. Public Health 122 (2), 113–124.

Gerschman, R., Gilbert, D.L., Nye, S.W., Dwyer, P., Fenn, W.O., 1954. Oxygen poisoning and X-irradiation: a mechanism in common. Science (Washington, DC) 119, 623–626.

Ghaly, M., Teplitz, D., 2004. The biologic effects of grounding the human body during sleep as measured by cortisol levels and subjective reporting of sleep, pain, and stress. J. Altern. Complement. Med. 10 (5), 767–776.

Gladwell, M., 2007. Blink: The Power of Thinking Without Thinking. Back Bay Books, New York, NY, 296 pp.

Goldman, L., Ausiello, D., 2004. Cecil Textbook of Medicine. 22nd ed. Saunders, Philadelphia, PA, 2670 pp.

Harman, D., 1956. Aging: a theory based on free radical and radiation chemistry. J. Gerontol. 2, 298–300.

Haynes, W.M., 2014. CRC Handbook of Chemistry and Physics, 95th ed. CRC Press, Boca Raton, FL.

James, R.G., 2001. Pulsed plasma radiation device for emitting light in biologically significant spectral bands. United States Patent 6,328,760, issued December 11, 2001.

Jamieson, K.S., ApSimon, H.M., Jamieson, S.S., Bell, J.N.B., Yost, M.G., 2007. The effects of electric fields on charged molecules and particles in individual microenvironments. Atmos. Environ. 41 (25), 5224–5235.

Johannessen, B., 2013. Nurses experience of aromatherapy use with dementia patients experiencing disturbed sleep patterns. An action research project. Complement Ther. Clin. Pract. 19 (4), 209–213.

Just, A., 1903. Return to Nature: The True Natural Method of Healing and Living and The True Salvation of the Soul. B. Lust, New York, NY.

Kantrowitz, B., 2006. Why women can't sleep. Newsweek Cover Story, April 25 issue.

Lee, R.P., 2005. Interface: Mechanisms of Spirit in Osteopathy. OR, Stillness Press, Llc., Portland.

Meinig, G.E., 1994. Root Canal Cover-Up, Second ed. Bion Pub, Ojai, CA.

Nelson, R., 1997. In-vitro activities of five plant essential oils against methicillin-resistant *Staphylococcus aureus* and vancomycinresistant *Enterococcus faecium*. J. Antimicrob. Chemother. 40, 305–306.

NIH State-of-the-Science Conference on Manifestations and Management of Chronic Insomnia in Adults, 2005. http://consensus.nih.gov/2005/insomniastatement.htm, June13–15, 2005.

Ober, A.C., 2003. Grounding the human body to earth reduces chronic inflammation and related chronic pain. ESD Journal, July issue.

Ober, A.C., 2004. Grounding the human body to neutralize bioelectrical stress from static electricity and EMFs. ESD Journal, February 22 issue.

Ober, A.C., Coghill, R.W., 2003. Does grounding the human body to earth reduce chronic inflammation and related chronic pain? In: Presented at the European Bioelectromagnetics Association Annual Meeting, November 12, Budapest, Hungary.

Ober, C., Sinatra, S.T., Zucker, M., 2014. Earthing: The Most Important Health Discovery Ever? Second ed. Basic Health Publications, Laguna Beach, CA.

Olson, S.F., 2013. http://www.kauaiyogaandfitness.com/the-awesome-benefits-of-walking-on-the-earth-barefoot/ (accessed 13.12.2013).

Oschman, J.L., 2003. Energy Medicine in Therapeutics and Human Performance. Butterworth Heinemann, Edinburgh pp. 180–181.

Oschman, J.L., 2007. Can electrons act as antioxidants? A review and commentary. J. Altern. Complement. Med. 13 (9), 955–967.

Oschman, J.L., 2008. Perspective: assume a spherical cow. The role of free or mobile electrons in bodywork, energetic and movement therapies. J. Bodyw. Mov. Ther. 12, 40–57.

Oschman, J.L., 2009. Charge transfer in the living matrix. J. Bodyw. Mov. Ther. 13, 215–228.

Oschman, J.L., 2013. Functional role of quantum coherence in interfacial water. In: Water Conference Sofia, Bulgaria. www.waterconf.org.

Oschman, J.L., Chevalier, G., Brown, R., 2015. The effects of grounding (earthing) on inflammation, the immune response, wound healing, and prevention and treatment of chronic inflammatory and autoimmune diseases. J. Inflamm. Res. in press.

Ostwald, W., 1909. Grosse Mdnner. Akademische Verlagsgesellschaft GMBH, Leipzig.

Owens, C., Baergen, R., Puckett, D., 2014. Online sources of herbal product information. Am. J. Med. 127 (2), 109–115.

Pall, M.L., 2013. Electromagnetic fields act via activation of voltage-gated calcium channels to produce beneficial or adverse effects. J. Cell. Mol. Med. 17 (8), 958.

Partnership to Fight Chronic Disease, 2011. Online document at: www.fightchronicdisease.org/issues/about.cfm (accessed 19.01.11).

Platt, R.J. Undated, personal communication to Albert Szent-Györgyi.

Popp, F.-A., Beloussov, L.V., 2003. Integrative Biophysics: Biophotonics. Springer, Berlin pp. 401–402.

Quinton, R., 1904. L'eau de Mer Milieu Organique (Seawater, Organic Matrix).. In: Paris, Masson et Cie. Libraries de L'Académie de Médicine, Éditeurs.

Rand, W., 1997. Reiki in hospitals. Winter 1997 issue of the Reiki Newsletter (precursor to Reiki News Magazine).

Reuters, London, November 14, 2013, cited from Huffington Post, http://www.huffingtonpost.com/2013/11/14/diabetes-worldwide-global-record-cases_n_4269979.html.

Rossi, W., 1989. The Sex Life of the Foot and Shoe. Wordsworth Editions, Hertfordshire, UK p. 61.

Selye, H., 1953. On the mechanism through which hydrocortisone affects the resistance of tissues to injury; an experimental study with the granuloma pouch technique. JAMA 152 (13), 1207–1213.

Selye, H., 1956. The Stress of Life. Mc-Graw Hill Book Company, New York, NY.

Sokal, K., Sokal, P., 2011. Earthing the human body influences physiologic processes. J. Altern. Complement. Med. 17 (4), 301–308.

Standing Bear (Chief Luther Standing Bear), 1971. Quoted from McLuhan TC Touch the Earth. Outerbridge & Dienstfrey, New York, NY.

Swartz, K., 2011. Projected costs of chronic diseases. Health care cost monitor. The Hastings Center. Online document at: http://healthcarecostmonitor.thehastingscenter.org/kimberlyswartz/projected-costs-of-chronic-diseases/ (accessed 18.01.11).

Szent-Györgyi, A., 1957. Bioenergetics. Academic Press, New York, NY, pp. 38–39.

Szent-Györgyi, A., 1968. Bioelectronics. A Study in Cellular Regulations, Defense, and Cancer. Academic Press, New York, NY.

Szent-Györgyi, A., 1972. Dionysians and apolionians. Science 176, 966.

Takaku, S., Osono, E., Kurigbayashi, H., Takaku, C., Hirami, N., Takahashi, H., 2013. A case of migraine without aura that was successfully treated with an herbal medicine. J. Altern. Complement. Med. 19 (12), 970–972.

Thut, W., 2013. Water, frequencies and harmonics. On the web at http://walterthut.com/media-coverage.html.

Tilden, J.H., 2010. Impaired health its cause and cure: a repudiation of the conventional treatment of disease. Kessinger Publishing, LLC Whitefish, MT. 370 pps.

White, G.S., 1929. The Finer Forces of Nature in Diagnosis and Therapy. Phillips Printing Company, Los Angeles, CA.

Williams, E., Heckman, S., 1993. The local diurnal variation of cloud electrification and the global diurnal variation of negative charge on the Earth. J. Geophys. Res. 98 (3), 5221–5234.

Clarity and Consensus Continue to Emerge from a Historic Tangle of Controversy and Confusion

After completing the first edition of this book in the year 2000, we decided to include an afterword to explain why the book was written and to summarize what it all meant. The result was a satisfying synopsis of the state of energy medicine at the time. Research done since then has not altered the conclusions that were reached, but has strengthened them and revealed new details.

There are two converging themes that provide a modern overview. The first is research confirming what many in the energy medicine community have long recognized: the human body is remarkably sensitive and responsive to tiny energy fields in its surroundings. This sensitivity enables skilled therapists from many disciplines to interact with their patients in effective ways using energetic techniques. This is a delicate issue, however, because this is the same sensitivity that enables electromagnetic pollution or 'electro-smog' to create health issues for a growing number of sensitive individuals, as was documented in Chapter 16. The delicacy of the issue arises because of the rapid spread of wireless technologies and the huge vested interests involved.

The second theme is increased understanding of the systems that enable the body to be so sensitive to energies in the environment, and the cellular systems that process incoming energetic signals of all kinds. These energetic signals are not mysterious or mystical – they are the same energies that are measured by physicists, except that we change the words slightly when they relate to a living system, such as biomagnetism and magnetobiology, or bioelectricity and electrobiology. Biomagnetism and bioelectricity refer to measurable magnetic and electric fields generated by a living organism; magnetobiology and electrobiology refer to the measurable effects of magnetic or electric fields on living things. Each of these is an academic discipline within the overall theme of energy medicine. There is a lot of confusion about the nature of these fields, for example:

An article on the web page of the US-based National Center for Complementary and Alternative Medicine (NCCAM) distinguishes between methods involving scientifically observable energy, which it calls "Veritable Energy Medicine", and methods which invoke physically undetectable or unverifiable or yet to be measured energies, which it calls "Putative Energy Medicine". Practices based on putative energy fields (also called biofields) generally reflect the concept that human beings are infused with subtle forms of energy; QiGong, Reiki, and Healing Touch are examples of such practices.

To refer to biofields (such as biomagnetic and bioelectric fields) as 'physically undetectable' or 'putative' is inappropriate because they are in fact measurable (see Chapter 8). The use of the phrase 'infused with subtle forms of energy' is likewise inappropriate, because 'infused' suggests that these energies arise from outside of the body. *Infuse: to cause a person or thing to be filled with something or for something to be added or introduced into a person.* These energies are not introduced or infused; they are produced within the body by well-known physiological processes taking place in organs such as the heart, brain, muscles, retina, glands, etc.

One result of our increased understanding is a deepening scientific basis for holism or wholism – the philosophy that defines and guides many of the complementary, alternative, and integrative therapies and that has a firm scientific foundation from energy medicine. This was discussed in Chapters 9 and 10.

The living matrix is a holistic system that provides a basis for 'systemic cooperation' – the mechanism that enables all of the diverse parts of the organism to function in complete harmony with all of the others to carry forward the moment-to-moment goals of the organism (Oschman, 2003). These vital systems operate 'behind the scenes' every moment of our lives, enabling us to do what we do without conscious awareness of the myriad processes that support us. The distinguished regulatory physiologist, E. Edward Adolph (1982), extensively quoted in Chapter 10, stated the situation eloquently:

> *The biology of wholeness is the study of the body as an integrated, coordinated, successful system. The integrated human body is the sum of thousands of physiological processes and traits working together. Each breath and each heartbeat involves the working together of countless events. Huge numbers of functions are carried on simultaneously. The parts and processes within an organism are woven together with great intricacy. Coordination occurs at a thousand points … All of the systems interdigitate. This is possible because of communication. Messages are indispensable because the parts are segregated in space. Communication is required by division of labor. The more activities present in an organism, the more messages needed.*

The brilliant German biophysicist, Fritz Albert Popp, referred to the phenomenon as Gestaltbildung – the mechanism of global communication and control. An excellent summary of his work on biophotonics can be found in McTaggart (2008). Further details can be found in Bischof (1995) and Chang et al. (2010).

> *It is now well established that all living systems emit a weak but permanent photon flux in the visible and ultraviolet range. This biophoton emission is correlated with many, if not all, biological and physiological functions. There are indications of a hitherto-overlooked information channel within the living system.*
>
> AMAZON SUMMARY OF CHANG ET AL. (2010)

Cells maintain their organized society by 'whispering together' in a faint and private language (Adey, 1996). The 'whispers' travel as chemical, electromagnetic, electronic, photonic, thermal, and phononic (sound) messages. Some messages are in material form (chemicals such as hormones, neuropeptides, neurohormones, electrons, or protons) while some are in the form of waves of different kinds, including transverse and longitudinal electromagnetic waves and scalar or soliton waves (Davydov, 1987; Meyl, 2012; Rebbi, 1979). There are also spin or torsion waves (Swanson, 2009). At a fundamental level all matter is actually composed of energy:

> *Concerning matter, we have been all wrong. What we have called matter is energy, whose vibration has been so lowered as to be perceptible to the senses. There is no matter.*
>
> ATTRIBUTED TO ALBERT EINSTEIN

Sensitivity of Living Systems to Tiny Energy Fields

The most important conclusion from modern biophysical and energy medicine research is that living systems are astonishingly sensitive to tiny environmental signals of all kinds. Hence very low levels of energy coming from the hands of a therapist or an energy medicine device or a cell telephone tower or other wireless technology or a toxic chemical in the environment (see the section on allergies in Chapter 16) can have profound effects on cell and tissue functions. These sensitivities enable us to benefit from very subtle inputs from a therapist or therapeutic device or an essential oil (Chapter 17); and, tragically, the same sensitivities cause some people to be disturbed and even made very ill by wireless technologies and electrical appliances. We need to stop arguing about whether or not these sensitivities are real, because they are real. They have been documented in double-blind studies (see for example Rea et al., 1991). Anyone who doubts this can watch presentations by Professor Johansson (2013) and Pall (2014); and read the BioInitiative Report (Sage 2012). We need to phase out harmful frequencies and substitute frequencies that are known to be beneficial. Those who have thought deeply on this subject have recognized that cellular communications and Wi-Fi, for example, could be operated at beneficial or health-promoting frequencies. Before this can happen, some basic research is essential. Such research should have very high priority because of the growing epidemic of electromagnetic sickness.

If the history of science has a lesson for us, it is that 'consensus among experts' is always changing – much faster in some areas than in others. And these changes are usually strongly resisted until the evidence for a new paradigm is overwhelming (see, for example, *The Structure of Scientific Revolutions* by Thomas S. Kuhn, 1962). Even overwhelming evidence can be slow to change opinions, as inaccurate concepts persist long after the crucial research has been done, simply because of the challenge of keeping up with the constantly changing scientific literature and because of vested interests that maintain that important discoveries are controversial, even after there is ample evidence to the contrary.

Energy medicine provides an example of a collection of completely reasonable and sound ideas that have been widely researched but are still resisted, because skeptics believe the whole endeavour is utter nonsense, and incorrectly state that there is no scientific evidence. This book documents the fact that there is an abundance of scientific evidence supporting energy medicine. This evidence is hidden in plain sight in medical libraries around the world. It is recommended that those who have formed their opinions without considering the data related to energy visit a good medical library, where they can enjoy an incomparable intellectual adventure as they explore the abundance of scientific reports on the energetic aspects of nature. There is enough evidence supporting energy medicine to fill many more books like this one. This evidence is fascinating, important and tremendously exciting, and is leading to a complete reversal of opinion in many areas, as well as to important new approaches to medicine. To summarize, the science of energetic interactions is providing valuable new insights into how the human body functions in health and disease.

Consensus Continuing to Emerge

New discoveries in energy medicine do not require us to abandon our sophisticated understandings of physiology, biochemistry or molecular biology. Instead, they extend our picture of living processes, and of healing, to finer levels of structure and function. Our definition of living matter is being expanded to incorporate the physics and chemistry of the solid state, including semiconduction, quantum mechanics, liquid crystals, and biological coherence (see for example Ho, 1998; Ho et al., 1994; Musumeci et al., 2002). These important topics are rarely presented in conventional texts or taught in medical schools. This means that relatively few physicians and medical researchers are aware of these phenomena that are affecting an increasing portion of the population and that have enormous potential to contribute to clinical medicine.

As a whole, energy medicine as a discipline is opening up new vistas as biomedical science and complementary medicines learn how to talk to each other. The physics and biophysics of energy is a major topic and language for this conversation. Much is known about energetics from various perspectives that have been kept separate from medicine for reasons that no longer serve us. A major force in this exploration is the public's justifiable insistence that there be a careful and thoughtful exploration of popular and successful therapeutic strategies that have traditionally been isolated from biomedical research, practice, and teaching; and that there be a comparable exploration of the health effects of our chemical and electromagnetic environment.

Each chapter of this book represents a major piece of the puzzle that will have its own evolution as new data and conceptual breakthroughs emerge. I have no illusion that any part of this book contains the last word on any of these subjects. When anyone tells you that science has spoken the 'last word' on any topic, be suspicious. This book is, of course, a 'work in progress'. The study is multidisciplinary, involving collaborations between physical, biological, and molecular sciences, including quantum physics and quantum chemistry. Each day, each visit to the library, each chat with a colleague, and each question or comment from a student or experienced therapist brings in a new piece of the puzzle, a new perspective.

References

Adey, W.R., 1996. A growing scientific consensus on the cell and molecular biology mediating interactions with environmental electromagnetic fields. In: Ueno, S. (Ed.), Biological Effects of Magnetic and Electromagnetic Fields. Pelnum Press, New York, NY, pp. 45–62, Ch. 4.

Adolph, E.F., 1982. Physiological Integrations in Action. Physiologist 25 (2), (April), Supplement.

Bischof, M., 1995. Biophotonen. Das Licht in unseren Zellen. Zweitauseneins, Frankfurt am Main.

Chang, J.-J., Fisch, J., Popp, F.-A., 2010. Biophotons. Springer, New York, NY.

Davydov, A.S., 1987. Excitons and solitons in molecular systems. Int. Rev. Cytol. 106, 183–225.

Ho, M.-W., 1998. The rainbow and the worm: the physics of organisms, second ed. River Edge, Singapore, New Jersey, NJ.

Ho, M.-W., Popp, F.-A., Warnke, U. (Eds.), 1994. Bioelectrodynamics and Biocommunication. World Scientific, Singapore, pp. 81–107.

Johansson, O., 2013. Health effects of electromagnetic fields. A Neuroscientist's view. At a Technical Seminar on Environment and Health, Barcelona, Spain, November 23, 2013. https://www.youtube.com/watch?v=I5udG8OCZWY.

Kuhn, T., 1962. The Structure of Scientific Revolutions. University of Chicago Press, Chicago, IL.

McTaggart, L., 2008. The Field. Harper Perennial, New York, NY.

Meyl, K., 2012. DNA and cell resonance: magnetic waves enable cell communication. DNA Cell Biol. 31 (4), 422–426.

Musumeci, F., Brizhik, L.S., Ho, M.-W. (Eds.), 2002. Energy and Information Transfer in Biological Systems: How Physics Could Enrich Biological Understanding. 18 -22 September 2002, In: Proceedings of the International Workshop Acireale. World Scientific, Catania, Italy, New Jersey, NJ.

Oschman, J.L., 2003. Energy Medicine in Therapeutics and Human Performance. Butterworth Heinemann, Amsterdam.

Pall, M.L., 2014. Elektrotåka - den nye helse- og miljøgiften? Presentation in Oslo, Norway on October 18 at https://www.youtube.com/watch?v=_Up8bqiJN2k.

Rea, W.J., Pan, Y., Fenyves, E.J., Sujisawa, I., Suyama, H., Samadi, N., Ross, G.H., 1991. Electromagnetic field sensitivity. J. Bioelectricity 10 (1&2), 241–256.

Rebbi, C., 1979. Solitons. Sci. Am. 240, 92–116.

Swanson, C., 2009. Life Force, the Scientific Basis: volume 2 of the Synchronized Universe, second ed. Poseidia Press Inc., Tucson, AZ.

The Regulation of Devices Used in the Practice of Energy Medicine

JUDY KOSOVICH, J.D., WASHINGTON, DC

A variety of devices are used in the practice of energy medicine. They include, for example, devices that measure electrical resistance of meridians, devices that provide electrical current or magnetic pulses to relieve pain or to stimulate the bodily functions, and devices that monitor physiological parameters as the input for training the body (biofeedback).

The Roles of FDA

The Food and Drug Administration (FDA) has the responsibility of protecting the public through its regulation of medical devices by determining whether the devices are safe and effective. The claims made in advertising and in instructions for use are usually the most important factor in determining whether FDA has jurisdiction and the standards that apply. The Federal Trade Commission (FTC) protects consumers from false or misleading advertising, deferring to FDA on findings related to safety and effectiveness. Not only must the claims be true (according to FDA's standards of truth), they must be 'substantiated' (kept handy in files) before the claims are made. Other agencies also defer to FDA's authority and technical expertise. For example, the Internal Revenue Service, in describing what is 'medical' for purposes of a deduction, uses the language of FDA's authorizing legislation – "diagnosis, cure, mitigation, treatment, or prevention of disease, or treatment affecting any structure or function of the body...".

This appendix describes laws governing devices that are used in the practice of energy medicine. For an overview of the issues faced under state law by the hundreds of thousands of energy practitioners who do not rely on devices, see http://www.midgemurphy.com/, especially her article "Legal Issues in the Practice of Energy Therapies." Laws that protect the freedom of consumers to choose a method of treatment don't necessarily protect practitioners. There are important risk management strategies that energy therapists can use to reduce their vulnerability. State laws vary greatly, so it is important to consult an attorney who is familiar with the issues faced by practitioners of energy therapies. The regulation of devices has much in common with the regulation of drugs, which came much earlier. The Federal Food, Drug, and Cosmetic Act (52 US Stat. 1040, 21 U.S.C.§301 et seq.) was passed by Congress in 1938 and gave FDA authority to oversee the safety of food, drugs, and cosmetics used for any one of the following – "diagnosis, cure, mitigation, treatment, or prevention of disease". FDA also has authority over drugs and devices that are used for "treatment affecting any structure or function of the body."

One additional area that has implications for energy medicine is homeopathic preparations (see Chapter 4). Products listed in the Homeopathic Pharmacopeia and sold over the counter are ordinarily exempt from FDA pre-market review. For details, see http://www.fda.gov/ICECI/ComplianceManuals/CompliancePolicyGuidanceManual/ucm074360.htm and its discussion of

CPG Sec. 400.400, Conditions Under Which Homeopathic Drugs May be Marketed. In 1976, the Medical Device Regulation Act (PL94-295, 90 Stat 539) was passed. The Act provided that all devices that were marketed before 1976 could be presumed to be safe and effective. Devices introduced after that had to be found to be safe and effective, as well as substantially equivalent to devices that were marketed before the device law was enacted, through the 510(k) process (named after the relevant section of the Act). In practice, it is not necessary to return to the marketplace of 1976 to meet the requirement of substantial equivalence. A device need only be substantially equivalent to a device that has already been 'cleared' for marketing. This allows device technologies to be improved gradually. In recent years, however, FDA has been increasingly strict about what constitutes 'substantial equivalence', requiring product-specific clinical trials to prove equivalence, even when peer-reviewed scientific literature or mere calibration might be sufficient for other legal purposes, e.g., to show due diligence or to provide patent protection. Further, devices that were once cleared for marketing may receive requests from FDA for costly clinical testing in order to remain on the market. Companies that want to remain in business quietly submit to these requests for data.

FDA law can require a more detailed review for products that present a significant risk or are significantly different in terms of design, material, chemical composition, energy source, manufacturing process, or intended use. When there is the possibility of significant risk or significant change in efficacy, premarket approval (PMA) is required. The level of detail required in a PMA approaches that of a new drug application. Only a small percentage of devices go this route, because it is very costly. Manufacturers with deep pockets may prefer PMA review in order to deter small businesses from entering their market. While FDA charges much less to small businesses for their first PMA, the cost of testing can easy exceed a million dollars. (One company is at $10 million and counting!)

There are five things that FDA looks at: (1) intended use, (2) claims made in advertising and in labelling, (3) substantial equivalence to a predicate, (4) safety, and (5) effectiveness. A concern regarding any one of these can be the basis for denying clearance to market a device. The FTC looks at studies in the context of the entire body of scientific literature, considers all relevant evidence, including contrary evidence, and has indicated that the weight of the evidence should support the claim: http://www.ftc.gov/news-events/press-releases/1998/08/ftc-staff-files-comment-fda-about-substantiation-dietary. For more information about FTC requirements and other restrictions on advertising, see http://www.ftc.gov/sites/default/files/attachments/press-releases/ftc-publishes-final-guides-governing-endorsements-testimonials/091005revisedendorsementguides.pdf and, for example, http://www.hpm.com/pdf/FLEDER082010FDLI.PDF.

As of 2007, devices are divided into three classes. Class I products do not require premarket clearance but the establishments that manufacture the products must be registered and must comply with general standards. Dental floss or bed sheets for hospital beds are examples of products in Class I. Class II products must go through the 510(k) process. Acupuncture needles and most noninvasive measuring devices are in Class II. Class III devices tend to be invasive (implants) or otherwise raise major safety concerns (defibrillators). Some products are a combination of drug and device. Whether drug law or device law applies is determined by which aspect predominates. FDA prefers to treat combination products as drugs. (See http://www.fda.gov/medicaldevices/deviceregulationandguidance/default.htm.)

For a 510(k), FDA may require data that demonstrates safety and effectiveness if the use or the novelty raises concerns. Increasingly, the data is clinical rather than the measurement or verification of design parameters. Certain categories of products (each device is given a 'product code' and a category) have guidance documents that describe what FDA will want to see in a 510(k) application. There is a collection of documents with the heading 'Guidance for Industry and FDA Staff: Class II Special Controls Guidance Document' on the FDA website.

For example, one can find a guidance document for 'Repetitive Transcutaneous Magnetic Stimulation Systems', document number 1728, on 26/7/2011. The FDA also publishes draft guidance documents. These are generally as applicable as guidance documents that are not 'draft', though comments submitted on draft guidance are more likely to be adopted than comments on final guidance.

Patents and Scientific Literature

The FDA treats patents as irrelevant to its device review because the focus of patents is novelty and utility, whereas FDA is concerned about safety and efficacy. It also treats scientific literature as largely irrelevant, and therefore requires product-specific clinical testing designed to show safety, efficacy, and substantial equivalence to the predicate(s).

The Anti-Alternative Press

While it has no official status, a website that often parallels FDA policies and enforcement priorities is the website Quackwatch. As might be surmised from the name Quackwatch, the website is not supportive of complementary and alternative medicine, including energy medicine. The assertions made on this website are often defamatory; Quackwatch was successfully sued for defamation in 2007 by Dr. Tedd Koren, a nationally known chiropractor.

Ethical Standards

In addition to regulation and certification, many professions have ethical standards. Standards have been developed and published for energy practitioners based on ethical standards of many other professionals (e.g., 'Professional Practice for the Energy Healing Practitioner', Melinda H. Connor, DD, Ph.D., AMP, FAM, Lulu Publishing ISBN # 978-0-557-11126-8). As of this writing, there is no certifying authority, so adoption of these standards is in its infancy.

Health Freedom Laws

The consumers' right to choose is distinct from a practitioner's right to practice. Alaska, Colorado, Georgia, Massachusetts, New York, North Carolina, Ohio, Oklahoma, Oregon, Texas, and Washington protect patient access to alternative therapies from licensed physicians. Because most practitioners of energy medicine are not licensed physicians, some states have gone much further in protecting the reality of health freedom. (See http://www.cancure.org/2-uncategorised/7-health-freedom-states and links therein.) As of this writing, Florida and Minnesota laws provide the greatest freedom, although other states may have a tradition of health freedom that is not codified and therefore harder to find. At least eight states have enacted health freedom laws or amendments to the state Constitution that allow consumers to choose any healthcare practice http://www.nationalhealthfreedom.org/InfoCenter/laws_passed.html). The impact of these laws on those who practice energy healing is still unknown.

Safety of Consumer Products

The regulations summarized above concern the regulation of therapeutic uses and wellness aspects of energy. There is another responsibility given to FDA related to energy medicine, namely, the protection of the public from energy from consumer products that are not for medical uses if the energy emissions are harmful to health (see Chapters 16 and 17 for a discussion of the effects of these harmful energies). Cell phones, cell towers, wireless routers, cordless phones, and more recently smart meters, are all subject to guidelines as to what is considered safe. The US standards for these radio frequency emitting technologies are among the most lax in the world and are based on outdated data and simplistic paradigms, failing to take into account pulsing of energy, frequent or prolonged exposure, and multiple sources. An excellent starting point with many references can be found at http://stopsmartmeters. org/2012/03/09/a-primer-on-the-fcc-guidelines-for-the-smart-meter-age/.

While the Federal Communications Commission has authority to set standards, its focus is on allocating specific frequencies to specific users and, as of this writing, its standards are based only on the heating of tissue, ignoring effects on DNA, blood-brain barrier permeability, cell membranes, sleep, etc. While it ostensibly relies on FDA for technical support, the consultations, if any, are not open to public scrutiny. Further, FDA has not published anything that reconciles its very conservative approach to medical devices that are used for short periods with much lower levels of energy, using beneficial frequencies, in contrast to its approach to consumer products that provide prolonged, multiple exposures at frequencies demonstrated to be harmful in a variety of ways.

Freedom of Religion

When a medical device is part of a spiritual practice, such as in the case of galvanic skin resistance measurements used in Scientology, the medical device is regulated but the spiritual practice is not. (See http://www.cs.cmu.edu/~dst/E-Meter/ for two perspectives.) Energy medicine, freedom of religion, and medical device law rarely intersect, but as people become ever more interested in happiness and wellness, this could change. This is an area of law worthy of attention and planning.

The World of Claims

Claims are statements about a product or technique that are used in marketing or labelling and that lead to expectations. Thus, disappointed consumers can be a major source of enforcement actions. One way to avoid irate consumers is money-back guarantees.

Not every tool of energy medicine is, by its intrinsic nature, a medical device, so claims can be pivotal. From the viewpoint of regulatory authorities, multipurpose objects like bells, tuning forks, fragrant oils, coloured lights, and jewellery are things that can be made into medical devices only by their use and the claims made about their use. The litmus test is whether a device will 'diagnose, cure, mitigate, treat, or prevent a disease or treat the body in a way that affects its structure or function'. If a device is claimed to do any one of these things, it will most likely be seen by FDA as a medical device.

Conversely, there are also some things that, by their nature, are undeniably medical devices regardless of the claims not made. The device that measures changes in the galvanic resistance of skin when current is applied, when routinely used in the practice of Scientology, is still considered a medical device by FDA. The practice is permitted to continue with certain stipulations that keep it legal and have to do with the claims about the device.

Substantiating Health Claims

Claims must be true and their truth must be substantiated. Even if a claim is substantiated but considered to be exaggerated, the FTC can bring an enforcement action for making false or misleading claims. Regardless of whether the claim is bold, vague, implied, or made by quoting a testimonial, it must not be false or misleading.

'Claims' can be made by using anecdotes or testimonials. The party who publicizes anecdotes or testimonials, as well as the parties who give them, share responsibility for making claims. Even though anecdotes or testimonials may be true and substantiated, FDA will not consider them to be scientific proof unless they are the result of a test design that meets the rigorous standards of science and statistics. The FTC defers to the FDA for matters involving science, so it is unlikely that the FTC would consider anecdotal evidence to be substantiation, although carefully drafted language that discloses the anecdotal nature of the evidence might satisfy FTC or be considered a showing of good faith. State law may be relevant as well.

Avoiding Health Claims to Avoid FDA Turf

Sometimes people deliberately avoid making health claims to avoid triggering FDA's authority. One can claim 'wellness' and assisting specific mechanisms of action. Whatever words are used, the implications to avoid are 'diagnose, cure, mitigate, treat, or prevent a disease or treat the body in a way that affects its structure or function'. Examples of words that have meaning in the realm of energy medicine and that might be safe (one can never be sure when FDA policies will change) as claims include:

Resonates with/enhances/supports the body's systems/performance/efficiency
Increases/enhances vitality/clarity/efficiency/well-being
Each person's response is unique
Reduces stress/influence of outside fields/forces/substances.

Modifying Claims, Reporting Problems

When a manufacturer makes claims about its device, it is natural for a practitioner who uses the device to make these same claims. Sometimes, either because of an FDA 'warning letter' or for other reasons, a manufacturer will change its claims. Broader or new claims will probably require a new application to be filed with FDA, even though the device is already cleared for marketing. Customers should be informed of these new claims if their device can be used according to the new claims.

A manufacturer also has an obligation to inform its customers of the change in claims if they are made narrower or more modest in response to a warning letter. Do the customers have an obligation to change their claims accordingly? Although FDA does not normally take action against practitioners, it can and has. FDA officials have confiscated equipment and records of practitioners. (See, for example, www.proliberty.com/observer/20091206.htm.) Contract clauses may require claims consistent with those of the manufacturer, as may due diligence standards in the industry.

If a practitioner discovers things about a medical device, unless there is an agreement to the contrary, he or she is under no obligation to inform the manufacturer of his or her discovery. So long as the practitioner keeps substantiation files and complies with FDA requirements and contract terms, a practitioner can make new claims. Most likely, the new use will require clearance from FDA before marketing, so involving the manufacturer may be the best strategy. If a practitioner sees 'significant adverse events or product problems', the requirements are different. A report must be made to MedWatch (www.fda.gov/MedicalDevices/Safety/ReportaProblem/default.htm).

The Regulatory Process: Getting FDA Clearance

The following is a brief overview of FDA's website (http://www.fda.gov/medicalDevices/). The website has links for industry, healthcare providers, and consumers.

If we look at the development of an energy medicine device or a practice, it almost always begins with research and testing. This phase is not immune from regulation. FDA requires the use of an institutional review board to safeguard human subjects, as well as the submission of an IDE, Investigational Device Exemption, in any situation involving risk. This IDE allows limited marketing (for example, devices can only be sold at cost). Use is limited to that covered by the protocol that has been submitted to FDA (http://www.fda.gov/MedicalDevices/DeviceRegulationandGuidance/HowtoMarketYourDevice/InvestigationalDeviceExemptionIDE/default.htm).

For devices developed in other countries, it is often possible to start with the application process if clinical data has already been collected. As discussed above, most widely used process is the 510(k) application, by which the applicant demonstrates to FDA's satisfaction that the product is safe and effective and that it is substantially equivalent to one or more existing products. In the process of granting clearance, the FDA can ask for clarification, design changes, or anything else it deems necessary. The easiest path forward is to comply with anything FDA suggests, although some have been successful in resisting FDA's opinions, either in the 510(k) process or the 'de novo' process. Once clearance for marketing is obtained, it is legal to sell and use the device, consistent only with the claims and information that have been reviewed and cleared by FDA.

In identifying the best 'predicate' devices, it is often necessary to search the FDA database for similar devices that have been cleared for marketing. Another approach would be to contact the manufacturer of a similar device and ask for the 510(k) number. Sometimes it is published on a manufacturer's website. The fact that a product is already being marketed does not necessarily make it a suitable predicate because there are many devices being marketed that have not obtained FDA clearance.

While searching FDA's database appears fairly straightforward the following things should be kept in mind. The name of the device or its manufacturer may have changed since the original application, in which case the original name is needed in order to find the 510(k) number. Sometimes, for reasons inscrutable, the 510(k) will not come up in a search of the FDA database using the correct product name or the correct manufacturer name. The best way to be certain that a device is not in the database is to look at every device in every product code that might apply. For large product categories and overlapping product categories, this is tedious.

Older 510(k) records have more information in the database than most recent 510(k)s. With older devices, there is some hope of determining which predicates are the most similar solely from what is in the FDA database. In the case of newer devices, the name may provide important clues as to similarities, but it will probably be necessary to visit websites for each candidate predicate to determine if there is substantial equivalence.

If a device is based on new technology or differs substantially in safety or effectiveness from what is on the market, the manufacturer needs a PMA (http://www.fda.gov/MedicalDevices/DeviceRegulationandGuidance/HowtoMarketYourDevice/PremarketSubmissions/PremarketApprovalPMA/default.htm). The 510(k) submission may be several inches thick and the application fee is more than $2000 for small manufacturers who file an application for the special fee many months in advance and more than $4000 for everyone else (prices change annually). The PMA may be several feet thick and the application fee is about 15 times more for small manufacturers and about 50 times more for others. Some large manufacturers seem to prefer to file a PMA because it makes it easier for them to dominate the market. FDA currently presumes that a device that has a PMA is not a suitable predicate for a 510(k). The fees are adjusted for inflation every year.

The Biofeedback Exemption

In the realm of energy medicine, there is one category of Class II devices that does not have to go through the 510(k) process, namely biofeedback devices that are consistent with the definition given under the biofeedback exemption.

Biofeedback first came to the attention of the scientific and regulatory community in the United States in the 1960s when measurements were taken to verify that practitioners of meditation were able to control bodily functions previously thought to be controlled only by the autonomic nervous system. It was later demonstrated that by providing data ('feedback') on biological parameters, e.g., heart rate or blood pressure, even a person not trained in meditation could learn to affect these functions. This became known as biofeedback. Although biofeedback as originally practiced involved a person providing instruction or coaching, the electronic age has allowed people to purchase inexpensive devices that they can use without a coach. The device must be battery operated (to limit the amount of electricity that the device can deliver should it malfunction), and it must otherwise comply with the following definition.

TITLE 21 – FOOD AND DRUGS

CHAPTER I – FOOD AND DRUG ADMINISTRATION DEPARTMENT OF HEALTH
  AND HUMAN SERVICES
SUBCHAPTER H – MEDICAL DEVICES
PART 882 – NEUROLOGICAL DEVICES
Subpart F – Neurological Therapeutic Devices
Sec. 882.5050 Biofeedback device.
  (a) *Identification.* A biofeedback device is an instrument that provides a visual or auditory signal corresponding to the status of one or more of a patient's physiological parameters (e.g., brain alpha wave activity, muscle activity, skin temperature, etc.) so that the patient can control voluntarily these physiological parameters.
  (b) *Classification.* Class II (special controls). The device is exempt from the premarket notification procedures in subpart E of part 807 of this chapter when it is a prescription battery powered device that is indicated for relaxation training and muscle reeducation and prescription use, subject to 882.9.
[44 FR 51730-51778, Sept. 4, 1979, as amended at 63 FR 59229, Nov. 3, 1998]

Consumer Products

Energy can be delivered to the body in many forms, including light, sound, electrical currents, magnetic fields, mechanical manipulation, and pressure. There is no threshold of energy intensity currently so low that it could not be regulated if the claims brought it within the realm of FDA. As discussed in this book (Figure 16.1), sometimes lowering energy intensity produces more results than raising intensity.

There is little consistency or coordination in the regulation or evaluation of consumer products and medical devices.

We are constantly surrounded by sources of energy. These sources of energy may affect us, but unless health claims are made, the FDA can intervene only if it can show that there is a significant risk. Its threshold for significant risk is many orders of magnitude different for medical devices versus consumer products. FDA oversight may provide a deterrent to the most reckless product designs, but it does not provide much protection. For example, there is increasing attention being given to the effects of smart meters on health, although not by FDA (http://electromagnetichealth.org/electromagnetic-health-blog/t-mobile-deutsche, http://www.bioinitiative.org/table-of-contents/, http://emfsafetynetwork.org/?page_id=872). An increasing number of local governments are giving customers a right to opt out of smart meters (http://emfsafetynetwork.org/wp-content/uploads/2012/01/Santa-Cruz-Public-Health-Official-Smart-Meter-report.pdf).

THE TENDENCY OF STATE LAW TO BECOME UNIFORM

Sometimes there are factors that move state law toward uniformity. For example, the nonprofit National Health Freedom Coalition is working to get health freedom laws adopted in every state. There are also commercial factors, for example, where people might cross state lines to obtain a particular service, governments may adopt similar policies to encourage local commerce. Where regulation of a profession requires a high level of expertise, e.g., the certification of acupuncturists, there is a movement toward making the California acupuncture license the national standard (http://www.acupuncture.ca.gov/). The biggest advantage of state laws gradually going national as a method of attaining a uniform standard to facilitate interstate commerce is that it avoids concentrated federal authority.

THE PRESENT AND THE FUTURE

There are forces contributing to the expanding use of energy medicine. These forces include rapidly rising costs of conventional medical care combined with ever-disappointing outcomes, a deepening understanding of why energy medicine works (through biophysics research summarized in this book and in many other sources), the development of techniques that validate its success and explain its mechanisms, and an increasing awareness among consumers and healthcare professionals of the value of these less costly and less risky alternatives. Many of these biophysical tools are noninvasive and employ energy levels so low that they cannot be felt. Many of them affect causes rather than suppressing symptoms, and may therefore prevent the development of costly chronic disease.

Before considering recommendations for the future, it is useful to first have clarity about the present. The following is a partial list of conjectures and observations about the present.

(1) Although science has provided considerable information about how the body works, it has barely scratched the surface of the complexity that surrounds us. For example, science may be unable to fully explain why certain modalities or practices work though it may be able to prove that they do work. Science cannot explain what differentiates living and non-living matter though it can manipulate life.

(2) While the scientific method has the possibility of preventing bias, it provides useful conclusions only if a hypothesis is well-formulated, the conditions are appropriately controlled for all relevant factors (with emphasis on all), the scientist understands as well as practitioners do what they are testing, and the results are evaluated without bias. These are all very difficult to achieve and wrong conclusions can be drawn despite the best of intentions. There is also the profound ethical problem of experiments designed to show a particular result rather than to find truth.

(3) Science does not yet have a decent explanation of why the placebo effect is stronger than most drugs. So long as this is the case, the design of experiments involving a placebo will be unreliable because conclusions will have no statistical significance.

(4) Science cannot adequately account for the roles of attitude and intention, as well as the mechanisms by which they work, which may or may not be related to the placebo effect.

(5) There are many non sequiturs, gaps, misconceptions and contradictions in the scientific literature.

(6) There are dichotomies and flaws in the formulation of public policy and little effort is being made to address these things.

(7) Personal freedom to make health care decisions varies greatly from state to state. Awareness of options is even more variable.

(8) There is no way to take into account in the evaluation of medical practices and devices the personal preferences people have for risk-taking, cost, discomfort, and what constitutes disease versus aging, yet these are important aspects of safety and effectiveness at the personal level.

(9) The insurance system provides a safety net, but it also puts a very large burden on personal finance with worse average outcomes in the US than in countries that spend less on health care. It does, however, provide an expanded, growing economy that benefits certain sectors that influence public policy. Insurance biases health care decisions toward what is covered, not what is effective.

Considering where we are, where should we go from here?

(1) Create an institution that would provide quality control and coordination among disciplines in the area of energy medicine, with responsibilities and authorities similar to those of FDA. This institution should be independent of FDA because FDA has too many biases and little relevant expertise in the field. The NIH Institute for Complementary and Alternative Medicine is a potential federal resource. Various professional organizations also have relevant expertise.

(2) Give this institution the responsibility for coming up with safety standards for consumer products as well as for medical devices.

(3) Incorporate holistic training, physics and biophysics into the standard curriculum for doctors and nurses.

Legal, Ethical, and Other CAM Resources

Legal, Ethical, and Other CAM Resources

Cohen, M.H., 1998. Complementary & Alternative Medicine: Legal Boundaries & Regulatory Perspectives. Johns Hopkins University Press, Baltimore, MD.

Cohen, M.H., 2000. Beyond Complementary Medicine: Legal & Ethical Perspectives on Health Care & Human Evolution. University of Michigan Press, Ann Arbor, MI.

Cohen, M.H., 2002. Future Medicine: Ethical Dilemmas, Regulatory Challenges & Therapeutic Pathways to Health Care. University of Michigan Press, Ann Arbor, MI.

Crellin, J., Ania, F., 2002. Professionalism & Ethics in Complementary & Alternative Medicine. Haworth Integrative Healing Press, New York, NY, Reviewed online at http://www.mun.ca/univrel/gazette/2002-2003/dec12/books5.html.

Murphy, M., 2012. Legal Issues in the Practice of Energy Therapies. http://www.midgemurphy.com/.

Wilson, L., 2003. Legal Guidelines for Unlicensed Practitioners. L.D. Wilson Consultants, Prescott, AZ.

Web Sites for Further Research

American College of Forensic Examiners International: http://www.acfei.com/.

American College of Legal Medicine: http://www.aclm.org.

American College of Wellness: http://www.collegeofwellness.com/.

American Naturopathic Medical Association: http://www.anma.net.

American Psychotherapy Association: http://www.americanpsychotherapy.com.

Annals of Internal Medicine: Advising: http://www.acponline.org.

Chiropractic Diagnosis & Referral: http://www.worldchiropracticalliance.org.

Complementary and Integrative Medicine: an Update for Texas Practitioners by Walter G. Mosher. http://www.law.uh.edu/healthlaw/perspectives/homepage.asp.

Council on Chiropractic Practice: http://www.ccp-guidelines.org.

Ethics and Policy Integration Center: http://www.ethicaledge.com/page8.html.

Legal, Ethical & Professional Issues in Psychoanalysis/Psychotherapy: http://www.academyprojects.org.

National Academies: http://www.iom.edu/reports/2005/complementary-and-alternative-medicine-in-the-united-states.aspx.

National Center for Complementary and Alternative Medicine: http://nccam.nih.gov.

National Institute for Science, Law and Public Policy: http://www.swankin-turner.com/nislapp.html.

Psychoanalytic WebRing: http://h.webring.com/hub?ring=lacan.

INDEX

Note: Page numbers followed by *b* indicate boxes, *f* indicate figures, *t* indicate tables and *np* indicate footnotes.